FIRST RESPONDER CARE Essentials

Second Edition

Text © Richard Pilbery and Kris Lethbridge 2024

All rights reserved. Without limiting the rights under copyright reserved above, no part of this publication may be reproduced, stored in or introduced into a retrieval system, or transmitted, in any form or by any means (electronic, mechanical, photocopying, recording or otherwise) without the prior written permission of the publisher of this book.

The information presented in this book is accurate and current to the best of the authors' knowledge.

The authors and publisher, however, make no guarantee as to, and assume no responsibility for, the correctness, sufficiency or completeness of such information or recommendation.

Printing history
Preliminary edition published 2016
First edition published 2016. Reprinted 2017, 2019 (twice), 2020, 2021 (thrice), 2022, 2023 and 2024
This second edition first published 2024, reprinted 2025.

The authors and publisher welcome feedback from the users of this book.

Please contact the publisher:

Class Professional Publishing
The Exchange, Express Park, Bristol Road, Bridgwater TA6 4RR
Telephone: 01278 427 800
Email: info@class.co.uk
www.classprofessional.co.uk

Class Professional Publishing is an imprint of Class Publishing Ltd

A CIP catalogue record for this book is available from the British Library

Paperback ISBN: 9781801611381

ePDF: 9781801611404

ePub ISBN: 9781801611398

Line illustrations by David Woodroffe and S4Carlisle
Cover design by Hybert Design Limited, UK
Typeset by Innodata
Printed in the UK by Hobbs the Printers Ltd.

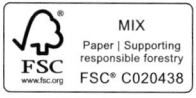
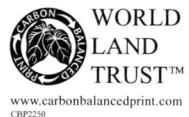

Product safety information can be found at https://www.classprofessional.co.uk/terms-of-use/gpsr-statement/

FIRST RESPONDER CARE Essentials

SECOND EDITION

Richard Pilbery
and
Kris Lethbridge

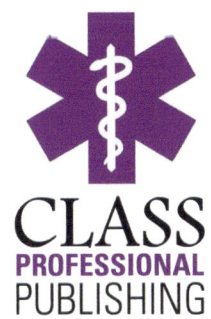

Contents

List of Abbreviations — xii
Acknowledgements — xiv
Foreword — xvi

1: Introduction — 1

1. Textbook guide — 1
   1.1 Introduction — 1
   1.2 Textbook — 1
   1.3 Getting started — 1
2. Anatomy of an emergency call — 1
   2.1 Introduction — 1
   2.2 The emergency operations centre (EOC) — 1
   2.3 Arriving on scene — 2
   2.4 Principles of communication — 2
   2.5 Patient assessment — 3
   2.6 Patient history — 3
   2.7 Cardiac arrest — 3
   2.8 Basic life support and defibrillation — 3
   2.9 Crew arrival — 4
   2.10 Clean up and prepare for the next call — 4
3. Extended skills — 4
   3.1 Scope of practice — 4

2: The Ambulance Service — 5

1. Response to a 999 call — 5
   1.1 Learning objective — 5
   1.2 Introduction — 5
   1.3 Call for help and triage — 5
   1.4 Ambulance service response — 5
   1.5 Onward care — 6
2. Roles within the ambulance service — 7
   2.1 Learning objectives — 7
   2.2 Introduction — 7
   2.3 Clinical roles — 7
   2.4 Clinical leadership roles — 9
   2.5 Command and control roles — 9
   2.6 Support structures — 11
   2.7 Working relationships — 11
3. Caring for yourself and colleagues — 11
   3.1 Learning objectives — 11
   3.2 Introduction — 11
   3.3 Mental well-being — 12
   3.4 Building resilience — 12
   3.5 Seeking help — 12
   3.6 Supporting a colleague — 13

3: Communication — 15

1. Principles of communication — 15
   1.1 Learning objectives — 15
   1.2 Introduction — 15
   1.3 Who you will be communicating with — 15
   1.4 Basics of communication — 15
   1.5 Social context — 18
   1.6 Barriers to communication — 18
   1.7 Summary — 19
2. Practical communication — 19
   2.1 Learning objectives — 19
   2.2 Record-keeping — 19
   2.3 Handover — 19
   2.4 Discussing with a remote clinician — 21
   2.5 Electronic communication devices — 21

4: Legal and Ethical Issues — 23

1. Being a healthcare volunteer — 23
   1.1 Learning objectives — 23
   1.2 Introduction — 23
   1.3 Values-based healthcare — 23
   1.4 Duty of care — 24
   1.5 Negligence — 25
   1.6 Scope of practice and standards — 25
   1.7 When things go wrong — 26
2. Consent and capacity — 27
   2.1 Learning objectives — 27

		2.2	Introduction	27
		2.3	Consent	28
		2.4	Mental capacity	28
		2.5	Summary	30
	3	Confidentiality and information governance		30
		3.1	Learning objectives	30
		3.2	Introduction	30
		3.3	Maintaining confidentiality	31
		3.4	Making a disclosure	32
		3.5	Key points	33
	4	Equality and diversity		33
		4.1	Learning objectives	33
		4.2	Introduction	33
		4.3	Equality in healthcare	33
		4.4	Discrimination	34

5: Health and Safety — 37

	1	Health and safety policies and legislation		37
		1.1	Learning objectives	37
		1.2	Introduction	37
		1.3	Health and Safety at Work etc. Act 1974	37
		1.4	Management of Health and Safety at Work Regulations	38
		1.5	Manual Handling Operations Regulations	38
	2	Risk assessment		38
		2.1	Learning objectives	38
		2.2	Introduction	39
		2.3	Structured risk assessments	39
		2.4	Dynamic risk assessments	39
	3	Infection prevention and controls		40
		3.1	Learning objectives	40
		3.2	Introduction	40
		3.3	Regulations and legislation	40
		3.4	Micro-organisms	41
		3.5	Chain of infection	41
		3.6	Standard infection control precautions (SICPs)	42

	4	Fire safety		55
		4.1	Learning objectives	55
		4.2	Introduction	55
		4.3	Fire prevention	56
		4.4	What to do in case of fire	56
	5	Stress		57
		5.1	Learning objectives	57
		5.2	Introduction	57
		5.3	Signs of stress	57
		5.4	Managing stress	58

6: Safeguarding Adults and Children — 59

	1	Safeguarding adults and children		59
		1.1	Learning objectives	59
		1.2	Introduction	59
		1.3	Learning from previous cases	59
		1.4	Vulnerability	60
		1.5	Forms of abuse	61
		1.6	Managing abuse or disclosures of abuse	63
		1.7	Safeguarding referrals	64
		1.8	Summary	64

7: Manual Handling — 65

	1	Principles of manual handling		65
		1.1	Learning objectives	65
		1.2	Introduction	65
		1.3	Consequences of poor manual handling	65
		1.4	Risk assessment	66
		1.5	Biomechanics	68
		1.6	General principles	68
		1.7	Handling aids	70
	2	Moving and handling equipment and techniques		71
		2.1	Learning objectives	71
		2.2	Introduction	71
		2.3	Patients on the floor	71

| | | 2.4 | Patients who need to be transferred to the floor | 76 |

8: Scene Assessment — 79

1. Scene assessment and safety — 79
   - 1.1 Learning objectives — 79
   - 1.2 Introduction — 79
   - 1.3 Safety — 79
   - 1.4 Cause — 79
   - 1.5 Environment — 80
   - 1.6 Number of patients — 80
   - 1.7 Extra resources — 80
2. Major incidents — 81
   - 2.1 Learning objectives — 81
   - 2.2 Introduction — 81
   - 2.3 Classification of incidents — 81
   - 2.4 Types of major incident — 81
   - 2.5 Role of the ambulance service — 82
   - 2.6 M/ETHANE model — 82
   - 2.7 Ten second triage — 83
3. Hazardous materials — 84
   - 3.1 Learning objectives — 84
   - 3.2 Introduction — 85
   - 3.3 Labelling of hazardous substances — 85
   - 3.4 Responder actions at scene — 86

9: Patient Assessment — 87

1. Patient assessment process — 87
   - 1.1 Learning objectives — 87
   - 1.2 Introduction — 87
   - 1.3 Primary survey — 87
   - 1.4 History taking — 89
   - 1.5 Secondary survey — 91
   - 1.6 Reassessment — 92

10: Airway — 93

1. Airway anatomy — 93
   - 1.1 Learning objective — 93
   - 1.2 Introduction — 93
   - 1.3 Upper airway — 93
   - 1.4 Lower Airway — 95
2. Assessing and managing the airway — 96
   - 2.1 Learning objectives — 96
   - 2.2 Introduction — 96
   - 2.3 Assessing the airway — 96
   - 2.4 Step-wise approach to the airway — 97
   - 2.5 Manual airway manoeuvres — 97
   - 2.6 Suction — 103
   - 2.7 Airway adjuncts — 104
3. Tracheostomies — 107
   - 3.1 Learning objectives — 107
   - 3.2 Introduction — 107
   - 3.3 Tracheostomy tubes — 108
   - 3.4 Management of the tracheostomy patient — 108
   - 3.5 Management of the laryngectomy patient — 110
4. Choking in adults — 111
   - 4.1 Learning objectives — 111
   - 4.2 Introduction — 111
   - 4.3 Recognition — 111
   - 4.4 Management — 111
5. Choking in the paediatric patient — 112
   - 5.1 Learning objective — 112
   - 5.2 Introduction — 112
   - 5.3 The paediatric airway — 113
   - 5.4 Recognition — 113
   - 5.5 Management — 113

11: Breathing — 115

1. Respiratory system physiology — 115
   - 1.1 Learning objective — 115
   - 1.2 Introduction — 115
   - 1.3 Respiration — 115
   - 1.4 The lungs — 115
   - 1.5 Mechanics of breathing — 116
   - 1.6 Gas exchange — 117
   - 1.7 Control of breathing — 118

2	Using medical gases safely	118	3	Cardiovascular system disorders	164

2 Using medical gases safely — 118
  2.1 Learning objectives — 118
  2.2 Introduction — 118
  2.3 Medical gas cylinder storage — 119
  2.4 Anatomy of a medical gas cylinder — 119
  2.5 Safety first — 121
  2.6 Preparing a new cylinder for use — 121
  2.7 Oxygen delivery devices — 122
  2.8 Assisted ventilation — 124
  2.9 Oxygen administration — 129
  2.10 Entonox administration — 134

3 Assessment of breathing — 137
  3.1 Learning objectives — 137
  3.2 Respiratory rate — 137
  3.3 Oxygen saturations — 138

4 Common respiratory conditions — 140
  4.1 Learning objectives — 140
  4.2 Asthma — 140
  4.3 COPD — 142
  4.4 Pneumonia — 143
  4.5 Pulmonary embolism — 144

12: Circulation — 147

1 Cardiovascular system anatomy and physiology — 147
  1.1 Learning objectives — 147
  1.2 Introduction — 147
  1.3 Heart — 147
  1.4 Blood — 150
  1.5 Blood vessels — 150
  1.6 Cardiac cycle — 151
  1.7 Electrocardiograms — 152

2 Assessment of circulation — 153
  2.1 Learning objectives — 153
  2.2 Introduction — 153
  2.3 Pulse — 153
  2.4 Capillary refill time (CRT) — 156
  2.5 Blood pressure (BP) — 158

3 Cardiovascular system disorders — 164
  3.1 Learning objectives — 164
  3.2 Introduction — 164
  3.3 Coronary artery disease (CAD) — 164
  3.4 Angina — 164
  3.5 Acute coronary syndrome (ACS) — 165
  3.6 Heart failure — 166
  3.7 Shock — 167

13: Disability — 169

1 Nervous system anatomy and physiology — 169
  1.1 Learning objectives — 169
  1.2 Introduction — 169
  1.3 Anatomy and physiology — 169
  1.4 Brain — 170
  1.5 Spinal cord — 171
  1.6 Somatic nervous system — 171
  1.7 Autonomic nervous system (ANS) — 172

2 Assessment of disability — 173
  2.1 Learning objectives — 173
  2.2 Introduction — 173
  2.3 FAST test — 173

3 Disorders of the nervous system — 174
  3.1 Learning objectives — 174
  3.2 Introduction — 175
  3.3 Convulsions — 175
  3.4 Stroke — 176
  3.5 Meningococcal disease — 177
  3.6 Paralysis — 179
  3.7 Coma — 179

14: Exposure — 181

1 Extremes of temperature — 181
  1.1 Learning objectives — 181
  1.2 Introduction — 181
  1.3 Hypothermia — 181
  1.4 Heat-related illness — 182
  1.5 Assessment of temperature — 183

2	Drowning	185	2	Integumentary system anatomy and physiology 206
	2.1 Learning objective	185		2.1 Learning objective 206
	2.2 Introduction	185		2.2 Introduction 206
	2.3 Pathophysiology	185		2.3 Epidermis 206
	2.4 Management	185		2.4 Dermis 206

15: Medical Emergencies — 187

- 1 Anaphylaxis — 187
  - 1.1 Learning objectives — 187
  - 1.2 Introduction — 187
  - 1.3 Signs and symptoms — 187
  - 1.4 Management — 187
- 2 Sepsis — 190
  - 2.1 Learning objectives — 190
  - 2.2 Introduction — 190
  - 2.3 Risk factors for sepsis — 190
  - 2.4 Recognition and management — 190
- 3 Endocrine system disorders — 192
  - 3.1 Learning objectives — 192
  - 3.2 Introduction — 192
  - 3.3 Anatomy and physiology of the pancreas — 192
  - 3.4 Diabetes — 194
  - 3.5 Glycaemic emergencies — 194
  - 3.6 Hypoglycaemia — 194
  - 3.7 Severe hyperglycaemia — 195
  - 3.8 Blood sugar measurement — 196
- 4 Poisoning — 199
  - 4.1 Learning objectives — 199
  - 4.2 Introduction — 199
  - 4.3 Toxidromes — 199
  - 4.4 Management — 201

16: Trauma — 203

- 1 Mechanism of injury (MOI) — 203
  - 1.1 Learning objectives — 203
  - 1.2 Introduction — 203
  - 1.3 Mechanisms that cause injury — 203
- 2 Integumentary system anatomy and physiology — 206
  - 2.1 Learning objective — 206
  - 2.2 Introduction — 206
  - 2.3 Epidermis — 206
  - 2.4 Dermis — 206
  - 2.5 Hypodermis — 207
  - 2.6 Physiology — 207
- 3 Wounds and bleeding — 207
  - 3.1 Learning objectives — 207
  - 3.2 Introduction — 207
  - 3.3 Bleeding — 207
  - 3.4 Wounds — 213
- 4 Assessment and management of the trauma patient — 214
  - 4.1 Learning objectives — 214
  - 4.2 Introduction — 214
  - 4.3 Scene assessment — 215
  - 4.4 Primary survey — 215
  - 4.5 Head injuries — 217
  - 4.6 Spinal injuries — 217
  - 4.7 Thoracic injuries — 217
  - 4.8 Abdominal injuries — 219
  - 4.9 Pelvic injuries — 220
  - 4.10 Musculoskeletal injuries — 220
- 5 Skeletal immobilisation — 223
  - 5.1 Learning objective — 223
  - 5.2 Introduction — 224
  - 5.3 First-aid techniques — 224
  - 5.4 Splints — 227
  - 5.5 Spinal immobilisation — 238
- 6 Burns — 247
  - 6.1 Learning objectives — 247
  - 6.2 Introduction — 247
  - 6.3 Assessment of burns — 247
  - 6.4 Thermal burns — 248
  - 6.5 Chemical burns — 250
  - 6.6 Radiation burns — 250
  - 6.7 Electrical injuries — 251

17: Children and Infants — 253

1. Why paediatric patients are different — 253
   - 1.1 Learning objective — 253
   - 1.2 Introduction — 253
   - 1.3 Anatomy and physiology — 253
   - 1.4 Cognitive development — 255
2. Initial assessment and management of the paediatric patient — 256
   - 2.1 Learning objectives — 256
   - 2.2 Introduction — 256
   - 2.3 Developmental approach to the paediatric patient — 256
   - 2.4 Recognising the sick infant and child — 257
   - 2.5 Primary survey — 258

18: Learning Disabilities — 263

1. Supporting the care of people with learning disabilities — 263
   - 1.1 Learning objectives — 263
   - 1.2 Introduction — 263
   - 1.3 Learning disabilities legislation and rights — 263
   - 1.4 Causes of learning disabilities — 264
   - 1.5 Categories of learning disabilities — 265
2. Disabilities and healthcare — 265
   - 2.1 Introduction — 265
   - 2.2 Inequality in healthcare — 265
   - 2.3 Communication — 266
   - 2.4 Learning disabilities and vulnerability — 266
   - 2.5 Further support — 267

19: Older People — 269

1. Ageing — 269
   - 1.1 Learning objective — 269
   - 1.2 Introduction — 269
   - 1.3 Anatomy and physiology of ageing — 269
2. Caring for older patients — 271
   - 2.1 Learning objectives — 271
   - 2.2 Age-related conditions — 271
   - 2.3 Attitudes to ageing — 273
   - 2.4 Patients with co-morbidities — 273
3. Dementia — 274
   - 3.1 Learning objectives — 274
   - 3.2 Introduction — 274
   - 3.3 Dementia — 274
   - 3.4 Communication — 278
   - 3.5 Challenging behaviour — 279

20: Cardiac Arrest — 281

1. Basic life support (BLS) and defibrillation — 281
   - 1.1 Learning objectives — 281
   - 1.2 Introduction — 281
   - 1.3 Chain of survival — 281
   - 1.4 Defibrillation — 282
2. Paediatric BLS — 284
   - 2.1 Learning objectives — 284
   - 2.2 Introduction — 284
   - 2.3 Infant BLS with AED — 285
   - 2.4 Child BLS with AED — 288
3. Adult BLS — 292
   - 3.1 Learning objectives — 292
   - 3.2 Causes of cardiac arrest in adults — 292
   - 3.3 Adult BLS with AED — 292
4. Cardiac arrest in special circumstances — 295
   - 4.1 Learning objectives — 295
   - 4.2 Introduction — 295
   - 4.3 Cardiac arrest in pregnancy — 295
   - 4.4 Cardiac arrest in hypothermic patients — 295
   - 4.5 Cardiac arrest in drowned patients — 295
5. Post-resuscitation care — 296
   - 5.1 Learning objectives — 296
   - 5.2 Introduction — 296
   - 5.3 Management — 296

6	Cardiac arrest decisions	296
	6.1 Learning objective	296
	6.2 When to start and stop resuscitation	296
	6.3 End of life decisions	297

References **299**

Glossary **319**

Index **323**

List of Abbreviations

AAP	associate ambulance practitioner
ABC	airway, breathing, circulation
ABCDE	airway, breathing, circulation, disability, exposure/environment
ABG	arterial blood gas
ACP	advance care plan
ACS	acute coronary syndrome
ADRT	advanced decision to refuse treatment ('living will')
AED	automated external defibrillator
AF	atrial fibrillation
ANS	autonomic nervous system
ATMIST	age, time of incident, mechanism of injury, injuries, signs and symptoms, treatment given/immediate needs
ATP	adenosine triphosphate
AVPU	alert, voice, pain, unresponsive
BLS	basic life support
BVM	bag-valve-mask
CBRNE	Chemical, biological, radiological, nuclear, explosive
CFR	Community First Responder
CNS	central nervous system
CO	Carbon monoxide
COPD	chronic obstructive pulmonary disease
CPR	cardiopulmonary resuscitation
CRT	capillary refill time
CSF	cerebrospinal fluid
DNA	deoxyribonucleic acid
DNACPR	do not attempt cardiopulmonary resuscitation
ECA	emergency care assistant
ECG	electrocardiogram
ECSW	emergency care support worker
ED	emergency department
EOC	emergency operations centre
ET	endotracheal
FB	foreign body
FGM	Female genital mutilation
GCS	Glasgow Coma Scale
HART	hazardous area response team
HCAI	healthcare-associated infection
HCPC	Health and Care Professions Council
HIV	Human immunodeficiency virus
ICP	intracranial pressure
ICU	intensive care unit
IR	infrared
IV	intravenous
kPa	kilopascal
LAD	left anterior descending artery
LCA	left coronary artery
LOC	level of consciousness
METHANE	major incident, exact location, type of incident, hazards, access, number of casualties, emergency services
MI	myocardial infarction
MILS	manual in-line stabilisation
MIU	minor injuries unit
MOI	mechanism of injury
MTC	major trauma centre
NAI	non-accidental injury
NHS	National Health Service
NIBP	non-invasive blood pressure measurement
NICE	National Institute for Health and Care Excellence
NOI	nature of illness
NSTEMI	non-ST-segment elevation myocardial infarction
OPA	oropharyngeal airway
PDA	posterior descending artery
PEA	pulseless electrical activity
PND	paroxysmal nocturnal dyspnoea
PPE	personal protective equipment
PPV	positive pressure ventilation
RCA	right coronary artery

RNA	ribonucleic acid		history, last oral intake, events leading to current illness/injury
ROM	range of movement		
ROSC	return of spontaneous circulation	**SARS**	severe acute respiratory syndrome
RTC	road traffic collision	**SC**	subcutaneous
SA	sino-atrial	**SCENE**	safety, cause including NOI/MOI, environment, number of patients, extra resources needed
SAD	supraglottic airway device		
SAMPLE	signs and symptoms of presenting complaint, allergies, medications, past medical		
		SCI	spinal cord injury
		SIRS	systemic inflammatory response syndrome

Acknowledgements

Class Professional Publishing would like to thank the following for their co-operation in the production of this book and others in the Ambulance Care series:

- Paul Maskell, Iris Murch, Mervyn Murch, Sarah Petter, Steven Petter, Karina Pilbery, Megan Pilbery, Vicky Pilbery, James Short, Peter Williams, the students at Coventry University and the University of Gloucester, and the teams at SWAST, WMS and YAS for modelling
- Charles L. Till and colleagues at Coventry University for the use of their facilities and equipment
- Martin Hilliard and colleagues at the University of Gloucestershire for the use of their facilities and equipment
- Cornwall Air Ambulance for the use of their facilities and equipment
- Tasnim Ali at YAS for sourcing volunteers for photoshoots
- Nigel Wilson for photography work
- Daniels, Ferno, Reflex Medical, Safeguard Medical, SP Services, University of the West of England and Zoll for the loan of equipment
- Mike Page for consulting
- Ken Wenman and Claire Warner at SWAST for the loan of the ambulance

We would like to thank the following for their invaluable feedback on earlier drafts of this book:

- Nic Morecroft, who deserves special thanks
- Rob Horton
- Jamie Todd
- Emma Scott
- Derek Flint
- Richard Rolfe
- Georgina Dunbar
- Ken Wheeler
- Steve Knowles

We would like to thank the following for their kind permission to publish material:

Chapter 5 Alcohol Handrub Procedure. Based on the 'How to Handrub' poster © World Health Organization 2024. All rights reserved.

Chapter 5 Handwashing Procedure. Based on the 'How to Handwash' poster © World Health Organization 2024. All rights reserved.

Figure 5.4 Clinell wipes. Republished with permission of GAMA Healthcare Ltd. Best practice guidance for infection control wet wipes developed by Clinell and GAMA Healthcare Ltd. © 2016

Figure 7.3 A mechanically powered ambulance stretcher. Republished with permission of Ferno.

Figure 7.5 Help Fall checklist. Reproduced with kind permission from Felgains.

Figure 8.1 Dynamic Risk Assessment model. Image reproduced by the kind permission of the National Ambulance Resilience Unit (NARU).

Figure 8.2 M/ETHANE model. Image reproduced by the kind permission of JESIP.

Figure 8.3 Ten Second Triage. Image reproduced by NHS England.

Figure 10.11, 10.12, 10.13 and 10.14 Tracheostomy tubes. Images reproduced by the kind permission of Kapitex Healthcare Ltd.

Figure 10.16 The FBAO algorithm for adults. Reproduced with kind permission of the Resuscitation Council (UK).

Figure 10.17 The FBAO algorithm for paediatrics. Reproduced with kind permission of the Resuscitation Council (UK).

Figure 11.11 A Firesafe. Image reproduced by kind permission of BPR Medical.

Figure 11.13 Bag-valve-mask with oxygen reservoir bag attached and inflated. Image reproduced by the kind permission of Ambu A/S.

Figure 12.14 An aneroid sphygmomanometer. Image reproduced by the kind permission of Welch Allyn.

Figure 13.5 Petechial non-blanching rash and Figure 13.6 Maculopapular rash with scanty Petechiae are courtesy of the Meningitis Research Foundation.

Chapter 15 Procedure for Jext auto-injector. Images reproduced with the kind permission of ALK.

Figure 19.3 The Abbey pain scale. Source: Abbey, Piller, De Bellis, Esterman, Parker, Giles and Lowcay (2004) 'The Abbey pain scale: a 1-minute numerical indicator for people with end-stage dementia', International Journal of Palliative Nursing. 10:1, 6–13. Copyright 2004 MA Healthcare Ltd. Reproduced by permission of MA Healthcare Ltd.

Figure 20.1 The chain of survival. Image reproduced by the kind permission of Laerdal Medical.

Every effort has been made to secure permission to republish copyright images. If any have been inadvertently overlooked, the copyright holders are invited to contact Class Professional Publishing and the omission will be rectified in the next printing as well as all further editions.

Foreword

The Association of Ambulance Chief Executives welcomes the second edition of *First Responder Care Essentials* to its portfolio of endorsed publications. This comprehensive textbook will continue to assist many in learning essential skills for their role as a volunteer community first responder. The progressive manner of introducing the basics of how an ambulance service functions, the ambulance service context, clinical skills and also how to provide optimum and inclusive patient care gives the reader a complete understanding of what is required. The second edition has been brought up-to-date with current guidance and introduces a new section on poisoning. We thank you for your interest in ambulance volunteering and trust this publication will support you to build confidence and skill.

Helen Vine, Assistant Director, the Association of Ambulance Chief Executives

The National Education Network for Ambulance Services welcomes the second edition of *First Responder Care Essentials* to its portfolio of endorsed publications written by Richard Pilbery and Kris Lethbridge. This innovative textbook will continue to assist ambulance first responders in learning essential skills. The second edition has been brought up-to-date with current guidance. We look forward to future editions. This textbook provides essential underpinning learning for first responder programmes in place across the UK ambulance services. The emergency and urgent care systems are undergoing significant and continual change and the development of a suite of resources for UK ambulance services will ensure that the ambulance workforce is able to continue working at the heart of these changing systems. The textbook will assist learners to develop their knowledge and skills as a part of taught programmes and will provide a strong understanding of what is required of today's ambulance workforce and a solid foundation for continued learning.

Pauline Cranmer, Chair, National Education Network for Ambulance Services (NENAS) and Chief Paramedic Officer, London Ambulance Service

Chapter 1 Introduction

1 Textbook guide

1.1 Introduction

This textbook is designed to help prepare you to work as a volunteer responder (sometimes referred to as community first responder, or first/emergency responder) or similar, but will also be of interest to readers who already have completed a first-aid or first-response emergency care course and wish to expand their knowledge.

1.2 Textbook

This textbook is designed to be read from start to finish on the first reading because concepts introduced later on in the book assume that you already have knowledge of the content that has been covered in earlier chapters. However, this textbook will also be a useful reference to which you can return again and again, reflecting on the learning points that are highlighted.

Each chapter comprises a number of different topics centred on a theme, such as health and safety, or the airway. The learning objectives for each chapter have been mapped to objectives from a range of courses that are used to prepare volunteers to become responders.

1.3 Getting started

To help get you orientated to the topics covered in this textbook and their relevance to clinical practice, the next section, 'Anatomy of an emergency call', will take you step by step through an emergency call, highlighting the variety of knowledge and skills that you will require in order to be an effective responder.

Each chapter is split into sections, which are typically laid out in the following way:
- learning objectives: to clearly highlight what you are expected to learn in the chapter
- introduction: setting the scene for the theme of the chapter
- content: the content!

2 Anatomy of an emergency call

2.1 Introduction

The topics covered in the chapters of this textbook are an essential part of your role as a responder. It can be helpful to find out WHY you need to learn something. In order to see this in context, let's review a typical clinical scenario that you may be faced with when responding on the behalf of the ambulance service (Figure 1.1).

2.2 The emergency operations centre (EOC)

When Mrs Brown makes a 999 call, she speaks to a telephone operator, who asks her which service she requires. She asks for the ambulance service and is put through to her local ambulance service's EOC (Figure 1.2).

Since the call has been triaged as an emergency, an ambulance and responder are allocated to it.

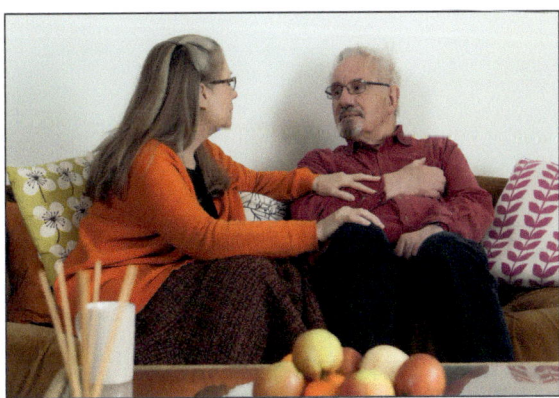

Figure 1.1 Mr James Brown, a 59-year-old man who has chest pain, with his wife, Patricia

Chapter 1 – *Introduction*

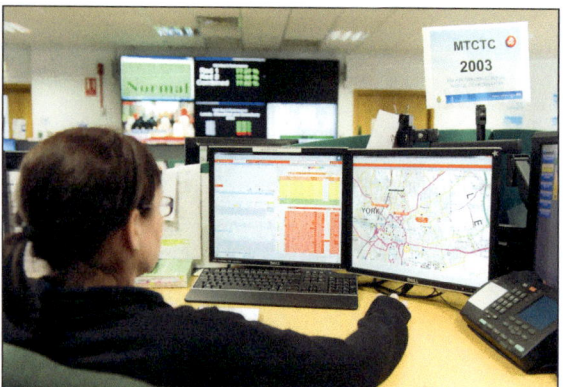

Figure 1.2 A dispatcher in the EOC

As a responder, you are tasked to incidents that can benefit from your knowledge and skills, and which are close to where you are located, meaning that you may well arrive before the ambulance crew.

You will learn more about the ambulance service, including the roles and responsibilities of its staff, and ambulance and clinical quality indicators in Chapter 2, 'The Ambulance Service'.

2.3   Arriving on scene

You will have been conducting a scene assessment, even before arriving at the address. This will include considering the location, time of day and type of incident, and is a dynamic process, i.e. should be constantly reviewed, as the scene can change rapidly. You will learn more about this in Chapter 8, 'Scene Assessment'.

In addition to scene safety, you will consider the need for personal protective equipment (PPE). At a residential address, this may be limited to a pair of disposable gloves, but other PPE may be required if there is severe bleeding, for example (covered in Chapter 5, 'Health and Safety').

You retrieve the response bag and automated external defibrillator (AED) from your vehicle and head towards the front door, where Mrs Brown is anxiously waiting (Figure 1.3).

2.4   Principles of communication

You are shown into the living room where Mr Brown is sitting on the sofa, clutching his chest and looking rather grey and sweaty. You introduce yourself to Mr and Mrs Brown and clarify what Mr Brown prefers to be called. He tells you to call him Jim (Figure 1.4).

Communication is a fundamental aspect of all ambulance work and your role as a responder. It is not always easy as you will have to communicate with patients, friends and family members, as well as other healthcare professionals, and adapt your approach and style appropriately. In addition, you cannot communicate the same way with an elderly person as you would a teenager. Some patients will not, or cannot, communicate with you, because they are depressed or don't speak English, for example. Chapter 3, 'Communication', will cover this in more detail.

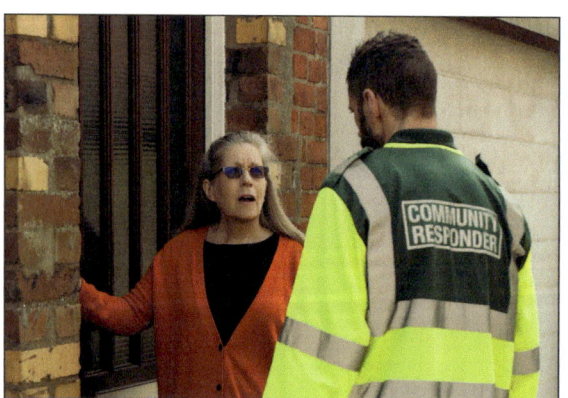

Figure 1.3   The responder arrives at the address

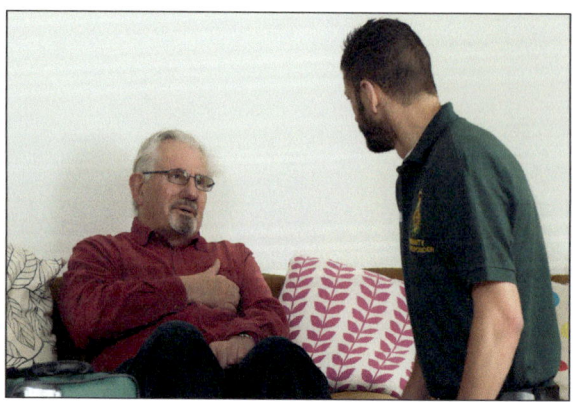

Figure 1.4   The responder talking to Jim

Anatomy of an emergency call

2.5 Patient assessment

You complete an initial catastrophic haemorrhage (bleeding), airway, breathing, circulation, disability, exposure (<C>ABCDE) assessment of Jim (reviewed in Chapter 9, 'Patient Assessment') and obtain a set of baseline observations to support this. Jim's airway is patent; he is breathing at a rate of 16 breaths per minute, which is in the normal range. After obtaining permission (correctly termed 'consent', an important legal concept, covered in Chapter 4, 'Legal and Ethical Issues') from Jim, you apply a pulse oximeter to one of his fingers. His oxygen saturations are 93% on air so you administer oxygen (covered in Chapter 11, 'Breathing'). Continuing with the assessment of Jim's circulation, you check his pulse and measure his blood pressure.

2.6 Patient history

Jim explains that he experienced a sudden onset of central chest pain radiating to his jaw, back and both arms an hour prior to his wife's 999 call. It feels like a heavy pressure, which he scores as 7 out of 10, and is associated with shortness of breath, nausea and sweating. His wife states that he has been very pale since the onset of the pain.

You ask about Jim's past medical history and he tells you that he has high cholesterol and high blood pressure; he takes medication to treat both. You ask for his medication so you can pass it on to the crew (Figure 1.5). He has never had a heart attack (myocardial infarction, MI), but does admit to experiencing occasional chest pain on exertion over the past month or so.

2.7 Cardiac arrest

You continue to talk to Jim and reassure him and his wife while you wait for the ambulance to arrive. Suddenly, Jim becomes unresponsive. After calling his name and then gently shaking his shoulders, you realise that he may be in cardiac arrest (Figure 1.6). After conducting a rapid Task, Individual, Load, Environment, Equipment (TILEE) assessment (covered in Chapter 7, 'Manual Handling'), you move Jim on to the floor.

2.8 Basic life support and defibrillation

After confirming that Jim is not breathing and is showing no signs of life, you instruct Jim's wife to start chest compressions while you update the EOC and get the AED ready (covered in Chapter 20, 'Cardiac Arrest'). You expose Jim's chest and ensure that the defibrillator pad sites are free from jewellery, piercings, medication patches, wounds and tumours. Luckily, there is no need to shave his chest.

The AED instructs everyone to stand clear while it analyses Jim's heart rhythm before instructing

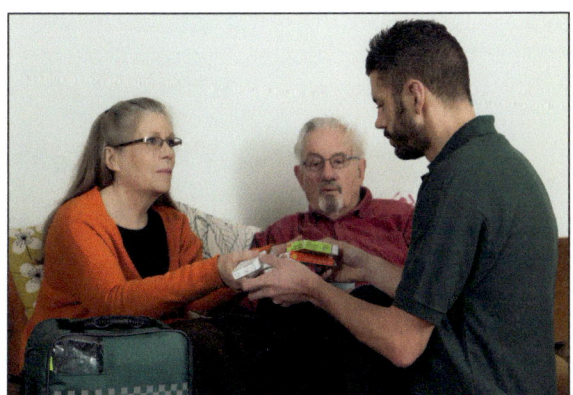

Figure 1.5 Gathering the patient's medication for the ambulance crew

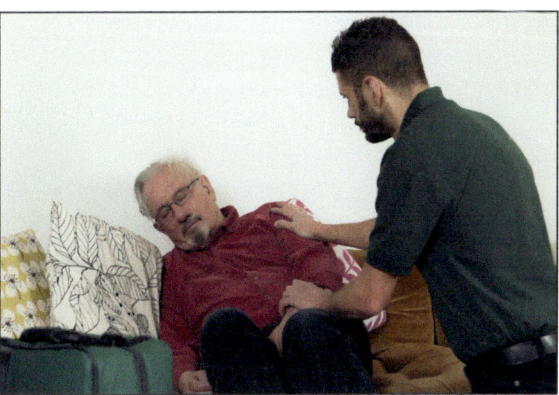

Figure 1.6 Jim collapses and is unresponsive

Chapter 1 – Introduction

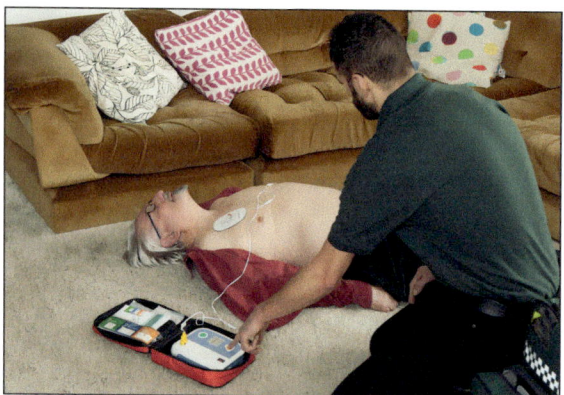

Figure 1.7 Using an AED safely is an important responder skill

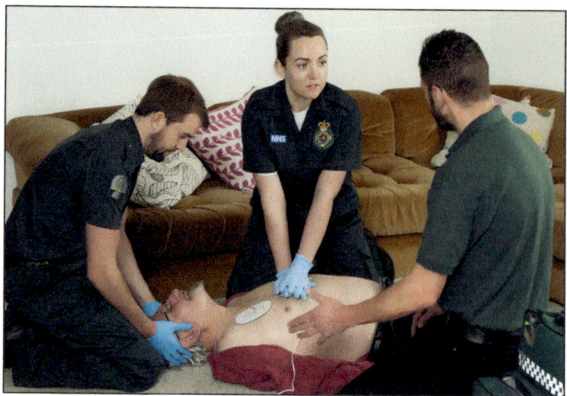

Figure 1.8 Providing a structured handover to the ambulance crew is important to ensure good continuity of care

you to resume chest compressions. Jim's wife is looking tired, so you take over. A shock is advised, so once the AED has charged you ensure that Jim's wife and you are clear of Jim before pressing the shock button (Figure 1.7). As soon as the shock is delivered, you immediately resume chest compressions.

After 2 minutes of cardiopulmonary resuscitation (CPR), the AED instructs you to stand clear, so you briefly pause chest compressions to allow it to assess the rhythm. Another shock is advised, which you deliver before immediately resuming chest compressions.

2.9 Crew arrival

The ambulance crew arrive and you provide a structured handover, explaining what has happened (Figure 1.8). The crew take over Jim's care but ask you to assist them while they reassess and then transfer Jim to the ambulance.

2.10 Clean up and prepare for the next call

After another 2 minutes of CPR, Jim shows signs of life and begins to breathe spontaneously. You assist the ambulance crew in loading Jim on to the ambulance before returning to the house to gather your equipment. You find out later that Jim had suffered a heart attack, but the blockage in his arteries was successfully removed and he is doing well.

3 Extended skills

3.1 Scope of practice

Look out for the ⊙ extended-skill icons throughout the book. These highlight where a skill may be outside of your scope of practice. If you are unsure, talk with your local co-ordinator about them.

Chapter 2 The Ambulance Service

1 Response to a 999 call

1.1 Learning objective

By the end of this section you will be able to:
- explain how the ambulance service manages an emergency call.

1.2 Introduction

The response to a 999 call can be complex and varies between each incident depending on the degree of need. The three main stages of a response are:
- call for help and triage
- ambulance service response
- onward care of patient.

1.3 Call for help and triage

When someone calls 999 (or 112) in the UK, they are connected to an operator from the national telephone network. Once the nature of the emergency has been established, the call will be forwarded to the police, fire, ambulance service or coastguard, depending on the most appropriate response(s).

Once the call is connected to the ambulance service EOC, a qualified call handler will ask a series of questions. Preset questions are designed to triage calls and identify those that need an ambulance most urgently. They can also identify those callers who do not need an ambulance and for whom an alternative care pathway, such as visiting the GP or self-presenting at a minor injuries unit (MIU), would be more appropriate.

As the call handler works through the questioning, the triage system will identify how urgently an ambulance is required and arrive at a triage code and a response category. Two systems are used for triage: NHS Pathways and the Advanced Medical Priority Dispatch System. Although there are significant differences between the two systems, they both ultimately generate a diagnostic code, which is then allocated to one of four priorities for response.

Following a large review of ambulance services responses in 2015/16 called the Ambulance Response Programme, the old categories of response were dropped and new response standards were introduced (Table 2.1) [NHS England, 2018].

During the triage process, a clinician is often available to assist in 'enhanced triage'. This is particularly useful when dealing with patients who have complex needs that the standard triage system may not be set up to deal with.

Also during triage, the call handler will identify if there is a need for other emergency services, or whether there may be any dangers to the responding ambulance clinicians present (such as an assailant still at the scene). Where required, other services will be contacted and ambulance crews and responders can be advised of the risks.

1.4 Ambulance service response

Based on the information gathered during the triage process, the most appropriate response can be determined. There are two main types of response, which are:
- hear and treat
- physical response.

1.4.1 Hear and treat

Hear and treat is where the patient is advised how to look after themselves, or recommended to self-present to a more appropriate care provider, such as a GP or MIU. Increasingly, clinicians working for the ambulance service, often specialising in urgent care or mental health, also provide remote treatment for patients who call 999. The percentage of 999 calls managed this way has steadily increased from around 5% in 2018 to 10–15% in early 2023 [NHS England, 2023a].

Chapter 2 – *The Ambulance Service*

Table 2.1 Ambulance Response Programme call categories

Category	Description	Details	Average response target	90th percentile response target
1	Life-threatening	A time-critical life-threatening event requiring immediate intervention or resuscitation	7 minutes	15 minutes
2	Emergency	Potentially serious conditions that may require rapid assessment and urgent on-scene intervention and/or urgent transport	18 minutes	40 minutes
3	Urgent	An urgent problem (not immediately life-threatening) that needs treatment to relieve suffering and transport or assessment and management at the scene with referral where needed within a clinically appropriate timeframe	None (mean indicator of 60 minutes)	2 hours
4	Less urgent	Problems that are less urgent but require assessment and possibly transport within a clinically appropriate timeframe	None	3 hours

1.4.2 Physical response

For the majority of 999 calls, the ambulance service will send a physical response.

Depending on the need of the patient and the scale of the incident, this may include:
- responder
- rapid response car
- emergency ambulance
- air- or ground-based critical care teams
- specialist practitioner in urgent care
- hazardous area response team (HART)
- ambulance service officer/commander
- specialist operations response team (SORT)
- joint mental health triage service
- medical support such as British Association for Immediate Care (BASICS).

1.5 *Onward care*

Where necessary, patients will be transported to hospital for emergency care and treatment. This is frequently to emergency departments (EDs) but now also includes an increasing number of specialist emergency care departments, such as stroke units or cardiac centres.

In addition to this, ambulance clinicians have a range of alternative care pathways available to them, in order to avoid hospital admission where appropriate. The number of patients being treated without being taken to hospital is increasing and will continue to rise as paramedics and other out-of-hospital clinicians receive more advanced training in the assessment and management of common conditions. During 2023, nationally only around 52% of 999 calls resulted in a patient being conveyed to an ED [NHS, 2023].

Alternative care providers may include:
- specialist or advanced practitioners in urgent care: clinicians with additional training who can manage a range of minor injuries and illnesses within the community
- GPs
- GP drop-in centres
- out-of-hours services
- mental health teams
- MIUs
- pharmacies
- 111
- social services
- 'Hospital at home' teams
- emergency residential care
- community hospitals.

2 Roles within the ambulance service

2.1 Learning objectives

By the end of this section you will be able to:
- identify a number of clinical roles within the ambulance service and briefly explain what the role entails
- describe the importance of good working relationships.

2.2 Introduction

There are 10 NHS ambulance trusts in England, as well as NHS ambulance services in Scotland, Wales and Northern Ireland, which are statutory providers of ambulance services for the government within the UK [AACE, 2023]. There are also a range of voluntary services, including St John Ambulance and the British Red Cross, and a variety of independent sector services, ranging from the very small to national-scale organisations.

Each service is structured differently, so it is not possible to give a definitive list of the different roles. However, over the following pages are descriptions of some of the roles you may find, which could be broadly divided into:
- clinical
- clinical leadership
- command and control.

2.3 Clinical roles

2.3.1 Community first responders

Community first responders (also referred to as first/emergency responders) come from a variety of backgrounds and volunteer their time for the ambulance service. They respond to incidents close to where they live or work, often in remote settings, which can take longer for an ambulance to reach. Responders carry basic life-saving equipment including an AED and devices for managing a patient's airway, and are trained in the initial management of emergency incidents and how to deliver life-saving skills such as CPR and control of major bleeding.

In recent years as pressure on ambulance services has increased, responders have become an ever increasingly important part of ambulance service response. Delays during periods of high demand in ambulance response means responders are often having to provide care for longer than was previously the case and so their training to assess and care for patients has increased to support this.

In some services responders may work in partnership with remote clinicians to decide on a course of action for a patient, and some schemes have taken on additional roles, such as using lifting chairs to help get patients who have fallen off the ground instead of waiting for an ambulance to be available to do this.

Chapter 2 – *The Ambulance Service*

Responders are an integral part of the ambulance service response in that they are normally the first person to arrive on scene and their role is essential for many services in providing prompt, effective help.

2.3.2 Support worker (SW)

SWs work under the supervision of registered clinicians on front-line ambulances. They are trained in providing emergency care, basic emergency interventions and life support, and are qualified emergency drivers. SWs normally work under the supervision of a qualified clinical colleague. They may also work on support vehicles that are used to transport patients to hospital when these have been assessed by another healthcare professional and are viewed as needing a less urgent admission to hospital. SWs have different names in different places, though common names are emergency care assistants (ECAs) or emergency care support workers (ECSWs).

2.3.3 Associate ambulance practitioners

Associate ambulance practitioners (AAPs, sometimes referred to as emergency medical technicians, EMTs) are non-registered clinicians who normally work alongside a registered clinician, but may also work on their own. They have a range of skills relevant to emergency and urgent care and can undertake a number of pre-hospital procedures and administer a limited range of medications. There is national variation in the skill sets of AAPs and the way in which they are deployed by different services.

AAPs are similar to, but not the same as, the previous role of Institute of Healthcare and Development (IHCD) ambulance technicians, who may still be found in some ambulance trusts. They are also unregistered clinicians who may work independently to a limited scope of practice.

2.3.4 Paramedic

Paramedics are qualified and registered clinicians who specialise in working in the urgent and emergency care setting. They are trained in the examination and treatment of emergency conditions, have a wide range of skills and treatment options, and are considered specialists in emergency care. Registered with the Health and Care Professions Council (HCPC), paramedics have a degree of autonomy in their practice and can be held accountable to the HCPC for their actions and omissions that arise from providing clinical care to patients.

2.3.5 Specialist practitioner – urgent care (SPUC)

Specialist practitioners have been known by a range of titles including emergency care practitioner and paramedic practitioner. They have undertaken an enhanced course of learning, usually at post-graduate level, along with a range of placements that equip them with the skills and knowledge to treat urgent care patients. These patients include those with acute illnesses such as respiratory tract and urinary tract infections or minor injuries and wounds. Specialist practitioners have a broad range of skills in the management of urgent patients and can administer a greater variety of medications [CoP, 2023].

2.3.6 Specialist practitioner – critical care

Also known as critical care practitioners (CCPs), like their SPUEC colleagues these clinicians have also undertaken enhanced study, but with a focus on dealing with the most critically ill or injured, normally at postgraduate level [CoP, 2023]. Specialist practitioners in critical care will often work as part of a multidisciplinary team alongside a doctor who specialises in emergency pre-hospital care.

2.3.7 Advanced practitioner

Advanced practitioners are experienced paramedics or nurses who have completed master's level study relevant to their practice. They will be very experienced, most likely having worked in a number of different clinical settings, and will be able to demonstrate an expert knowledge base, complex decision-making, and clinical leadership in their area of practice. Advanced practitioners may have roles that mix clinical practice and clinical leadership or education and research. Advanced practitioner roles are generally new to ambulance services, but as services transform to meet the ever increasing demands on them, advanced practitioners are likely to play an increasing role [CoP, 2023].

2.3.8 HART

HART teams are groups of ambulance service clinicians who have been specially trained to work in difficult situations and alongside the police and fire services at large and dangerous incidents. They have a special set of skills and equipment, which can enable swift water rescues, working at heights, and use of breathing apparatus among others. This allows them to safely access patients in remote and difficult settings. There is a network of HART bases around the country and their help can normally be requested through the EOC when required [NARU, 2024].

2.4 Clinical leadership roles

Running any ambulance service requires a large range of clinical leaders. Some of the common roles include:
- consultant paramedic
- clinical development manager
- pharmaceutical adviser
- medical director.

2.4.1 Consultant paramedic

The consultant paramedic is a relatively new role in some ambulance trusts throughout the UK. The role of the consultant is to act as a senior clinical leader involved in service development, clinical leadership, research and evaluation, and education and professional development. Consultant paramedics will normally work in a mixed role providing advanced clinical support to operational staff while also undertaking their other responsibilities. After the medical director, a consultant paramedic is normally the most senior clinical leader in an ambulance trust.

2.4.2 Clinical development manager (CDM)

The CDM is responsible for ensuring that clinical policies and procedures are up to date. They also consider what new procedures and medication may be beneficial for patients.

2.4.3 Pharmaceutical adviser

Most organisations will have a pharmacist working for them at least part-time. This is to ensure that the use of medications by the service is safe and appropriate and that the relevant laws are being followed.

2.4.4 Medical director

The medical director, normally a doctor with a background in emergency and/or critical care, is the ultimate person responsible for the clinical care inside an organisation. They are a very senior clinical leader and are answerable for clinical errors and omissions within an organisation.

2.5 Command and control roles

Inside every large organisation is a command and control structure. This structure is required to co-ordinate and effectively deliver the functions of the organisation, but it becomes particularly relevant in emergency services at times of complex or major incidents. All commanders receive specific training relevant to their role. Different command roles do not necessarily indicate rank or seniority within an organisation, but are instead allocated so that those involved understand their role in managing an incident. Previous reviews of major incidents have identified weaknesses in the ways in which different emergency services interact and use different processes and protocols for responding, deploying and communicating. National programmes, such as the Joint Emergency Services Interoperability Programme (JESIP), seek to ensure that all emergency services can work effectively together at large-scale incidents through a series of common principles which all commanders, regardless of background, will be familiar with [JESIP, 2024].

2.5.1 Operational commanders

Operational commanders, broadly equivalent to what were formerly known as 'bronze' commanders, have responsibility for the activities undertaken during an incident and will be located at the scene, ideally collocated with commanders from other emergency agencies. They are responsible for organising the delivery of care and the safety of those working at a scene. They have to assess what resources are available to them, or have been made available to them by tactical and strategic commanders, and utilise those resources in the most effective way possible.

Depending on the size of the incident, operational commanders work alongside a number of other officers from both the ambulance and other emergency services to ensure services are being provided in an effective and co-ordinated manner.

Operational commanders receive direction from tactical commanders, with whom they have to constantly liaise closely to ensure they have the resources they require to manage an incident [NARU, 2019].

2.5.2 Tactical commanders

Formerly known as 'silver' commanders, tactical commanders are individuals with thorough working knowledge of NHS ambulance service operations. They are responsible for ensuring that all the tactical resources an operational commander requires for the management of an incident are in place. They will communicate closely with other emergency services and agencies and may or may not be present at the scene, depending on the scale and nature of the incident as well as the amount of time it goes on for.

At some incidents there may be multiple operational commanders, each dealing with different sections of the scene, in which case the tactical commander will be responsible for co-ordinating their actions.

The tactical commander achieves a level of oversight for an incident which cannot normally be achieved by an operational commander on the ground. From this position, the tactical commander can ensure there is effective joint working of agencies and that the deployment of resources and the tactics being used to manage an incident are appropriate [NARU, 2019].

2.5.3 Strategic commanders

Strategic, formerly known as 'gold', commanders are responsible for devising and making available the resources to implement a strategy for managing an incident. They will have executive level decision-making ability for their organisation and have overall responsibility for command response and recovery of an incident. The strategic commander has control over all the organisation's resources and is responsible for making them available to the tactical and operational commanders as appropriate.

Strategic commanders, like tactical commanders, have oversight of the management of an incident and are responsible for ensuring the tactics being used are appropriate, that all services are working effectively together and that clear lines of communication are in place.

Where necessary, strategic commanders are responsible for national-level communication to make available further resources if they are required [NARU, 2019].

2.5.4 National inter-agency liaison officer (NILO)

The NILO is a nominated person who has had specific training and experience to ensure that agencies such as fire, police and ambulance services can communicate effectively during a major or serious incident [NARU, 2019].

2.5.5 Hospital ambulance liaison officer (HALO)

The HALO is a hospital-based member of ambulance service staff whose role it is to help co-ordinate hospital handovers. This involves liaising with hospital and ambulance service managers around capacity and timeframes for offloading patients. They can also warn the hospital of any incoming patients and provide support to ambulance crews waiting to hand over. The increasing delays at hospital which have been present over recent years have made the role of the HALO more important and turned it into one that is much more frequently now seen [NARU, 2019].

2.6 Support structures

As a responder you will be an integral part of the ambulance service workforce and you should be aware of the support structures around you. Every service will operate in a slightly different model, but you should be allocated a line manager whom you can approach with any challenges or difficulties you have. This line manager will typically be responsible for ensuring you have appropriate equipment and for leading training and regular assessment sessions, and will also be a point of contact if you find you need to discuss any incidents you have attended.

It is likely that you will be given key contact information by the organisation you respond for, but if you are unclear, make sure you ask and become familiar with those who are there to support you in your role.

In addition, there will likely be a variety of services available to support your well-being. These vary from organisation to organisation, but may include some of the below:
- occupational health teams
- Staying Well teams
- mental health first-aiders
- trauma risk management (TRiM) practitioners
- physiotherapy
- counselling services.

Although responders are typically volunteers, organisations have the same responsibility to care for them and ensure their well-being and safety as employed members of staff. You should be made aware of the services available to you on induction, but further information will also likely be available via your line manager or organisation communication channels such as the intranet or bulletin.

2.7 Working relationships

As you can see, there is a wide range of roles in the ambulance service and it is likely that you will need to work collaboratively with many of them at some time or another. Key to successful collaborative working will be building successful working relationships.

A good relationship with your manager is particularly important. Key principles of good working relationships are:
- knowledge of the responsibilities and limits of your own role
- regular face-to-face meetings
- performance feedback sessions
- opportunities to ask questions so you can develop your skills.

Should you have a problem with or encounter bullying from your manager, escalate this to your organisation. The NHS Constitution details that all staff, paid or voluntary, have a right to 'a good working environment' [DHSC, 2023]. NHS trusts must strive to provide 'a positive working environment for staff and to promote supportive, open cultures which help staff do their job to the best of their ability' and this includes volunteers such as responders as well as paid staff.

3 Caring for yourself and colleagues

3.1 Learning objectives

At the end of this section you will be able to:
- define mental well-being
- list factors that may have an impact on mental well-being
- define resilience in terms of mental well-being
- describe how to improve personal mental well-being and resilience
- list sources of help for mental well-being
- describe how to support a colleague's mental well-being.

3.2 Introduction

As a responder, your role is to help and support other people during times of crisis, but this constant exposure can have a detrimental impact on your own mental health and well-being. Research suggests that emergency service workers and volunteers are more likely to experience mental health problems than the general workforce but are less likely to take time off work or seek help [Mind, 2016].

3.3 Mental well-being

Mental well-being describes your overall mental state and considers how the way you are feeling impacts on how you can cope with day-to-day life and what feels possible at the moment [Mind, 2024a]. People with good mental well-being can:
- feel confident and have positive self-esteem
- build and maintain positive relationships
- live and work productively
- cope with the stresses of daily life
- adapt to changes around them.

3.3.1 Impact on mental well-being

Mental well-being can be impacted by several factors, both inside and outside of work, including:
- repeated exposure to traumatic incidents
- impact of physical injuries
- workload pressure
- suffering personal loss
- relationship problems
- financial worries
- loneliness.

3.4 Building resilience

Dealing with more difficult times in life, whether they be due to personal or work-related issues, can be challenging. The capacity to stay mentally well during these periods relies on your personal mental health 'resilience'. You can try to build resilience to deal with these difficult times by [Mind, 2024b]:
- talking about the way you feel
- developing your interests and hobbies
- looking after your physical health
- doing something you enjoy regularly
- setting yourself a challenge
- spending time in nature
- identifying triggers.

3.5 Seeking help

There will be times when you recognise, either in yourself or a colleague, that personal resilience is not enough and that further help is required. Often this decision is difficult to arrive at and can be left longer than it really should have been; emergency service staff often feel they should be the ones who stay strong, as it is their role to help others. Left unsupported, poor mental well-being can lead to anxiety, depression and post-traumatic stress disorder (PTSD).

Help can be sought from a range of sources, including:
- employer support
- medical support
- charities.

3.5.1 Employer support

Your employer is likely to have a form of internal service for supporting staff, which may include peer counselling, a multi-faith chaplain, or schemes such as TRiM or external counselling support.

3.5.2 Medical support

Your GP will be able to help. While a GP may be able to give a diagnosis and medications, this is rarely the first step. They have a range of options, including just listening to your situation, and can refer you to other treatments, such as talking therapies or counselling if appropriate.

If you are facing a more urgent situation or crisis, you can also call 111 or visit an ED or call 999.

3.5.3 Charities

The **Samaritans** provide 24-hour emotional support for anyone struggling to cope. You can call anonymously if you want, with no need to give personal details, and telephone numbers are not tracked. The Samaritans are available 24/7 via their freephone telephone number 116 123.

The Ambulance Staff Charity (TASC) is a service specifically for supporting the mental health, physical rehabilitation and financial well-being of UK ambulance service employees, including volunteers [TASC, 2024]. Among the services it offers is a 24/7 crisis phoneline for any ambulance staff experiencing suicidal thoughts. It also has a range of mental health support services including talking therapies and self-care resources. More information can be found on their website at www.theasc.org.uk.

3.6 Supporting a colleague

There may be occasions when you think the mental well-being of a colleague is suffering and you may want to try and help them. The charity Mind produces information on how to do this specifically for people working in the ambulance service, which you should look at [Mind, 2024c]. In summary, you should:
- show support by asking them how they are
- ask if you can help in any way
- treat them as you normally would
- don't just talk about mental health
- show trust and respect.

It may be helpful to remind them what support and services are available to them. If there is another colleague you know they respect who has been through a similar situation in the past, it may be useful for them to talk to each other.

Your colleague may not be ready to seek help yet, so be there for them, be patient and continue to offer support and reassurance. Remember that there will be an additional emotional stress on you, so continue to look after yourself and your own resilience.

3 Communication

1 Principles of communication

1.1 Learning objectives

By the end of this section you will be able to:
- identify the different reasons why people communicate
- explain how communication affects relationships in the work setting
- describe the factors to consider when promoting effective communication
- explain how people from different backgrounds may use and/or interpret communication methods in different ways
- identify barriers to effective communication
- explain how to access extra support or services to enable individuals to communicate effectively.

1.2 Introduction

As a responder, you will frequently have to engage and communicate with a diverse range of people at every incident you attend. In the pressure of an emergency situation communication can be very challenging, so understanding the basics of communication in advance can be very beneficial.

As inter-personal communication forms such a fundamental aspect of our daily lives, we rarely stop to think about how we do it, but, as will be discussed throughout this chapter, effective communication, especially in a high-stress environment, is a skill that requires development and practice.

Poor communication is one of the most frequently received complaints for healthcare organisations, including the NHS [NHS Digital, 2022], and poor communication is a well-known cause of disastrous medical and surgical errors, including the removal of incorrect organs and limbs [WHO, 2009].

1.3 Who you will be communicating with

When working as a responder, either at emergency incidents or just as part of your day-to-day activity with the ambulance service, you will interact with a large range of people, which may include:
- service users
- health and care professionals
- colleagues
- members of the public
- staff in the EOC
- other professional services (police, fire etc.).

This communication is likely to occur through a variety of methods, including:
- verbal
- body language
- written
- electronic written (email or electronic patient record)
- radio
- telephone.

This will often be under pressure or personal stress, where poor communication or misinformation can have a detrimental effect on patient outcomes. Therefore, mastering communication in the emergency environment is a core skill of anyone working for an ambulance service.

1.4 Basics of communication

Traditionally, communication has been regarded as the sending of a message from one person to another (Figure 3.1). In World War II, Shannon and Weaver [1949] created a communication model which considered how messages were sent. The original theory relied on radio traffic, but the principles have been widely applied since to all forms of communication. They identified five steps to communication:

1. **Sender:** The person who originally has the message to send.

Chapter 3 – *Communication*

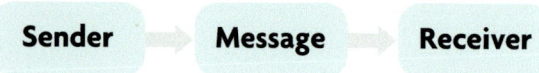

Figure 3.1 Basic model of communication

2. **Channel:** The route through which a message is sent, for example through speech or email.
3. **Encoding:** The process of converting the message into a suitable form for transmission, for example selecting the words to be used, the grammar, the emphasis, tone or even facial expression.
4. **Decoder:** The process of receiving and interpreting the message.
5. **Receiver:** The intended final recipient of the message.

In this model, the sender (person A) has a message they wish to pass on to the receiver (person B). The message exists within the consciousness of the sender initially, before they decide on a method of transferring that message. Before it can be passed on it must be 'encoded'. This encoding may be the selecting of certain words, certain emphasis during part of the sentence, or other verbal or non-verbal features. The receiver must then 'decode' the message as they receive it and try to interpret the original communication from all the verbal and non-verbal information they have received. The complexities of this and the multiple opportunities for misunderstanding to occur along that process are immediately evident.

First, this model implies that communication is a one-way process and does not consider the importance of checking that the message received by the recipient was that intended by the sender. We all communicate in the context of our own beliefs and experience. The words we use, the emphasis we place, the tone or even pace when speaking can all have a dramatic effect on the message being conveyed. While in the mind of the encoder the message is clear and unambiguous, it may well not be the case for the decoder.

Second, another issue this model identified was interference in communication. Initially this largely referred to 'noise source' for radio signals and how that used to impede radio communication, but the

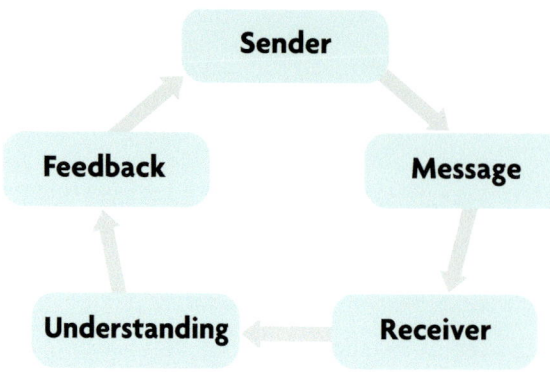

Figure 3.2 Modified model of communication

same concept can be considered as the wider issue of barrier to communication, which we will discuss below in more detail. This could be a technical issue, such as poor radio or mobile signal, but could equally be as complex as a previous inter-personal disagreement between two people impacting on how they communicate information.

A modified model includes the variables of understanding and feedback and is a cyclic process (Figure 3.2). This inclusion of checking the understanding of the message given, and receiving feedback, is fundamental to ensure that messages have been understood in the way in which they were intended.

This is particularly important in high-stress situations or when communicating information a person may not understand well (such as a medical complaint), to ensure that the correct message has been received and understood. In these situations it is very easy for a message to be misinterpreted, with potentially disastrous consequences.

1.4.1 Verbal skills

Verbal communication can be divided into two broad areas:
- language and vocabulary
- paralinguistic features of communication.

Language and vocabulary
Working in healthcare, you must be able to adjust your language and vocabulary so that it is suited to the person you are communicating with. When communicating with colleagues and other health

professionals, you will need to use more complex and professional language. However, there will be times when you need to adjust what you say in order to communicate with those who have a narrower range of language skills, which may include children or those with cognitive impairment, such as dementia patients or those with learning difficulties.

Guidance for ensuring clear verbal communication includes:
- Do not try to say too much at one time; people can process only a certain amount of new information at once.
- Avoid using jargon or 'medical speak'.
- Frequently check that what you are trying to communicate is being understood by asking the person to explain what you have told them
- Plan your communication, think about what you want to say and then the easiest way to communicate that to someone else.

Paralinguistic features

Paralinguistics refers to the modification of the way in which we speak and place emphasis in communication. This includes:
- volume
- rhythm
- pitch
- pace
- emphasis
- tone.

1.4.2 Non-verbal communication

Non-verbal communication can have a dramatic impact on the message you are sending and the way that it is then interpreted. It can be possible to communicate entirely by non-verbal means, for example when giving someone a look or a hand gesture. This can become vital for patients who are unable to communicate verbally due to foreign language, learning difficulties or previous injury.

Examples of non-verbal communication include:
- eye contact
- facial expression
- gesture and posture
- personal space and touch.

All of these should be used in a manner that is appropriate to the situation. For example, when gathering a history from a patient, if you are head down and writing as they speak then the patient may get the impression you are not paying attention to them and might leave out key details. In contrast, if you are making eye contact, nodding your head and acknowledging their communication with small verbal cues, such as 'OK' and 'yes' as they are speaking, known as active listening, then they are more likely to continue communicating and reveal all the information you need in order to assess them properly.

Equally, you should observe the body language of those you are communicating with. If the person you are talking to looks as though they are becoming increasingly agitated and frustrated, you should respond to this and change the conversation or method of communication.

1.4.3 Written communication

It is likely that every patient contact you have will involve some form of written communication, most commonly as part of the patient record. Increasingly, written records are completed as part of an electronic record system, but your service should make you familiar with the record system you are required to complete and how this should be undertaken. In addition, you should be provided with on-going feedback about your documentation. It is important that all written communication is neat, legible, concise, and follows a logical structure. Some key pointers for achieving this include:
- Avoid unnecessary abbreviations
- Ensure that your writing is legible, and that it has transferred through to the carbon copy if you're using one
- Diagrams can be beneficial, but they need to be clear and labelled appropriately.
- Ensure you follow a structure; most organisations use some form of standardised 'medical model' to aid this.

1.5 Social context

Communication relies heavily on the social context in which it takes place. Consider the two following scenarios and how the changing social context may influence how you communicate:

- **Scenario A:** You attend a small child who has fallen and injured their wrist. As part of your assessment you need to look at the wrist, but the child is wary of letting you get close, due to fear that you will cause more pain.
- **Scenario B:** You are called to give evidence in court at the case of a serious assault you attended. You are placed in the witness box and asked a series of questions by the prosecution, prior to cross-examination by the defence.

In both these scenarios, effective communication is critical to ensure that others receive the message you intended to send. However, the way in which you communicate these messages will be vastly different. Your role is to ensure you encode the message, using both verbal and non-verbal features of communication, in such a way that it is likely it will be decoded in the manner you intended.

This concept extends well beyond the extreme examples cited above and into your daily role as a responder. You will meet people from a wide range of social and cultural backgrounds. Every one of these people will have a different social context in which they exist, and you will need to be mindful of modifying your communication, based on the needs of the individual, to ensure that accurate messages are passed on and misunderstanding does not occur.

1.6 Barriers to communication

Barriers to communication are anything that influences your ability to effectively pass on and receive the message you need. You will frequently encounter difficult-to-manage barriers to communication and will need to think of ways of dealing with them. Here are some examples of barriers to communication and how they can be overcome:

- **Sensory problems:** Many patients will have sensory impairments to their hearing, sight or speech, making communication more challenging. Speak slowly; listen carefully. Don't shout at someone who has a hearing impairment – just pronounce your words clearly and make sure the person can see your lips. Make use of communication aids such as a patient's hearing aids and think about alternative methods of communication such as writing things down.
- **Language:** You will inevitably meet people with whom you cannot communicate in their native language. Many simple issues can be communicated through imitating and actions – such as eating and drinking. For more complex messages, using a family member as a translator can be helpful. Alternatively, your service may have provided you with other tools such as phrase books or access to Language Line, a telephone service that provides translators for a wide range of languages over the phone.
- **Emotions:** You will frequently encounter patients and situations where those involved are experiencing extreme emotions. At these times people are less able to understand what is being said to them or asked of them. Use of your verbal and non-verbal skills of communication will be key here to ensure clarity of message.
- **Age:** Young patients in particular will need to be communicated with in a way that is suitable to them and that they can understand. Using pictures, drawings and other props can be an effective means of overcoming barriers to communication.

Other examples of communication barriers include [Ali, 2017]:

- time constraints
- environmental issues such as noise
- pain and fatigue
- embarrassment or anxiety
- value and beliefs
- information overload.

It is not possible to give an exhaustive list of barriers to communication, or how each should be overcome; instead it is important that within your role you are constantly mindful of the risk of barriers developing and consider in each situation how a barrier may be impacting on communication and what, if any, steps you can take to overcome that barrier. For example, in some scenarios it may be possible to overcome environmental noise issues by moving the patient to another location. Sometimes though this may not be possible, and you may have to do your best with written communication, or even gestures and motions to communicate for a period of time.

It is worth noting that whenever you adapt your communication to overcome such difficulties there is an increased risk of your message being misinterpreted, so you should make doubly sure that what you wanted to communicate is the message the person has received.

As with all elements of your practice, you should constantly reflect on your communication skills to learn from both positive and negative experiences to continue improving your abilities.

1.6.1 Clarify misunderstandings

In the emergency and urgent care setting it is inevitable that, at times, you will be communicating large quantities of information in a short space of time and subsequently misunderstandings can develop. To combat misunderstandings you should:
- Observe for non-verbal cues that the person you are talking to has not understood what you are trying to communicate.
- Confirm the person understands what you are saying to them.
- Repeat what you are trying to communicate in a different manner if you suspect misunderstanding.

1.7 Summary

Communication is a natural skill that we all use on a daily basis. However, in your front-line role you will routinely be faced with challenging and demanding communication scenarios. To help overcome these, having an understanding of the theory of communication and a strong working knowledge of what resources are available to you locally will be helpful. You will also need to be adaptive, creative, responsive and innovative in overcoming barriers to communication on a daily basis.

2 Practical communication

2.1 Learning objectives

By the end of this section you will be able to:
- explain the importance of clear, concise reporting of findings to the clinician
- explain the importance of recording patient observations
- describe the procedure for clinical handover to medical professionals.

2.2 Record-keeping

In your role it is likely that you will frequently need to undertake examinations and record observations. Keeping accurate records and gaining accurate observations is critical to safe patient care as it forms a part of the continuity of their care. Changes in observations can indicate a deteriorating or improving patient, so if there are errors in the recorded observations it can create a false perception of the patient's changing state of health.

The following tips will help to ensure patient safety when undertaking this part of your role:
- Pass on, or record, all the information you obtain (even if you are not sure of its relevance) to the clinician responsible for the patient's care.
- If you are asked to undertake procedures, observations or interventions that are outside your skill set, politely inform the responsible clinician that you are not able to do this
- Make your supervising clinician aware if you are struggling or are unsure.
- Never fabricate, estimate or make up observations; doing so not only exposes the patient to risk, but would also be considered as unprofessional conduct when identified.

2.3 Handover

As a responder, it is likely you will often arrive at an incident first and on your own. Your initial observations and history gathering is very important and you must be familiar and prepared to hand over this information in an effective and concise manner to all other healthcare staff that may arrive at an incident after you; this will be done via a structured handover.

Chapter 3 – Communication

The process of a handover is passing on the care of your patient to another healthcare provider(s). During handover all information relevant to the care of the patient should be provided in a concise and effective manner. It is well recognised that handovers are a high-risk aspect of a patient's care, where significant amounts of important information are frequently forgotten or missed out [Merten, 2017]. This can lead to errors or omissions on the part of the receiving clinician and then harm to the patient as a result. This risk of error is increased in high-stress situations, for example when patients are critically ill or injured: just the time when that information needs to be passed on accurately.

There are many models to help facilitate clinical handover and thereby reduce the risk of key information being forgotten. It may be necessary to use different models in different circumstances. You should use your organisation's preferred models, as they will be familiar to your colleagues and the other health professionals you encounter. Two that are particularly common are SBAR for medical cases and ATMIST for traumatic injuries.

2.3.1 Medical handover

SBAR is usually the most appropriate tool when conducting a handover of a patient whose primary concern is a medical problem [NHS Institute for Innovation and Improvement, 2010]:

S: Situation
- identify yourself and your role
- identify the patient by name and the reason you have come into contact with them
- outline your concerns.

B: Background
- describe the reason the patient has called for help
- describe the history of the presenting condition
- list any other pertinent information about the patient's background, which may include: medical history, previous illnesses, current medications, allergies, social situation etc.

A: Assessment
- relate details of the patient's vital signs
- pass on your clinical impressions and concerns.

R: Recommendations
- explain what you need – be specific about the request and timeframe
- make suggestions (if appropriate).

In some scenarios you may not need to make a recommendation. For example, when handing over to an ambulance crew, it may not be appropriate to recommend action to them, but you may still want to share your thoughts or any discussion you have had with the patient about what might happen next.

2.3.2 Trauma handover

The UK Ambulance Services Clinical Practice Guidelines recommend the use of the ATMIST model as a quick and easy way of conducting a handover for trauma patients [JRCALC, 2023]:
- **A:** Age of patient (include a name and date of birth, if you know it)
- **T:** Time of incident
- **M:** Mechanism of injury
- **I:** Injuries sustained
- **S:** Signs and symptoms
- **T:** Treatment given/immediate needs.

Other principles to consider when conducting a handover include the following:
- Make sure the person to whom you are handing over is the person responsible for the patient's care.
- Have your handover ready: make notes in advance to help if necessary and consider rehearsing elements of it in your mind
- Make it concise: you will have a very limited period of time (often less than 60 seconds) in which to provide a handover, especially for the critically ill and injured patient.
- Make sure you have everyone's attention prior to beginning your handover.
- Provide written copies of all information as well as a verbal account whenever you hand over the care of your patient.

2.4 Discussing with a remote clinician

As ambulance services evolve and change the way they deliver care in response to increasing demand, it is becoming more common for clinicians working remotely to contact others at scene to perform a remote assessment and decide on clinical management plans. Increasingly, responders are also involved in this process. Your ambulance service may have a process whereby once you have reviewed a patient, you contact a remote clinician in order to decide on an appropriate management plan.

Being involved in remote triage is a challenging process and increases the potential for error to occur. You are acting as the eyes and ears of the clinician on the phone, so your observations and findings need to be accurate and presented in such a way as to avoid ambiguity or potential for confusion or misunderstanding.

Prior to becoming involved in a remote discussion, ensure you have all the relevant information; this should include:
- medical history, including drug history and allergies
- events that led up to the call for help
- current signs and symptoms
- recent set of observations (taken within the last 10 minutes).

When on the phone to a remote clinician, consider how the language you use can help to paint a picture for that clinician to better understand the patient's condition. For example, describing a patient as looking 'tense, anxious and restless, like they are in pain' creates a very different image from one described as 'relaxed, comfortable and freely engaging in conversation'.

It may help to make notes in advance and highlight any specific points you want to raise with the remote clinician to ensure when the time comes you cover all the vital information.

It is common for those present with a patient and those remote to form different views of the same patient. If this happens and you are concerned that the plan put in place is not suitable for the patient, you should politely highlight this to the remote clinician. As the person on scene with the patient, your observations are vital in forming a gut instinct that is very difficult to share with someone remotely. Any concerns you have over the appropriateness of the plan should be discussed openly and honestly to help ensure the patient remains safe.

2.5 Electronic communication devices

Being able to communicate with the EOC is essential, not just so you can be dispatched to incidents, but also for your own personal safety. It is likely you will have one of two electronic ways of doing this, either:
- mobile phone
- airwaves pager.

Your organisation should train you in the use of the relevant device and you must be familiar with its operation, otherwise you may miss being dispatched to an incident or find you're not able to request help when you need it. You also need to ensure it is kept charged!

4 Legal and Ethical Issues

1 Being a healthcare volunteer

1.1 Learning objectives

By the end of this section you will be able to:
- explain what it means to have a duty of care
- explain how duty of care contributes to the safeguarding or protection of individuals
- describe how to respond to complaints
- explain the main points of agreed procedures for handling complaints
- explain expectations about your work role as expressed in relevant standards
- describe how your values, belief systems and experiences may affect working practice
- describe why it is important to adhere to the agreed scope of the job role
- explain why it is important to work in partnership with others.

1.2 Introduction

This section will describe what it means to be a healthcare volunteer, with a focus on:
- values-based healthcare
- duty of care
- negligence
- scope of practice
- standards
- complaints.

1.3 Values-based healthcare

Working as a member of the ambulance service is an extraordinarily privileged role. As a responder, you will often be caring for people when they are at their most vulnerable. The majority of people have less than a handful of contacts with the ambulance service throughout their lifetime, so when they do call, during extreme life events, patients will look to you for help and support in whatever situation they find themselves in. Being in this privileged role, it is important to recognise that you should be patient focused and that the attitudes and beliefs that you hold can influence the care you provide to your patient.

1.3.1 What influences your values and attitudes?

Being aware of what influences our own attitudes, and how our attitudes impact on the management of our patients, is important to understand. Everyone harbours pre-judgements about certain people or groups of people. These can be positive or negative, and these stereotypes are used as a form of mental shortcut [Amodio, 2014]. However, this can also be dangerous, as it can lead to judgements being made about people based on limited information. These judgements can even influence the way in which a patient is treated, which in turn can lead to errors.

Consider the following scenario:

You are on call overnight on a Friday evening. You have had a long week at work, and already have been out to one incident earlier in the night. Around 02:00 you are awoken by your pager dispatching you to an incident around half a mile away from your home address. You recognise the address on the pager: it is an elderly female who frequently calls the ambulance service saying she has chest pain. Despite lengthy tests and examinations, no-one has ever found any medical issues with the patient and it is thought that her calls are more due to loneliness and panic attacks than any critical medical need.

Is there a risk of stereotyping influencing your practice in this scenario? The answer is almost certainly yes, particularly if you approach the incident thinking 'here we go again', and wondering how long it will be until you can get back home to bed.

A degree of pre-judgement in this scenario is probably unavoidable, but you should recognise that this is the case, and not allow these judgements to bias your thinking, which may in turn lead to you providing less than optimal patient care.

1.3.2 NHS values and attitudes

The NHS Constitution was introduced in 2013, setting out the key principles and values that the NHS embodies. The key principles include that the NHS is a comprehensive service available to all and available based on an individual's need, not their ability to pay for services. The patient is at the heart of the NHS, which is committed to providing the highest standards of excellence and professionalism.

The 6Cs are a set of values all healthcare staff should adopt into their role (Figure 4.1) [NHS Professionals, 2024]. They are:

- **Care:** Care is our core business and that of our organisations; the care we deliver helps the individual person and improves the health of the whole community. Caring defines us and our work. People receiving care expect it to be right for them consistently throughout every stage of their life.
- **Compassion:** Compassion is how care is given through relationships based on empathy, respect and dignity. It can also be described as intelligent kindness and is central to how people perceive their care.
- **Competence:** Competence means all those in caring roles must have the ability to understand an individual's health and social needs. It is also about having the expertise and clinical and technical knowledge to deliver effective care and treatments based on research and evidence.
- **Communication:** Communication is central to successful caring relationships and to effective team working. Listening is as important as what we say. It is essential for 'No decision without me'. Communication is the key to a good workplace with benefits for those in our care and staff alike.

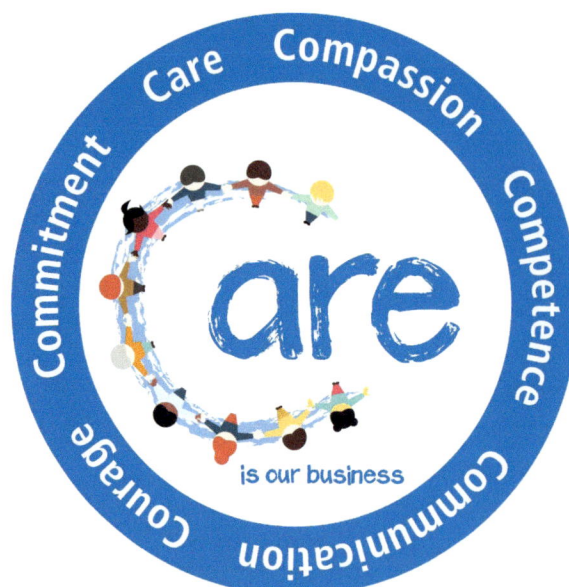

Figure 4.1 The 6Cs describe the core values of a caring, safe and effective healthcare culture
Source: NHS England, 2019: https://www.england.nhs.uk/leadingchange/about/the-6cs/.

- **Courage:** Courage enables us to do the right thing for the people we care for, to speak up when we have concerns. It means we have the personal strength and vision to innovate and to embrace new ways of working.
- **Commitment:** A commitment to our patients and the populations we serve is a cornerstone of what we do. We need to build on our commitment to improve the care and experience of our patients.

As a healthcare volunteer, you have an important part to play to make this vision and strategy a reality for the patients you help care for.

1.4 Duty of care

Duty of care is a civil law concept within the UK and exists to ensure that one party does not allow 'reasonably foreseeable' harm or loss to occur to another [RCN, 2023].

Like all other healthcare providers, as a responder you owe a duty of care to your patient from the point at which they are accepted as a service user. From that point onwards you must act in a way to prevent harm where a reasonable person could see that harm might occur. If you breach this duty of care and someone suffers as a result, this can lead to the civil wrong of negligence.

1.5 *Negligence*

Negligence occurs when duty of care is breached and reasonably foreseeable harm occurs as a result. If a party is guilty of negligence, they can be pursued through the civil courts for damages. There are four stages for negligence to be proven [NHS Resolution, 2023]. Establish:
1. a duty of care
2. breach of duty
3. harm occurred
4. causation.

Establishing a duty of care is usually straightforward, since as a responder you owe a duty to any patient you encounter.

Breach of duty occurs when a reasonably foreseeable consequence of a person's action leads to harm. The difficult part to measure in this section is what counts as 'reasonably foreseeable' and this is a point that the courts may have to decide upon.

Harm can take many forms including physical injury, but may also include:
- mental or emotional distress
- loss of earnings or loss of potential future earnings.

Causation is the final step in proving negligence. It is not enough for a duty of care to exist and for that duty to be breached. That breach of duty must result in harm and it should be evident that this breach was the cause of that harm. Also sometimes referred to as the 'but for' principle, it is applied by asking 'But for the action (or omission) would harm have occurred?' If the answer to this is 'yes', then negligence is not proven; if the answer is 'no', then it is likely that negligence exists.

If negligence is proven, it is likely that the person suffering harm will receive damages for the harm they suffered. This money, likely to run to thousands, if not hundreds of thousands, of pounds or more, depending on the nature and severity of the harm caused, will be paid by the ambulance service under their responsibility of vicarious liability (the ambulance service is responsible for your actions and omissions). However, you should note that in certain exceptional circumstances you can also be found guilty of certain criminal charges if you are criminally negligent in caring for your patient. Therefore it is important to ensure you act within your scope of practice to ensure your own safety.

1.6 *Scope of practice and standards*

Your scope of practice as a responder will be established by the service you are linked to through a series of standards. Such standards are treated as the benchmark for determining whether or not a person is working within their scope of practice and also whether or not they are fit to be a responder.

Standards cover a wide range of topics and not just clinical skills. It is not possible to list the standards for responders here, as they will vary from organisation to organisation, but you should be aware of the standards expected of you and what your scope of practice is, i.e. what can you actually do when responding to a patient. Not everything included in this book will be within the standard scope of practice for all responders. A number of skills through this text have been marked as 'extended' and it is the decision of your organisation as to exactly what examination and management skills, including medications, are available to you as a responder.

You should not attempt to undertake any activity outside your scope of practice, as you are not likely to have the knowledge, skill or experience to perform these activities safely and would therefore be putting the patient and yourself at risk.

What constitutes negligence was outlined earlier, and it should be noted that any activity undertaken outside your scope of practice that leads to harm is likely to be grounds for a negligence claim.

1.7 When things go wrong

All ambulance services strive to be a 'no harm' organisation, but it is probably an unavoidable fact that systems as large and complex as modern ambulance services will always have adverse incidents. However, these errors should not lead to patient harm, and lessons should be learnt from mistakes when they occur.

All health organisations should learn from their mistakes. They should also promote a learning culture, where staff are not unnecessarily blamed for mistakes and where people feel safe in reporting incidents so that the larger organisation can learn from those incidents, even small ones. Only when organisations can learn from their mistakes will they be able to prevent events from being repeated, meaning that, overall, a well-functioning complaints system plays a major role in service improvement and preventing patient harm.

It is a core part of the NHS Constitution that organisations learn from their incidents, and when mistakes occur they are investigated and learnt from. All staff should feel supported to identify errors or omissions and be supported in reporting these and learning from them [DHSC, 2023].

The Patient Safety Incident Response Framework (PSIRF) sets out the NHS's approach to developing and maintaining effective systems and processes for responding to patient safety incidents for the purpose of learning and improving patient safety.

1.7.1 Failure to achieve standards

This concept of reporting extends to you and your own practice as well. If you recognise that in the course of your duty you have failed to achieve the expected standards for someone in your role, then you should make this known. Different organisations will have different methods of reporting, but most now have a central system for reporting incidents and a dedicated team that deals with those reports.

1.7.2 Complaints

During the course of your duty it may be the case that someone wishes to make a complaint about you, the ambulance staff, your organisation or another organisation. This can be challenging, as the natural response is to be defensive, but remember that the principles of a learning organisation, together with opportunities to reflect, should be seen as a way of improving our services and should be welcomed as such. It is likely that your service will have specific guidelines or a policy on handling complaints, which you should be familiar with, but good general guidelines for the actions you should undertake include the following:

- Record facts and pass them on to appropriate people; do not undertake the investigation yourself.
- If someone wishes to make a complaint, take their details and pass them on to relevant parties, or give the person the contact details of the relevant people inside your organisation.
- Do not challenge details about a complaint; if necessary this can be done later on, once all the facts have been established.
- Provide contact details so that patients know how to get in touch should they wish to.

If you become involved in an investigation or complaint, you should do all you can to support the investigation. Withholding key information may be seen as a misconduct offence, which is likely to be handled very differently from learning from a genuine error.

1.7.3 Whistleblowing

Improving patient safety relies on staff identifying when things are not right, or when mistakes have been made, so that organisations can learn and prevent similar circumstances from arising again in the future. Whistleblowing is the act of reporting suspected wrongdoing at work. Whistleblowers should be supported and congratulated for speaking up and thereby providing an opportunity to remedy the problem. However, whistleblowers are not always treated fairly by their employers, with instances of bullying and dismissal occurring [Francis, 2013].

Changing an organisation's culture takes time, but all organisations should be committed to embracing a learning culture and taking staff concerns seriously, while treating the staff involved fairly.

1.7.4 Freedom to speak up

The NHS aims to ensure that everyone working for an NHS organisation feels safe and confident to speak up when necessary, and every organisation should have a freedom to speak up (FTSU) policy [NHS England, 2024a]. The purpose of the policy is to outline how concerns should be raised and handled inside NHS trusts. It includes safeguards for staff to protect them from bullying and harassment if they should raise a concern.

Several channels are normally available to raise a concern, including your manager or a formal written reporting process, but each trust should also have a FTSU Guardian. This is a senior person who can be confidentially contacted with concerns you do not feel you can raise with other managers.

You could also raise a serious concern directly with the regulator, most often the Care Quality Commission (CQC), but this should be an option of last resort in most situations. If it was necessary, it would be a sign of a major failure of leadership and the FTSU principle within an NHS organisation.

Ultimately, a culture that supports raising concerns should result in improving patient care and the safety of both patients and staff. Most managers and leaders want to hear concerns so that they can work to improve standards.

1.7.5 Duty of candour

Duty of candour is a legal obligation on healthcare providers to inform a patient if they have been harmed by the provision of healthcare and offered an appropriate remedy, regardless of whether a complaint has been made or a question asked. For healthcare organisations, this is a standard of their regulation by the CQC [CQC, 2022].

This extends to you as a responder. If you believe that the actions you have undertaken have caused a patient harm, or may cause harm at some future point, you should report this immediately (through the normal reporting channels) in an open and honest manner. If possible, you should also apologise to the patient at the time. For example, if you were to cause a minor injury to a patient's arm while wheeling them out of the house in a chair, then apologise for the mistake once the injury has been treated.

Do not wait for a complaint to be received or for a question to be asked before highlighting the issue. Ultimately, the longer a lot of mistakes are left, the worse the outcome may be for the patient. It is also likely that any wilful failure to observe your duty of candour would be a breach of your duty of care, contract of employment, and conditions of registration for registered clinicians.

1.7.6 Additional sources of support

Dealing with situations where things have gone wrong can be a challenging time and you may well need further advice and support. In those circumstances, you may find that some of the options below are able to assist you:
- organisational policy
- your line manager
- making experiences count (or similar) investigation team within your organisation
- FTSU Guardian.

2 Consent and capacity

2.1 *Learning objectives*

By the end of this section you will be able to:
- assess capacity
- gain consent
- maintain consent
- analyse factors that influence the capacity of an individual to express consent
- describe different ways of applying active participation to meet individual needs
- describe how to support an individual to question or challenge decisions concerning them that are made by others.

2.2 *Introduction*

As a responder in a front-line role, you will regularly have to seek consent to treat people and should have a basic understanding of mental capacity and how it impacts on patient treatment.

Chapter 4 – Legal and Ethical Issues

Having a good understanding of the basic principles will make this easier and help to remove doubt when tackling challenging and potentially confusing scenarios.

2.3 Consent

In the United Kingdom, case law has determined that adult patients with mental capacity must give consent before they are touched or treated. Failure to do this leaves the ambulance crew (or you as a responder) open to civil claims for trespass against the person, which includes assault and battery [BMA, 2019]; therefore you must seek valid consent to treat your patient. When a person is unable to consent, you may need to make decisions for them based on their best interests.

2.3.1 Valid consent

In order for consent to be valid, there are three criteria that must be met [BMA, 2019]; they stipulate that:

- **Consent must be given voluntarily:** i.e. free from pressure exerted by relatives, partners, ambulance staff or police officers, etc.
- **Consent must be informed:** The patient must understand what course of action is being proposed, what the benefits and risks are, what alternatives are available, and what the consequences are of doing nothing.
- **The person consenting needs to have the mental capacity to do so:** This is usually the patient but includes someone with parental responsibility in patients less than 18 years of age, or a person who has been given a lasting power of attorney (LPA) or authority by a court to make treatment decisions.

2.3.2 Communicating consent

Communicating consent may take many forms. Often for elective procedures in hospital it will be written. Working out-of-hospital, the majority of the time it will be verbal, but it may take another form, particularly if the patient has a disability that would make written or verbal communication impossible. Other forms that you may encounter include, but are not limited to:

- sign language
- use of props
- blinking
- movement of limbs
- use of technology, such as speech generators.

2.3.3 Maintaining consent

Gaining consent is not a one-time issue. You may need to gain consent several times during your contact with one patient. For example, while a patient consents to be examined, they may not consent to receiving treatment or being conveyed to hospital for further assessment.

You should gain consent for all interventions and actions you take, clearly explaining what you want to do and why, as well as any associated risks.

2.3.4 Best-interest decisions

Generally, if your patient is over 18 years of age, only they can consent to any intervention. Lying unconscious in the street after being involved in a road traffic collision does not imply consent. Prior to the Mental Capacity Act (MCA) 2005, you would have cared for this individual in the absence of consent as part of your duty of care for the patient and out of necessity in an emergency. Now this is covered by the MCA whereby you act in the patient's best interests if they lack the capacity to consent at the time.

2.4 Mental capacity

Case law has clearly laid out the right of a mentally competent adult to refuse treatment, including potentially life-saving interventions. In England and Wales, this framework is the MCA 2005, and in Scotland, the Adults with Incapacity (Scotland) Act 2000. The purpose of this legislation is to protect the rights of individuals from having treatment forced upon them in all but rare circumstances.

Central to capacity and consent is the concept of personal autonomy, that is, the right of an individual to 'govern themselves' according to their own set of personal values, preferences, commitments and character traits. This can come into conflict with an ambulance crew's tendency towards beneficence (i.e. serving the best interests of patients) and wanting to safeguard their jobs.

Mental capacity is the ability to make a decision, and covers everything from when to get up to how much alcohol to drink and whether to go to hospital as advised by an ambulance crew. A lack of capacity is defined as an inability of your patient to make a specific decision at the time they are required to make it, due to an impairment of, or disturbance in the functioning of, the mind or brain. It does not matter if this impairment or disturbance is temporary or permanent. Examples of impairment include:

- temporary:
  - post-ictal following a convulsion
  - a diabetic experiencing a hypoglycaemic event
  - ingestion of alcohol or drugs
- permanent:
  - dementia
  - significant learning disabilities
  - long-term effects of brain injury.

2.4.1 What to do if you suspect a lack of capacity

Assessing capacity is challenging. As a responder, it is unlikely you will receive the specific training required to undertake a full capacity assessment. Instead, if you have a patient who is refusing treatment and who you believe may lack capacity, you should contact the EOC as soon as possible and inform them about the situation. A clinician in the EOC may be able to assist you and they can make sure you are receiving appropriate backup.

Qualified clinicians that back you up should be able to undertake a capacity assessment and may, in certain circumstances, depending on the immediate risk facing the patient, decide to treat them against their will.

While you are waiting for backup, you should explain clearly and simply, in a way the patient will understand, why you want to treat them, what it is you want to do and what risks are associated with their refusing treatment. If capacity is in doubt and you can do so safely, then you should continue to act in the patient's best interests and give appropriate treatment, though consider your own safety in doing this.

2.4.2 Advance decision to refuse treatment (ADRT)

An ADRT is an order made by a person over the age of 18, when they still have capacity, to refuse specified medical treatment at a future point in time when they may lack the capacity to consent to or refuse treatment.

If faced with an ADRT, you should be confident that it is valid before working to it. For it to be valid you should, where possible, confirm whether the patient [NCPC, 2013]:

- has done anything that clearly goes against their advance decision since having made it, which suggests that they may have changed their mind
- has withdrawn their decision
- would have changed their decision if they had known more about the current circumstances
- has subsequently conferred the power to make that decision to an LPA.

Generally an ADRT does not have to be written – it can be verbal – but if it refers to life-saving treatment then it must:

- be in writing
- be witnessed and signed, and
- state clearly that the decision applies even if life is at risk.

If you believe an ADRT exists, is valid and applicable, you should follow the instructions contained within, though as a responder on your own it is possible that in some situations you may not be able to establish its validity prior to receiving backup. For example, if you arrive at a cardiac arrest and are presented with an ADRT but are not sure if it is valid, you should start CPR and continue resuscitation until backup arrives; once more people are available, time can be taken to safely establish whether the ADRT is valid and cease further care if appropriate.

2.5 Summary

As a responder, you are subject to the same laws as any other clinician in respect of consent. Be sure that, where possible, you seek valid consent from your patient and that you are not accidentally forcing unwanted treatment on them. You should also have a general understanding of what mental capacity is and what you should check for if you believe your patient may lack capacity. In this case, a clinician will undertake an assessment and decide on the best course of action; in the meantime you should act in the patient's best interests so long as it is safe for you to do so.

3 Confidentiality and information governance

3.1 Learning objectives

By the end of this section, you will be able to:
- explain the meaning of the term 'confidentiality'
- demonstrate ways to maintain confidentiality in day-to-day communication
- define information governance
- explain your role in information governance.

3.2 Introduction

All responders, like other healthcare professions, have a duty of confidentiality to their patients, whereby they must protect all patient information and handle it in an approved manner. Failure to follow strict organisation policies and, where relevant, codes of conduct in relation to handling information can be a source of distress for patients and embarrassment for organisations. It can also result in legal or disciplinary action for both organisations and individuals [NHS England, 2019].

Information governance is broadly defined as the framework organisations have in place to bring together all the legal rules, guidance and best practice that apply to the handling of information. Relevant legislation includes [NHS England, 2024b]
- NHS Act 2006
- Health and Social Care Act 2012
- Data Protection Act 2018 (the UK's implementation of the General Data Protection Regulation (GDPR))
- Human Rights Act 1998.

Within your role you will routinely have access to confidential, patient-identifiable information. This information, or data, should be protected: this means that you should record, handle and store this information in such a way that you are not likely to misplace any information or accidentally breach confidentiality by making an unauthorised or unnecessary disclosure, which could lead to civil or criminal legal proceedings being brought against you or the organisation you work for.

3.2.1 What should be considered patient-identifiable information?

Patient-identifiable information is anything that may enable a patient to be identified, either directly or indirectly [JRCALC, 2023]. This includes obvious personal information, such as name, address, date of birth, etc. However, it also includes less commonly considered things, such as:
- clinical record numbers
- images or voice recordings of a patient
- rare disease information.

Consider the following scenario:

You work in a small town with a population of around 25,000 people. In this town lives a patient with Addison's disease, a rare endocrine disorder. The patient frequently experiences Addisonian crises, and when this happens family members call for an ambulance. You attend this patient experiencing a crisis one day; as this is not a condition you are familiar with, next time you visit a local ambulance station you ask an ambulance crew for some information about the condition. You are mindful not to disclose the name or location of the patient (to prevent a breach of confidentiality), but instead describe the incident and ask for advice. Considering that Addison's is a rare disease and this one person, in a small community, frequently requires ambulance assistance, is it reasonable that, on the balance of probabilities, the crews would be able to identify who you are talking about, just by describing the condition?

Any information that has the potential to identify the patient, however remotely, should be considered as identifiable and managed in such a way as to help avoid a breach of confidentiality from occurring [JRCALC, 2023].

3.3 *Maintaining confidentiality*

Organisations should have policies in place to describe how they handle information and protect confidentiality. You have a legal obligation to maintain confidentiality so should have a good working knowledge of these policies.

During the course of your duties, it may be necessary to discuss or share patient-identifiable information on a number of occasions. Such occasions may include:
- discussing the care of your patient with another healthcare professional
- handing over the care of your patient to another health or care professional
- requesting support in clinical decision-making for your patient
- contacting other organisations or services to help provide care or support.

These communications can take many forms, including:
- face to face
- written
- telephone
- mobile data systems
- email.

Different systems will have different strengths and weaknesses in their security of managing data. Most records in the out-of-hospital setting are recorded either on paper or on electronic patient record devices. Below are some of the security features of each type of storage:
- electronic record-keeping:
  - All data is transferred and stored securely. No data is left 'hanging around' once it is no longer required.
  - No physical copies of records means it is less likely records will be 'misplaced'.
  - Records are easily accessed again in the future when required.
- physical records:
  - Once completed these should be submitted to a secure storage system.
  - Copies of the record are passed only to patients or patients' relatives with permission once completed.

Regardless of which system you use, you should consider how best to maintain confidentiality. Your employer or volunteer organisation should make a copy of its policy available, but some good practice guidelines include [NHS England, 2019]:
- **Seek consent before sharing information:** Before you share patient information you should seek consent from the patient to do so. However, in a limited range of situations it may be appropriate to share information without the patient's consent, for example:
  - It is not possible to gain consent.
  - There is a legal requirement to make certain disclosures.
  - It is in 'the public interest' to make a disclosure.
- **Share only that information which is necessary:** If you phone the EOC after an incident to book clear, you are probably going to speak to a dispatcher. It is unlikely that person needs to know all the medical details of the patient, so you should limit your discussion to relevant points and not disclose confidential information unnecessarily.
- **Maintain physical security of information:** Part of your role is likely to include making notes and records on the patients you attend. It is unlikely that you would keep these records once you have treated the patient; instead they should go with the patient to be passed on to the ambulance crew that backs you up.

You may decide to keep a record of incidents that you attend for your own development; however, this must not include any personal identifiable information: it must not be possible to identify any patients from such a log.

If you find following an incident that you have accidentally retained a copy of patient-identifiable information, you should immediately inform your line manager and follow their instructions on how to deal with it appropriately.

3.4 Making a disclosure

In the course of your role, you may be faced with the need to disclose information to other bodies or organisations. The primary principle here is that, wherever possible, consent should be gained prior to sharing information. However, in certain circumstances it may be necessary to make a disclosure without that consent [NHS England, 2019].

Below is an outline of some scenarios where it may be necessary to share information without patient consent [JRCALC, 2023; GMC, 2024]:

- **Police:** The police have the right to personal information (name, address, contact details, etc.) in the detection and prevention of a crime. However, this does not extend to personal health information unless it is part of the investigation or prevention of a serious crime (rape, arson, murder, etc.) or related to terrorism offences. On most occasions, this information can be requested by the police through locally agreed channels, and only information required immediately in the prevention and detection of a crime should be shared by ambulance crews.
- **Local authorities:** A local authority officer who believes a person to be at risk is allowed access to health, financial and other records to determine whether any action needs to be taken to protect them.
- **Coroner:** An ethical duty of confidentiality continues after a patient has died, but relevant information should be disclosed to a coroner or similar officer in the investigation of an inquest or fatal accident inquiry.
- **Risk to well-being:** In certain situations, there may be a risk to a patient's well-being by not informing other professionals and/or the relevant authorities, for example safeguarding concerns relating to vulnerable adults and children.
- **Unable to gain consent:** If a person lacks the capacity to consent to their information being shared, it is possible to share that information which is relevant to the situation. However, information should be shared cautiously; a proxy, guardian or parent should be consulted first, if available.
- **Public interest:** It may be permissible to share information if it is in the public interest. This may be to prevent or detect a serious crime or in cases where others are placed at risk. Examples include:
  - The release of information relevant to serious crimes. For example, if you were to attend an incidence of physical violence and the victim does not want the police contacted, but they or others remain at serious risk of further harm or injury, then contacting the police and giving details without their consent would likely be justified.
  - Releasing relevant confidential information to social services where there is a risk of significant harm to children. In all cases, consent should be sought prior to disclosure unless it is not practical to do so, or it would be inappropriate because, for example, they lack capacity to consent, or they are suspects who should not be informed that they are under criminal investigation.

Services should have policies in place that cover the majority of the above circumstances, and these policies should be studied and followed when making a disclosure. In the absence of a specific policy, wherever possible, the organisation's data protection officer/information governance manager/Caldicott Guardian should be consulted prior to releasing information, but this should not be at the cost of endangering patient care due to the delay in passing on information.

As a responder, you should seek the advice of your line manager whenever possible prior to making disclosure. However, if the disclosure is required urgently, then seeking advice from the EOC or requesting contact from a duty officer may be the best route to gaining urgent support and advice.

3.5 Key points

Remember these key points relating to confidentiality:
- Patients are the owners of information or data relating to them.
- Patient-identifiable information comes in many forms and is communicated in a range of ways.
- Patient-identifiable information should not be shared without consent except in specific circumstances.
- Only share information that is necessary.
- Consider how to maintain security of data in order to prevent accidental disclosures.
- Organisations should have policies in place for protecting information and you should be familiar with these.

4 Equality and diversity

4.1 Learning objectives

By the end of this section you will be able to:
- explain what is meant by diversity, equality, inclusion and discrimination
- describe the potential effects of discrimination
- explain how inclusive practice promotes equality and supports diversity
- explain how legislation and codes of practice relating to equality, diversity and discrimination apply to your own work role
- describe how to challenge discrimination in a way that promotes change.

4.2 Introduction

Promoting equality should be at the heart of a healthcare organisation's values. It ensures that organisations work in a way that is fair, so that no community, group or individual is left behind. This is well summarised as [NHS England, 2020]:

'The NHS must welcome all, with a culture of belonging and trust. We must understand, encourage and celebrate diversity in all its forms.'

It is helpful to understand what the terms 'diversity', 'equality' and 'inclusion' mean [HCPC, 2020]:
- **Diversity:** This involves recognising and valuing the differences between individuals and their different perspectives, while maximising the range of people who can contribute.
- **Equality:** This means treating people fairly in a way that reflects their needs, ensuring they have equal opportunity to achieve their desired outcomes, and eliminating discrimination.
- **Inclusion:** This involves positively striving to meet the needs of different people and taking deliberate action to create environments where everyone feels respected and able to achieve their full potential.

4.3 Equality in healthcare

At first glance, it may not be obvious how equality and diversity can have an influence on healthcare or influence outcomes. However, various health inequalities do exist [NHS England, 2024c]. Despite significant advances in health and social care in England, people living in the least deprived areas of the country can live up to almost ten years longer on average than those living in the most deprived areas [Kings Fund, 2024].

Healthcare inequalities are unfair and avoidable differences in health across the population, and between different groups within society [NHS England, 2024c]. People living in areas of high deprivation, those from Black, Asian and minority ethnic communities, and those from other vulnerable groups, such as the homeless, are most at risk of experiencing these inequalities.

The exact reasons for the inequalities are complex, but often include issues such as [NHS England, 2024c]:
- unavailability of local services
- lack of access to transport
- language barrier
- poor literacy
- poor experiences in the past
- fear
- misinformation.

As a responder, it is likely you will frequently encounter patients who are vulnerable to health inequalities, and while you will not be able to fully remove this risk there are some small things you may be able to do to help patients access services. These include:

- making patients aware of local services they did not know existed
- providing contact information for relevant services
- referring to other sources of local help as appropriate.

4.4 Discrimination

Discrimination occurs when someone treats one person less favourably than they would another, because of a personal characteristic. This is often due to stereotyping.

Under the Equality Act 2010, it is unlawful for a person to discriminate against another with respect to certain protected characteristics.

The nine characteristics are:
- age
- disability
- gender
- gender reassignment
- marriage and civil partnership
- pregnancy and maternity
- race
- religion and belief
- sexual orientation.

As well as the Equality Act, the Human Rights Act 1998 also provides for ensuring certain equalities, including:
- the right to life
- the right to a fair trial
- the right to education
- the right to participate in free elections.

4.4.1 Discrimination in your role

In order to make sense of society and those in it, we naturally group individuals together when they share common characteristics. Based on these characteristics, we may expect people within the group to act in similar ways or to have similar responses to the same situations; this is the process of stereotyping [Amodio, 2014].

Using these stereotypes is a natural process as it allows us to 'shortcut' our thinking, but often they are not accurate. Making such shortcuts in healthcare can be dangerous because we will make incorrect assumptions about our patients and fail to challenge our own thought processes.

Applying such stereotypes is probably unavoidable, but we must be prepared to challenge our own thinking and the assumptions made on the basis of that thinking. For example, elderly patients have very varied life expectancies. Some patients may live with a multitude of medical conditions in their early seventies and therefore have a relatively limited life expectancy, whereas many people will live late into their nineties and beyond with very few medical concerns. If all of these patients were treated the same purely on the basis of their age, you would not be treating patients as individuals and would be likely to provide poor care as a result, potentially even leading to the avoidable early death of a patient. Remember that age is a protected characteristic, and it is both unethical and unlawful to discriminate against someone on the basis of one of these characteristics.

Applying the same thought process to all patients is clearly inappropriate and could lead to your making unreasonable, unjustifiable and unethical decisions. You must actively practise treating all patients equally and base your care on their specific circumstances, rather than on those of a group they may fit into.

4.4.2 Challenging discrimination

When you observe signs of discrimination in practice it should be challenged, not least because, in healthcare, discrimination based on stereotypes, whether it be on purpose or unthinking, can lead to patient harm. If discrimination is allowed to continue unchallenged, it is likely to become a normal part of the way in which an organisation works and be embedded as part of the organisational culture. Therefore it is essential that people speak up and challenge any sign of discrimination.

Challenging discrimination can be difficult and could lead to conflict if not done in an appropriate manner. Each situation will be unique, so there

is no single solution that can be described here. However, some general guidance includes:
- Promoting discussion, rather than telling someone they have got it wrong; during discussion, most people will realise their mistakes.
- Encouraging an open environment, where people can feel safe to discuss a wide range of difficult and complex issues.
- Providing sources of further information.
- Avoiding appearing judgemental.

4.4.3 Further support

If you observe discrimination then you will need support in understanding how best to resolve the situation. In this instance help would normally be available from your:
- line manager
- organisation equality and diversity lead.

If a patient wishes to make a complaint in relation to being discriminated against, then you should support them in doing this.

Remember, everyone is responsible for promoting equality, recognising diversity and challenging discrimination. Only by doing this will you be able to ensure your patients are receiving the best care possible and that you are practising in a non-discriminatory manner. Do not assume that others will tackle the issue.

5 Health and Safety

1 Health and safety policies and legislation

1.1 Learning objectives

By the end of this section you will be able to:
- identify key legislation relating to health and safety in the ambulance service
- explain the main points of health and safety policies and procedures
- analyse the main health and safety responsibilities for:
  - yourself
  - your employer/volunteer organisation and manager
  - others in the work setting.

1.2 Introduction

A variety of the legislation that relates to the ambulance service has already been reviewed in Chapter 4, 'Legal and Ethical Issues', but it is also important that you are aware of the legislation relating to health and safety, and, in particular, that you know your and your employer's legal responsibilities.

1.3 Health and Safety at Work etc. Act 1974

All workers, including volunteers, have a right to work in places where risks to their health and safety are properly controlled. Health and safety is about stopping you getting hurt at work or ill through work. Your employer is responsible for health and safety, but you must help [HSE, 2009].

Employers must do the following in order to comply with the Act [HSE, 2009]:
- Decide what could harm you in your job and what precautions could prevent it; this is part of risk assessment.
- In a way you can understand, explain how risk will be controlled and tell you who is responsible for this.
- Consult and work with staff and the health and safety representatives to protect everyone from harm in the workplace.
- Provide (free of charge) health and safety training, and equipment and protective clothing that you need to do your job.
- Provide toilets, washing facilities, drinking water and adequate first-aid facilities.
- Notify the Health and Safety Executive in the event of any major injuries and fatalities at work.
- Have insurance that covers staff in the event of injury at work.
- Display a physical or electronic copy of the current insurance certificate where you can easily read it.
- Work with other employers or contractors sharing the workplace to ensure that everyone's health and safety is protected.

You have a number of responsibilities as an employee, even if you are a volunteer, too [HSE, 2009]:
- Follow the training you have received when using any work item your employer has provided.
- Take reasonable care of your own and other people's health and safety.
- Co-operate with your employer on health and safety.
- Tell someone (for example your employer, line manager or safety representative) if you think that a method of working or inadequate precautions are putting anyone's health and safety at serious risk.

1.4 Management of Health and Safety at Work Regulations

The Management of Health and Safety at Work Regulations 1999 require employers to put in place arrangements to control health and safety risks. These include [HSE, 2013a]:
- a written health and safety policy
- assessments of the risks to employees, contractors, customers, partners, and any other people who could be affected by work-related activities, and written records of significant findings
- arrangements for the effective planning, organisation, control, monitoring and review of the preventive and protective measures that come from risk assessment
- access to competent health and safety advice
- providing employees with information about the risks in the workplace and how those employees are protected
- instruction and training for employees in how to deal with the risks
- ensuring there is adequate and appropriate supervision in place
- consulting with employees about their risks at work and current preventive and protective measures.

1.5 Manual Handling Operations Regulations

Any transporting or supporting of a load (including the lifting, putting-down, pushing, pulling, carrying or moving thereof) by hand or by bodily force is considered to be a manual handling operation according to the Manual Handling Operations Regulations 1992.

Employers are required to make a suitable and sufficient assessment of the risks to the health and safety of their employees while at work. Where this assessment indicates the possibility of risks to employees from the manual handling of loads, the Regulations require a hierarchy of measures that must be adhered to. These are [HSE, 2016]:
- avoiding the need for hazardous manual handling, 'so far as reasonably practicable'
- assessing the risk of injury from any hazardous manual handling that cannot be avoided
- reducing the risk of injury from hazardous manual handling 'so far as reasonably practicable'.

No doubt you have noticed the term 'reasonably practicable' appearing a couple of times. This means that the employer's duty to avoid manual handling or to reduce the risk of injury can be limited, if they can show that the cost of any further preventive steps would be grossly disproportionate to their perceived benefit.

Employees are also expected to play their part by following appropriate systems of work laid down by their employer to promote safety during the handling of loads.

1.5.1 Emergency services

Preventing all potentially hazardous emergency service manual handling operations would result in an inability to provide the general public with an adequate rescue service. As a volunteer for an ambulance service, you may be asked to accept a greater risk of injury than someone employed to move inanimate objects (like boxes). In this case, additional relevant factors may include:
- the seriousness of the need for the lifting operation
- the ambulance service's duty to the public overall and the patient who requires assistance.

Taking these factors into account, the level of risk which an employer may ask an employee to accept may, in appropriate circumstances, be higher when considering the health and safety of those in danger, although this does not mean that employees can be exposed to unacceptable risk of injury, and they must still undertake all reasonably practicable steps to reduce the risk [HSE, 2016].

2 Risk assessment

2.1 Learning objectives

By the end of this section you will be able to:
- define the term 'risk'

- describe the process of carrying out a risk assessment
- explain the importance of carrying out a risk assessment
- compare different uses of risk assessment in health and social care
- explain why risk assessments need to be regularly reviewed and revised.

2.2 Introduction

All healthcare staff and responders have a duty to protect patients, their colleagues and themselves as far as is 'reasonably practicable', by minimising the chance that they are harmed by something, whether that be a procedure, drug administration or dangerous environment.

It is helpful to understand what is meant by the terms 'hazard' and 'risk' [HSE, 2024a]:
- **Hazard:** Anything that might cause injury or illness, such as chemicals, electricity, working from ladders, a viral infection, etc.
- **Risk:** The chance, high or low, that somebody could be harmed by these hazards, together with an indication of how serious the harm could be.
- **Clinical risk:** the chance of an adverse outcome resulting from clinical investigation, treatment or patient care; also known as a healthcare risk.

2.3 Structured risk assessments

Your employer is responsible for undertaking structured assessments of risks that it is reasonably foreseeable you will come across while undertaking your duties as a responder.

These assessments are usually completed using a structured risk assessment template and rating chart. Where possible your employer will then reduce the risk so far as is reasonably practicable. An example of this is your employer providing your equipment in bags, which are not too heavy or difficult to handle.

Copies of these risk assessments are available from your employer. Details of how and when your employer undertakes structured risk assessments will be available in your organisation's health and safety policy.

2.4 Dynamic risk assessments

As an operational member of staff you are responsible for undertaking a whole range of dynamic risk assessments. Dynamic risk assessments are undertaken in a less structured method, inasmuch as they are not usually formally recorded and documented, but they should still follow a process.

These dynamic risk assessments are a continual process to ensure your safety and the safety of those around you. Two of the dynamic risks assessments you will undertake, at every incident you attend, are the SCENE and TILEE assessments.

2.4.1 SCENE assessment

Every time you approach a scene you need to assess whether it is safe to continue and treat the patient, or if you should withdraw to protect yourself and others.

This is covered in detail in Chapter 8, 'Scene Assessment', but is highly dynamic as every situation is different, and even the same situation can change dramatically from having been safe to becoming unsafe after you have been there for a period of time.

2.4.2 Moving and handling assessment

Every time you perform a moving or handling task, you will need to undertake a risk assessment of how to safely perform the procedure. Although your organisation will have undertaken a general structured risk assessment for moving and handling, it is clearly not possible to formally assess every location you will be attending in advance. Subsequently you must undertake an assessment following the TILEE approach.

This is covered in detail in Chapter 7, 'Manual Handling', and is something you should be very familiar with, as you will need to perform this risk assessment very frequently.

Chapter 5 – *Health and Safety*

3 Infection prevention and controls

3.1 *Learning objectives*

By the end of this section you will be able to:
- explain what is meant by 'infection' and how infections can occur and be transmitted
- describe how to manage and dispose of sources of infection safely while avoiding causing harm to yourself or others
- outline the current regulations, legislation and responsibilities relating to infection control
- describe the different types of PPE and how to use them appropriately
- explain the role of regulators and other bodies in infection prevention and control
- describe the key principles of good personal hygiene
- describe the correct sequence for handwashing and when it should be carried out
- describe the services that occupational health provides to employees.

3.2 *Introduction*

Infection prevention and control is a collective term for the practical, evidence-based approach to preventing patients and health workers from being harmed by avoidable infections [WHO, 2024a].

An infection is the body's adverse response to the presence of a pathogen, or disease-causing micro-organism [Betsy, 2012]. Damage to tissues caused by an infection can either be limited to the site of infection (localised) or spread throughout the body, typically via the blood (systemic). Sometimes, however, a pathogen in or on the body may not lead to an infection. This is known as colonisation [Weston, 2014].

A healthcare-associated infection (HCAI) is any infection acquired as a result of a healthcare-related intervention or an infection acquired during the course of healthcare that the patient may reasonably expect to be protected from. The scale of the problem is staggering. In 2016/17 there were an estimated 834,000 HCAIs costing the NHS £2.7 billion and accounting for 28,500 patient deaths [Guest, 2020].

3.2.1 Your own and the patient's health

Health professionals and associated staff, including responders, not only pass disease and illness on to patients, but they themselves can be made unwell by poor infection and prevention control. Some diseases, such as norovirus, a viral infection which causes gastroenteritis [CKS, 2023], is very infectious and spreads easily from person to person. In winter, when it is most prevalent, it is likely you will come into contact with patients who are ill with this on a frequent basis. If you do not apply adequate infection prevention and control, it is likely that you may also become unwell and contract the illness. This could mean that you are off sick for several days or weeks from work, impacting not only your health, but potentially the health and well-being of family and friends as well.

Equally, you can spread illness to your patient. If you are not well, you should not make yourself available to respond, as you might spread illness to already unwell people. For many patients, including the elderly, those with chronic lung conditions or receiving chemotherapy, even a small infection will place a major strain on their immune system; an illness that may not be a major issue for a healthy person could kill someone who is already unwell.

3.3 *Regulations and legislation*

At the beginning of this chapter, some of the relevant legislation relating to infection prevention and control was reviewed, in particular the Health and Safety at Work etc. Act 1974. This requires employers to provide training and appropriate PPE to prevent harm. It also requires employees to follow the training that they have received, use the PPE provided, and report any situations where they believe that patients' and/or staff's health and safety are at serious risk.

However, the Health and Social Care Act [2008] specifically highlights health professionals' duty of care to implement effective infection prevention and control procedures and also makes the CQC responsible for ensuring that ambulance (and other care) services meet the requirements of the code of practice that accompanies the legislation.

3.4 Micro-organisms

Micro-organisms are very small organisms that live outside and inside larger organisms such as the human body. The four main types that enter the body and cause infection are:
- bacteria
- viruses
- fungi
- parasites.

3.4.1 Bacteria

These are probably the most important micro-organisms in relation to infection control as they are responsible for many opportunistic infections in healthcare. There are around ten times as many bacteria as there are cells in the human body and many have functions that are essential, such as *Escherichia coli* (*E. coli*), which aids digestion in the gut. However, it can cause a urinary tract infection (UTI) if it gains access to the urinary tract [Dougherty, 2015].

Bacteria are fairly simple, single-celled micro-organisms and are often classified by their shape. For example, they may be termed bacillus (rod-like), coccus (spherical or ovoid) or spiral (corkscrew or curved). Examples of common bacteria include Group A *Streptococcus*, which can cause throat and ear infections, and *Staphylococcus*, which can cause impetigo and pneumonia. You may have heard of a particularly troublesome strain of *Staphylococcus* that is resistant to many antibiotics and is called methicillin-resistant *Staphylococcus aureus* (MRSA) [NHS, 2023a].

3.4.2 Viruses

Viruses are even smaller than bacteria and have no cellular structure. They typically just consist of a core containing genetic material, such as deoxyribonucleic acid (DNA) or ribonucleic acid (RNA), and are sometimes surrounded by a membrane called an envelope. Viruses can reproduce only by using the cellular machinery of other organisms and so are rather like parasites [Tortora, 2017].

Common viruses include the rhinovirus, which is the most common cause for the common cold, and the varicella-zoster virus (VZV), which causes chickenpox and shingles [Betsy, 2012]. Coronavirus disease (COVID-19) is caused by the SARS-CoV-2 virus and as of early 2024 was responsible for over 7 million deaths and over 750 million recorded infections [WHO, 2024b] since its outbreak in late 2019.

3.4.3 Fungi

You are probably most familiar with fungi as mushrooms or as yeast used in bread-making and brewing. Some fungi are responsible for opportunistic infections, such as dermatophytes, which can cause athlete's foot, and *Candida albicans*, yeast that can cause vaginal thrush [Dougherty, 2015].

3.4.4 Parasites

Parasites are organisms that live at the expense of another organism or host. Pathogenic parasites include bacteria, viruses, protozoa (animal-like single-celled micro-organisms) and animals such as roundworms, flatworms and arthropods. Examples of parasitic infections include malaria and toxoplasmosis [Betsy, 2012].

3.5 Chain of infection

Transmission of infection is a complex process, involving a number of factors, which must all be present and are collectively known as the chain of infection (Figure 5.1) [NHS Scotland, 2024; Seventer, 2017].

3.5.1 Pathogen

An infectious agent is required, such as a bacterium, virus, fungus or parasite. This link can be broken by cleaning, sterilisation of equipment and the treatment of the patient, using antibiotics for bacterial infections, for example, to reduce the presence of pathogens.

Chapter 5 – *Health and Safety*

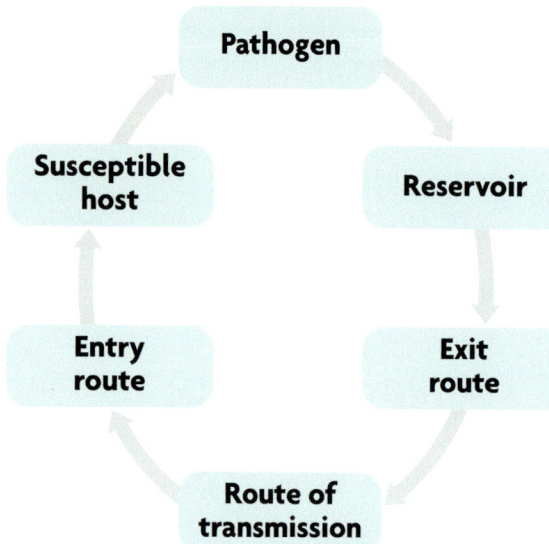

Figure 5.1 Chain of infection

3.5.2 Reservoir

A reservoir is a place where the pathogen can live and replicate; it includes the human body, but also animals, water and the soil, for example. This link can be broken by cleaning equipment and the environment (such as the ambulance) and removing stagnant water.

3.5.3 Exit route

The exit route is a method for the pathogen to leave its reservoir. In humans, this usually involves urine, faeces, vomit and sputum, as well as the aerosolised form, such as after sneezing or coughing. Asking a patient with a respiratory infection to wear a mask would help break this part of the chain.

3.5.4 Route of transmission

The transmission route can be direct, such as through touching, sexual intercourse and faecal–oral via ingestion, or indirect via contaminated bedding, clothing, blood and bodily fluids and then the hands of healthcare workers. One of the most effective ways of breaking this link is using good hand hygiene.

3.5.5 Entry route

Entry routes include the respiratory, gastrointestinal and genitourinary tracts, but also mucous membranes and via the skin. Direct access to the blood is also possible if the pathogen is inadvertently injected into a person. Covering an open wound with a plaster would be a good example of breaking this part of the chain by blocking the route of entry.

3.5.6 Susceptible host

Some people are more vulnerable to infection than others, for example those with a weak immune system due to old age, medication or pre-existing disease. Others may have their natural defences compromised by wounds, surgery, intravenous cannulas and urinary catheters. This link can be broken by ensuring that healthcare workers are vaccinated and that adequate nutrition and personal hygiene are provided to vulnerable groups.

3.6 *Standard infection control precautions (SICPs)*

SICPs are a range of measures to be used by all staff in all care setting at all times for all patients, whether infection is known to be present or not. They are basic measures necessary to reduce the risk of transmitting infection agents from both recognised and unrecognised sources. There are 10 elements to SICPs, which are [NHS England, 2023b]:

- assessment of infection risk
- hand hygiene
- respiratory and cough hygiene
- PPE
- safe management of the care environment
- safe management of care equipment
- safe management of healthcare linen
- safe management of blood and body fluids
- safe disposal of waste (including sharps)
- occupational safety: prevention of exposure, including sharps injury.

3.6.1 Assessment of infection risk

When you arrive with a patient, consider that they may be a source of infection. This is for the benefit of the patient, but also for healthcare staff and other patients.

Consider if the patient has a history and/or signs or symptoms suggestive of infection. These may include:
- unexplained fever, rash or respiratory symptoms
- diarrhoea and/or vomiting
- known history of a multi-drug resistant organism, i.e. MRSA
- recent exposure to a known infection, i.e. norovirus outbreak in a care home.

This information is useful as it may lead you to adopt a different level of PPE. In addition, by passing information about an infection risk to the ambulance crew, they will be able to protect themselves and notify the receiving hospital, who may care for the patient in a different area for the patient's own safety as well as the safety of others in the department.

3.6.2 Hand hygiene

Good hand hygiene is the primary measure to reduce HCAIs. It is a straightforward method and inexpensive, but poor compliance among healthcare workers remains a worldwide problem [WHO, 2024c].

You should clean your hands in the following circumstances [NHS, 2023a]:
- immediately before every episode of direct patient contact or care, including aseptic procedures
- immediately after every episode of direct patient contact or care
- immediately after any exposure to body fluids
- immediately after any other activity or contact with a patient's surroundings that could potentially result in your hands becoming contaminated
- immediately after removal of gloves.

In order to ensure that you can maintain good hand hygiene while at work, you should [NICE, 2017b]:
- be 'bare below the elbows' while delivering care
- not wear any wrist or hand jewellery

- ensure that fingernails are short, clean and free from nail polish
- cover cuts and abrasions with waterproof dressings.

Hand hygiene with soap and running water procedure

Take the following steps to wash your hands:

Note: This procedure assumes that you have adopted a 'bare below the elbows' dress code. The entire process should take around 40–60 seconds.

1. Wet hands with water.

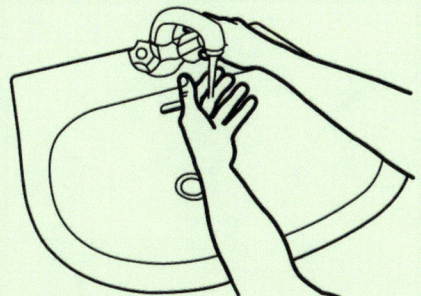

2. Apply enough soap to cover all hand surfaces.

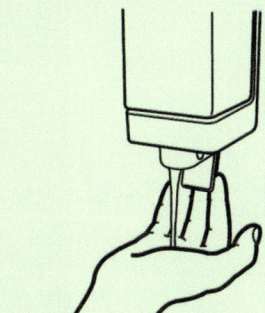

3. Rub hands palm to palm.

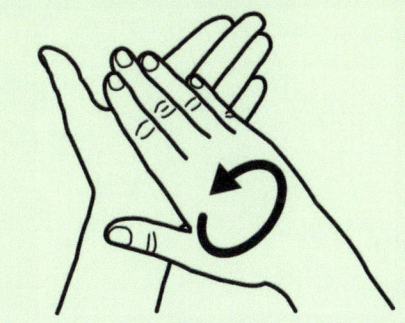

Hand hygiene with soap and running water procedure – *cont*

4. Rub your right palm over the back of the left hand with interlaced fingers and vice versa.

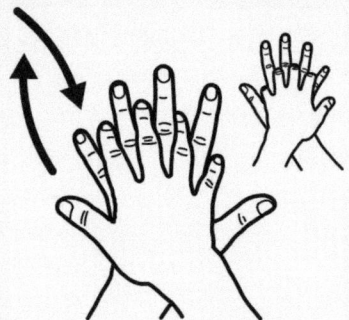

5. Rub palm to palm with fingers interlaced.

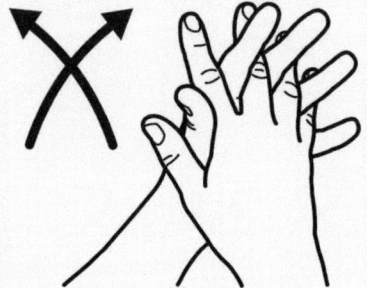

6. Rub the backs of your fingers to opposing palms with fingers interlocked.

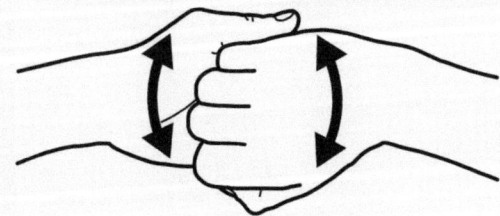

7. Rub the left thumb in your right palm in a rotational motion and vice versa.

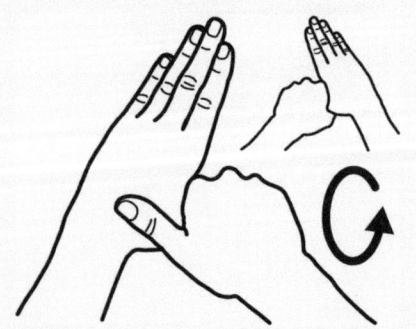

Hand hygiene with soap and running water procedure – *cont*

8. Clasp the fingers of your right hand in your left palm and rub in a rotational motion, backwards and forwards, and vice versa.

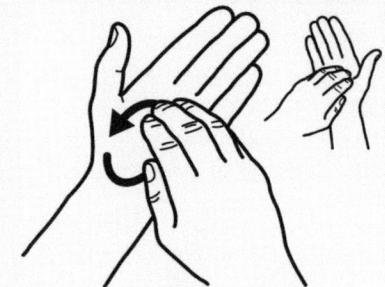

9. Rinse hands with water.

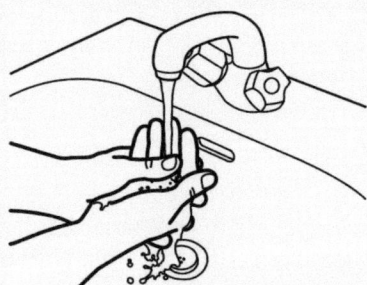

10. Dry thoroughly with a disposable towel.

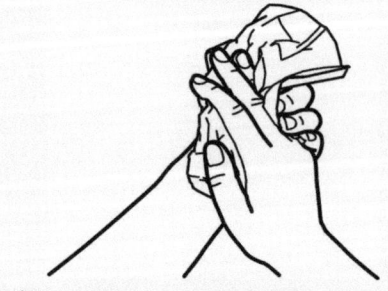

11. Where possible, use your elbows to turn off taps. However, if this is not possible, use a towel to turn off taps.

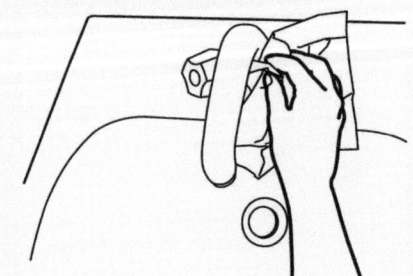

Infection prevention and controls

Hand hygiene with alcohol-based rub procedure

Take the following steps to clean your hands with an alcohol-based hand rub:

Note: This procedure assumes that you have adopted a 'bare below the elbows' dress code. The entire process should take around 40–60 seconds.

1. Apply a palmful of the product into a cupped hand and cover all surfaces.

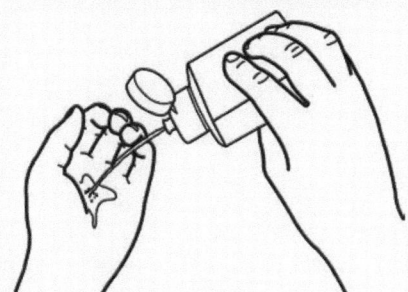

2. Rub hands palm to palm.

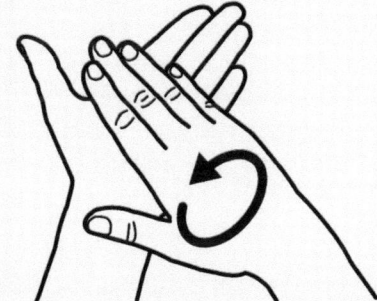

3. Rub your right palm over the back of the left hand with interlaced fingers and vice versa.

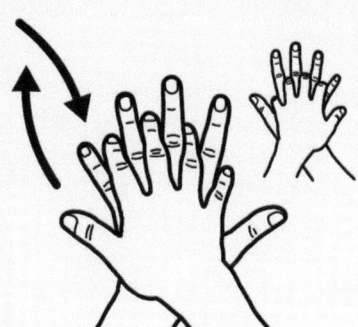

Hand hygiene with alcohol-based rub procedure – *cont*

4. Rub palm to palm with fingers interlaced.

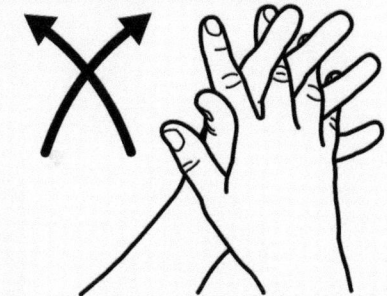

5. Rub the backs of your fingers to opposing palms with fingers interlocked.

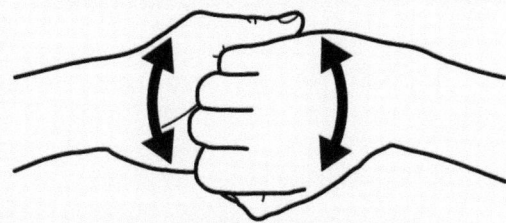

6. Rub the left thumb in your right palm in a rotational motion and vice versa.

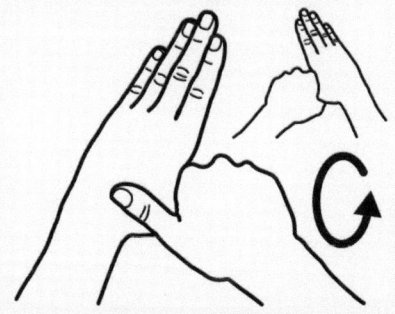

7. Clasp the fingers of your right hand in your left palm and rub in a rotational motion, backwards and forwards, and vice versa.

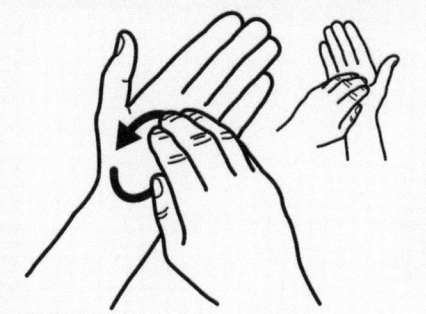

Chapter 5 – Health and Safety

Hand hygiene with alcohol-based rub procedure – *cont*

8. Once dry, your hands are safe.

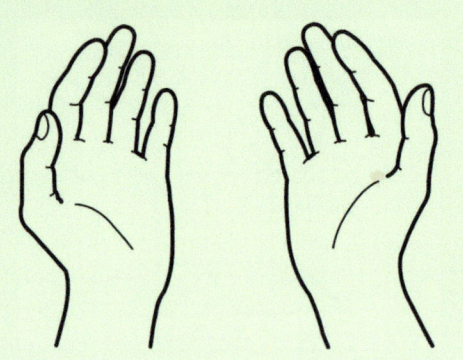

Skincare

Work-related skin problems are very common, with contact dermatitis being the most common form of work-related skin disease. It is more common in healthcare staff due to their need to wash their hands regularly, and skin frequently coming into contact with chemicals or rubber materials as used in PPE [HSE, 2015].

When washing your hands frequently it is important to use hand cream to replace the natural oils that are lost in the washing process [HSE, 2015] and to observe for signs of contact dermatitis developing. These signs include:
- dry itchy skin
- reddening
- flaking, cracks or blisters.

If you experience contact dermatitis, or any other form of skin disease, then you should see your GP or occupational health team to try to find a personal solution for improving your skincare.

3.6.3 Respiratory and cough hygiene

Airborne droplets from coughing and sneezing are a common route of transmission for HCAIs. The following steps should be taken to reduce the risk of airborne transmission with respiratory and cough hygiene [NHS, 2023a]:
- Cover the nose and mouth with a disposable tissue when sneezing, coughing or blowing the nose; if unavailable use the crook of the arm.
- Dispose of all used tissues promptly into a waste bin.
- Wash hands with liquid soap and warm water after coughing, sneezing, using tissues or contact with respiratory secretions or objects contaminated by respiratory secretions.
- Where running water is not available, use hand wipes followed by an alcohol-based hand rub and wash with soap and water at the first opportunity.
- Keep contaminated hands away from eyes, nose and mouth.

You should encourage patients to also practise good respiratory and cough hygiene with coaching and the provision of tissues as appropriate.

3.6.4 PPE

PPE is used to prevent the spread of infection to you, your colleagues, patients and other members of the public. During the COVID-19 pandemic, PPE was a major issue due to national shortages and subject to frequent changes in guidance. As services recover from the pandemic, guidance has been revised multiple times and there remains significant difference in organisations as to what PPE should be used at different times. Make yourself aware of your organisation's own risk assessment and policies on the use of PPE and ensure you are trained on the equipment made available to you.

Typical items of PPE to prevent HCAIs include:
- gloves
- aprons
- face masks
- eye protection
- sleeve protectors.

Gloves

Gloves should be worn (Figure 5.2) [NHS, 2023a]:
- if contact with blood, bodily fluids, non-intact skin or mucous membrane is anticipated or likely
- when sharp and/or contaminated items are handled.

Gloves should not be worn longer than necessary and never when driving to or from the scene. Don't forget that hand hygiene is required before and

Infection prevention and controls

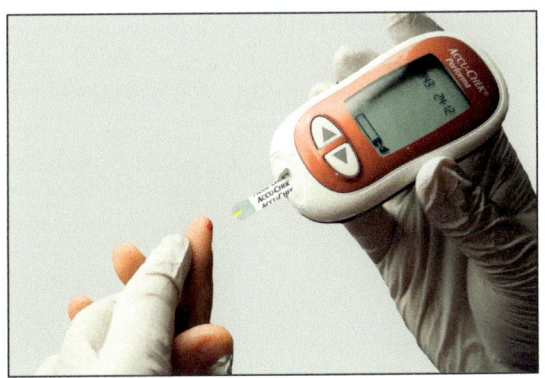

Figure 5.2 Non-latex disposable gloves should be worn when there is a risk of contact with blood, such as when checking a patient's blood sugar

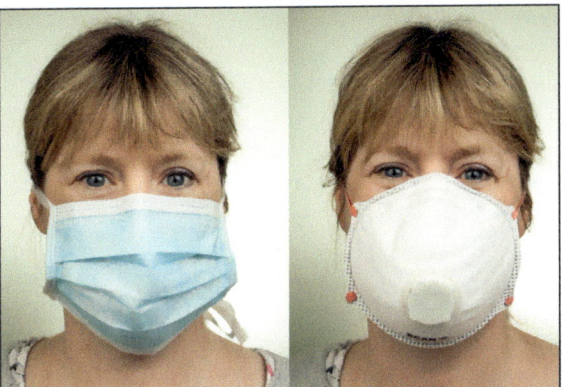

Figure 5.3 Surgical face mask (left) and FFP3 mask (right)

after wearing gloves. Put gloves on immediately prior to patient contact and change them between each patient task, when caring for different patients and as soon as they are contaminated. Once you have removed your gloves, discard appropriately and be sure to clean your hands with an appropriate method [NHS, 2023a].

Aprons
Aprons should be worn when:
- your clothing is likely to become contaminated with blood and/or other bodily fluids
- carrying out cleaning that may lead to contamination of your clothing.

Aprons should be disposed of appropriately following a single use [NHS, 2023a].

Face masks
There are two types of face mask in common use by ambulance services (Figure 5.3):
- fluid-resistant surgical face mask (FRSM)
- filtering face piece (FFP3) mask.

FRSMs are worn to protect the wearer when there is a risk of splashing or spraying blood, body fluids or secretions on to the respiratory mucosa. FRSMs are also an element of PPE for droplet precautions.

Some surgical face masks come with a clear shield to protect the eyes from splash contamination. They should be used if you believe there may be a risk of you being splashed by bodily fluids from the patient.

FFP3 masks, when fitted correctly, provide protection against airborne infections such as COVID-19. They need to be well fitted and users must be 'fit-tested' prior to wearing them. As a responder, it is unlikely your role will require you to undertake a procedure that requires the wearing of FFP3 masks and so you should only ever need to wear a FRSM. If locally there is a need to wear a FFP3, you should ensure you are appropriately fit-tested to ensure the mask works effectively for you.

Eye protection
Eye protection, such as goggles or FRSMs with eye covering, should be worn if a procedure being undertaken is likely to lead to splashing of bodily fluids, including blood, into the eyes, for example when trying to stop a major bleed. Eye protection used in the ambulance service should be single-patient use [NHS, 2023a].

Sleeve protectors
All ambulance services have a 'bare below elbows' policy, making contamination of long-sleeved clothing less likely. However, cross-contamination can occur if you are manual handling multiple patients while wearing long-sleeved clothing such as your hi-visibility jacket or fleece. Sleeve protectors can help protect your clothing from wrist to elbow.

They are for single-patient use, can be worn over the top of gloves and should be disposed of as clinical waste [NHS, 2023a].

Chapter 5 – Health and Safety

Wearing and removing PPE

The PPE required will vary depending on the patient and not all items are always necessary. As a responder, the level of PPE you are likely to need would be an apron, FRSM, eye protection and gloves. Adopt the following procedures for putting on and removing PPE [DoHSC, 2024]:

Donning PPE for SICP

Take the following steps to don PPE for SICP:
1. Ensure you have the required PPE in the correct sizes. This should include:
   - disposable apron
   - surgical face mask
   - disposable gloves
   - eye protection (goggles or visor, if required)
   - alcohol-based hand rub.
2. Remove any items from the pockets of your clothing, tie back hair and remove jewellery. Where possible, ensure you are adequately hydrated prior to donning PPE.
3. Perform hand hygiene using an alcohol-based hand rub.
4. Place your head through the neck loop of the apron and fasten it to your body by tying the ties behind your back. Try to cover as much of the front of your uniform as you can.

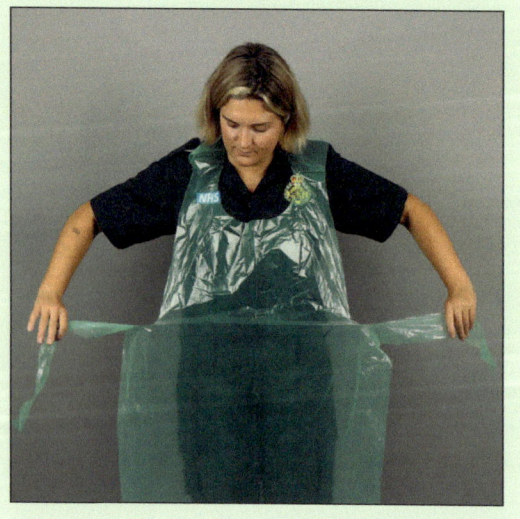

Donning PPE for SICP – *cont*

5. Put on the face mask:
   1. Place the mask over your nose, mouth and chin.
   2. If you have elastic ear loops, hook these over your ears.
   3. If you have ties, tie the upper straps on the crown of your head and the lower straps at the nape of the neck.
   4. Mould the nose piece over the bridge of your nose.
   5. Ensure the mask extends under the chin.

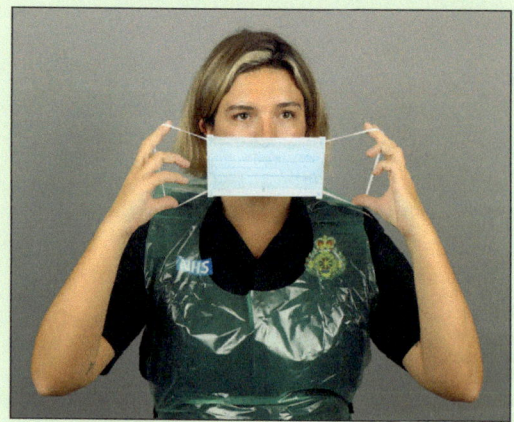

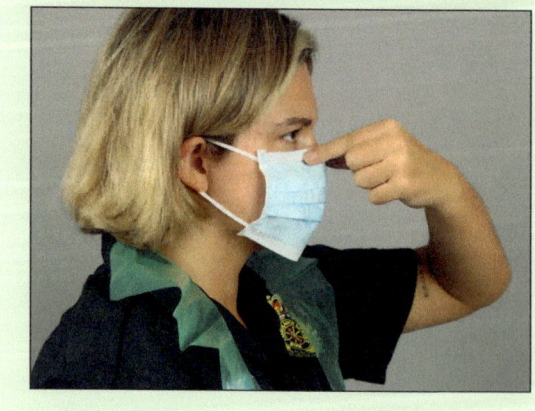

Infection prevention and controls

Donning PPE for SICP – *cont*

6. Apply eye protection and adjust as required to ensure a secure fit.

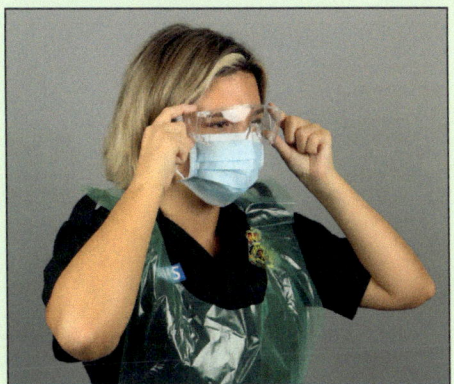

7. Put on disposable gloves.

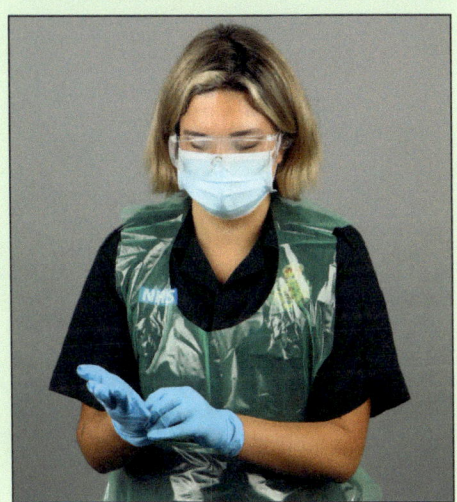

Doffing PPE for SICP

Take the following steps to doff PPE for SICP purposes:
1. Plan your movements: gloves, apron and eye protection should be removed prior to leaving the ambulance or the patient's immediate environment. Face masks should be removed after you have left the environment.

Doffing PPE for SICP – *cont*

2. Grasp the outside of a glove with the opposite gloved hand and peel off. Hold the removed glove in the hand that is still wearing a glove.

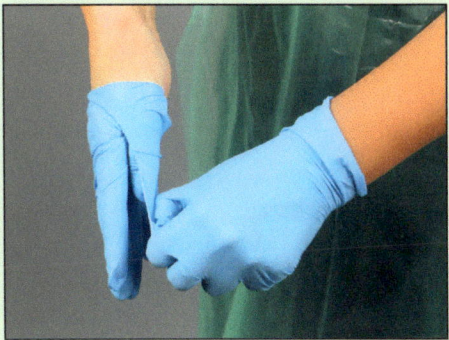

3. Slide a finger from the ungloved hand under the wrist of the gloved hand, hook the glove and peel it off over the glove being held in the hand.
   Discard both gloves into a clinical waste bag.

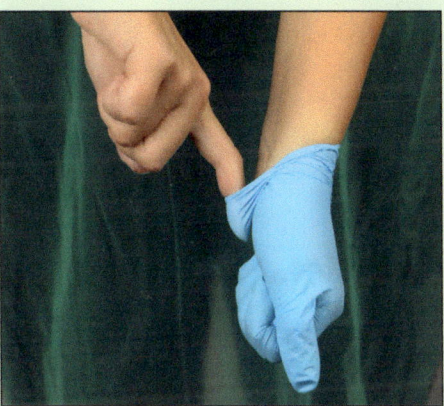

4. Perform hand hygiene using an alcohol-based hand rub.
5. Remove the disposable apron:
    1. Unfasten or break apron ties at the neck.
    2. Let the apron fall forward to fold on to itself.
    3. Break the ties at the waist.
    4. Fold the apron in on itself.
    5. Roll up apron sufficiently so that it can be discarded easily.
    6. Dispose of apron into clinical waste.

Doffing PPE for SICP – *cont*

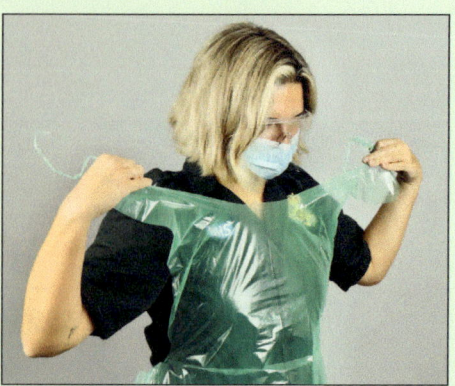

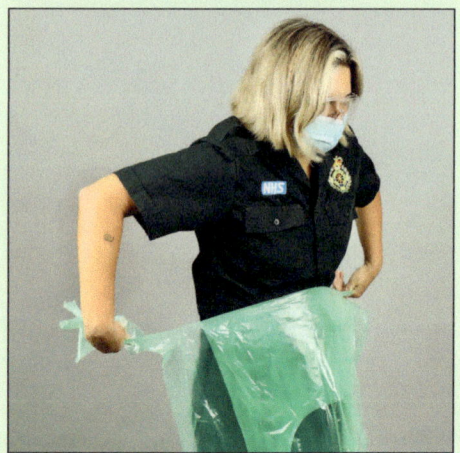

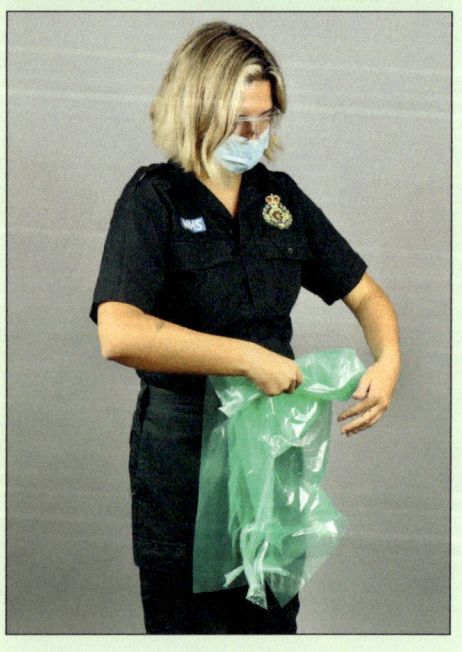

Doffing PPE for SICP – *cont*

6. Remove eye protection by holding both arms of the eye protection, then lift and pull it away from your face.

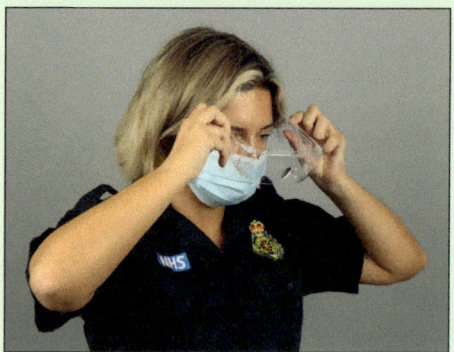

7. Dispose of eye protection into clinical waste.
8. Perform hand hygiene using an alcohol-based hand rub.
9. Once outside of the ambulance or the patient's immediate environment, remove the surgical face mask:
   1. Untie or break bottom ties.
   2. Untie or break top ties.
   3. Handling the mask by the ties only, lean forward and pull mask away from your face.
   4. Dispose of the mask into clinical waste.

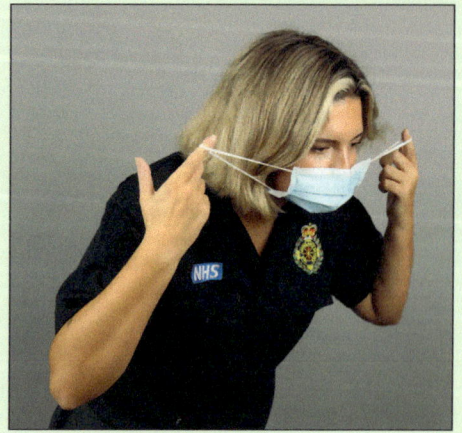

10. Perform hand hygiene with soap and water if available; if not, use an alcohol-based hand rub.

Infection prevention and controls

3.6.5 Safe management of the care environment

Where possible, the care environment should be kept clean, free of non-essential items and be maintained in a good state of repair with adequate ventilation. However, you will often have little control over the environment in which you provide care. Be mindful that the environment can be a significant hazard not only to you, but also to your patient from an infection control perspective. Consider what, if anything, you can do to minimise risks. For example, if a patient has fallen over in a dirty location and has a series of minor wounds that need dressing consider moving them to a clean location before cleaning and dressing the wounds.

Ensure that the waste produced while providing pre-hospital care is cleared away once the patient is removed, i.e. be sure to remove packaging, e.g. used dressings before leaving the scene.

3.6.6 Safe management of care equipment

The equipment used for providing healthcare as well as the environment itself can become a means of transmitting an infection if not appropriately cleaned and decontaminated. In this next section we will consider the process of cleaning and decontaminating. As a responder this will be most relevant to the equipment you use with a patient, such as a blood pressure cuff or a pulse-oximeter device, both of which could be means of transmitting a HCAI.

Cleaning and decontamination
Decontamination is a key principle of infection prevention and control. It prevents both healthcare workers and patients from contracting infectious diseases that could be avoided, preventing patient deaths and patient discomfort as well as reducing costs.

Decontamination is divided into three separate processes [HSE, 2024b]:
- Cleaning is defined as the process that removes physical dirt or visible contamination from surfaces, but without necessarily destroying potentially infectious micro-organisms.
- Decontamination or disinfection refers to the destruction of micro-organisms so that they no longer represent a danger of initiating infection, or any other harmful response.
- Sterilisation is the process that removes all viable micro-organisms including viruses.

Cleaning, decontamination and sterilisation may not all be required; it depends on the item and its use.

Think back to the chain of infection: decontamination is all about trying to break the transmission of potentially infective processes from reaching a new susceptible host.

Cleaning schedules
Your organisation should have a cleaning schedule, which will provide a schedule for the cleaning of ambulance stations, ambulance and equipment. Much of this is probably not relevant to your role as a responder, but you should seek out information about cleaning the equipment you use and the clothing you wear. It is likely that the following are guidelines that will be similar to those of your organisation:
- All patient equipment should be wiped clean after each use using an approved product, such as Clinell wipes.
- If equipment is visibly soiled and unable to be fully cleaned, it should be swapped.
- Bags and other equipment which doesn't frequently come into contact with patients should be cleaned regularly (weekly), by being wiped down.
- Clothing should be changed daily, or sooner if visibly soiled.

Cleaning and decontaminating procedures
Cleaning is the first step of effective decontamination and refers to removing visible dirt, including organic matter, and reducing the presence of micro-organisms. Cleaning should include the use of detergent and warm water to remove all visible contamination and items should then be allowed to thoroughly dry [HSE, 2024b].

Decontamination should be carried out after a detergent clean and uses a range of products to

Chapter 5 – Health and Safety

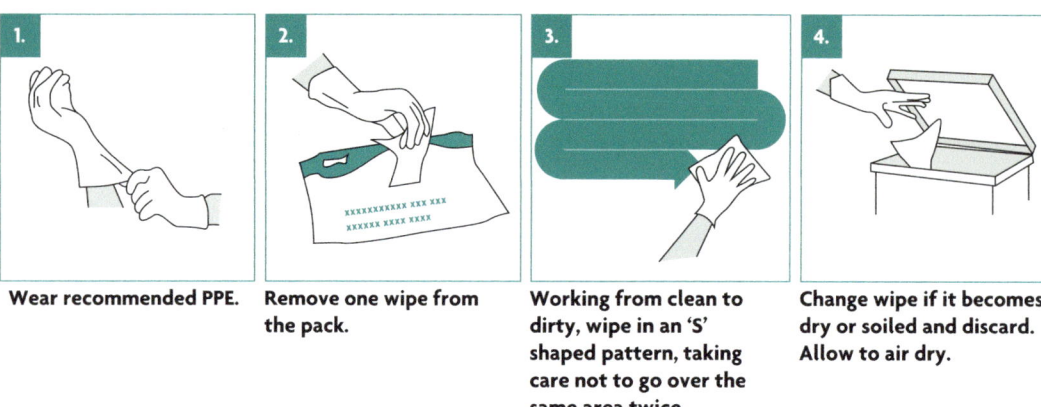

Figure 5.4 Clinell wipes
Source: Republished with permission of GAMA Healthcare Ltd. Best-practice guidance for infection control wet wipes developed by Clinell and GAMA Healthcare Ltd © 2016.

reduce the number of viable micro-organisms still remaining. A general principle is that disinfection should be minimised and instead single-use equipment used wherever possible.

Depending on what you are trying to clean, you may use different products, but one product you are likely to have available is some form of sanitising wipes. Clinell combined detergent-and-disinfectant wipes are found widely in healthcare settings for decontaminating solid items and surfaces; instructions for their use are shown in Figure 5.4.

PPE for decontamination

Chemicals involved in the procedure of decontamination can be harmful to health if you are exposed to them inappropriately or in high doses. Whenever you are decontaminating you should protect yourself from coming into direct contact with chemicals or any micro-organisms on surfaces that you may be attempting to clean. Be sure to use the appropriate PPE; this is likely to include:
- gloves
- apron
- sleeve protectors

- FFP3 face mask protection: if you are having to scrub something to clean it, then there is a high possibility the liquid will become aerosolised, meaning you could inhale associated micro-organisms.

3.6.7 Safe management of healthcare linen

In your role as a responder, handling linen should not be something that happens too frequently. It is unlikely you will have the need to frequently use linen or the facilities to safely store fresh linen. Despite this, you should still be aware of some basic points when it comes to the management and storage of linen, including the following [NHS, 2023a]:
- Hand hygiene should be performed prior to handling fresh linen.
- Clean linen should not be stored in plastic bags, to prevent growth of *Bacillus cereus*.
- Clean linen must always be separated from used/infectious linen.
- Wear PPE when handling used/infectious linen.
- Ensure used/infectious linen is disposed of appropriately. This will most likely mean being taken by an ambulance crew to hospital where appropriate facilities will be available.

3.6.8 Safe management of blood and body fluids

Any spillage of blood or body fluids may be a method of transmission and is sometimes referred to as a biological spillage. These can be accidental or malicious and include blood, urine, vomit and faeces. As a responder it is unlikely you will have the equipment to immediately deal with such a spillage, but an attending ambulance crew should have the necessary supplies including a spill pack. If you are waiting for backup, then you should isolate the area where the spill has occurred, if possible, and await support. It may be necessary to inform the clinical hub that you need help in managing a biological spill so that the EOC can warn the attending ambulance crew to ensure they have the equipment required to assist.

3.6.9 Safe disposal of waste (including sharps)

Healthcare waste must be segregated immediately by the person generating the waste into appropriate colour-coded waste disposal bags or containers and labelled, stored, transported and disposed of appropriately [NHS, 2023a].

You should be aware of your organisation's policy on managing healthcare waste, but below are a number of basic principles that apply to most healthcare organisations.

Types of healthcare waste
It's very important that all waste is segregated correctly as the way in which different waste is processed varies greatly based on the risk it presents. There are also significant cost variations with processing waste, with domestic waste being far cheaper to dispose of than infectious waste. Therefore, if infectious waste was filled with unnecessary packaging, it could lead to substantial unnecessary costs.

There are four main types of waste you will encounter as a responder; they are:

- **Mixed sharps:** Sharps are items that could cause cuts or puncture wounds, including needles, scalpels, knives, broken glass and open drug ampoules. They are disposed of in a yellow sharps bin with a yellow lid.
- **Clinical waste:** Waste from a healthcare activity that:
  - contains viable micro-organisms or their toxins which are known or reliably believed to cause disease in humans or other living organisms
  - contains or is contaminated with a medicine that contains a biologically active pharmaceutical agent.

  Given the emergency nature of ambulance work, it is rarely possible to confirm a patient is non-infectious, so much waste is handled this way. This would be disposed of in a UN-approved orange bag.
- **Offensive waste:** Non-infectious, non-hazardous waste, from human healthcare that is likely to include items contaminated by bodily fluids, but where the patient is known to not be infectious. This waste is disposed of in a yellow bag with a black stripe, also known as a 'tiger bag'.
- **Domestic/municipal waste:** This form of waste is non-hazardous and is similar to the domestic waste you would produce at home. Most of the packaging for products used in an ambulance which has not been contaminated can be disposed of this way.

Table 5.1 provides examples of typical waste arising from ambulance service activity.

Chapter 5 – Health and Safety

Table 5.1 Types of waste emerging from ambulance service activity

Activity	Waste type	Receptacle/bag	Justification	Disposal route
Injections	Contaminated sharps or syringes with medicine residue	Yellow-lidded sharps receptacle	Potentially contaminated with medicinal products	Incineration
Items/equipment for treating patients	Contaminated packaging, gloves, aprons, other PPE, dressings, airways, suction liners, laryngoscope blades	Infectious waste in orange waste receptacles	Due to lack of patient records/screening, unlikely to be able to classify as non-infectious	Alternative treatment or incineration
Items/equipment for treating patients	Uncontaminated aprons, other PPE, non-medicated intravenous bags, non-infectious urine, faeces, vomit and their containers	Offensive/unhygienic waste disposed of in yellow and black striped ('tiger') bags	Risk assessment to determine no possible contamination and non-infectious	Non-hazardous municipal incineration/energy from waste or landfill **Note:** Liquids (including body fluids) are banned from landfill
Refuse/rubbish	Uncontaminated packaging and refuse/rubbish	Non-infectious, black or clear bag	Used packaging, while patient treatment is being carried out in the vehicle, will usually not be infectious/clinical waste	Non-hazardous municipal incineration/energy from waste, materials recycling facilities or landfill

Storing and handling healthcare waste

All waste should be stored in appropriate receptacles, in line with your organisation's procedures. As a responder it is likely that you will pass any waste you have on to an ambulance crew that backs you up so they can dispose of it appropriately. You should not be carrying waste around in your own vehicle.

When handling healthcare waste, consider the risks it poses and protect yourself appropriately by using PPE. At minimum, when handling infectious or offensive waste bags, or containers, wear gloves and also use other appropriate PPE if you anticipate any leakage of waste contained within.

3.6.10 Occupational safety: prevention of exposure (including sharps injury)

The risk of blood-borne virus infection is associated with any significant occupational exposure. A significant occupational exposure is defined as [UKHSA, 2021]:
- a percutaneous injury, e.g. injuries from needles, instruments, bone fragments or bites which break the skin; and/or
- exposure of broken skin (abrasions, cuts, eczema, etc.); and/or

- exposure of mucous membranes including the eye from splashing of blood or other high-risk body fluids.

If handled correctly, there should be minimal risk of a sharps injury occurring, especially to responders. However, accidents do happen, so you should be aware of the action to undertake if you are injured by a sharp object. You should take particular care with any 'used sharps' as these present a risk for transmitting infection. To reduce the risk of sharps injury you should:

- Keep sharps covered whenever possible.
- Immediately dispose of used sharps into approved containers.
- Know where your sharps are stored and check the integrity of packaging frequently.
- Ensure that others around you are aware when you are using a sharp item.

If you do receive a sharps injury, then you should [NHS Choices, 2021a]:

- Encourage the wound to gently bleed, ideally holding it under running water.
- Wash the wound using running water and plenty of soap.
- Don't scrub the wound while you are washing it.
- Don't suck the wound.
- Dry the wound and cover with a waterproof plaster or dressing.
- Seek urgent medical attention as prophylaxis may be required.
- Report the injury – this is a legal requirement.

Sharps injuries from needles and cannulation equipment are considered to be high risk and can potentially spread infections of blood-borne viruses, including:

- hepatitis B
- hepatitis C
- human immunodeficiency virus (HIV).

You should seek expert medical help as soon as possible after a sharps injury. Your employing organisation will most likely have a procedure in place for doing this, which you should be aware of.

Splash contamination

There is a risk of diseases being transmitted if blood or other bodily fluids are splashed on to healthcare workers in a location where they can easily enter the body. These locations include:

- open cuts or wounds
- mucosal membranes including the eyes and mouth.

If this happens, you should immediately irrigate the area with copious amounts of tap water. Following this, you should attend an ED or MIU so that a risk assessment can be undertaken and post-exposure prophylaxis administered, if it is thought to be necessary, along with gathering blood samples.

4 Fire safety

4.1 Learning objectives

By the end of this section, you will be able to:
- describe practices that prevent fires from:
  - starting
  - spreading
- explain emergency procedures to be followed in the event of a fire in the work setting.

4.2 Introduction

Fire is a chemical reaction that requires three elements [HSE, 2024c]:
- heat
- oxygen
- fuel.

Together, they make up the fire triangle (or triangle of combustion, Figure 5.5). For combustion or

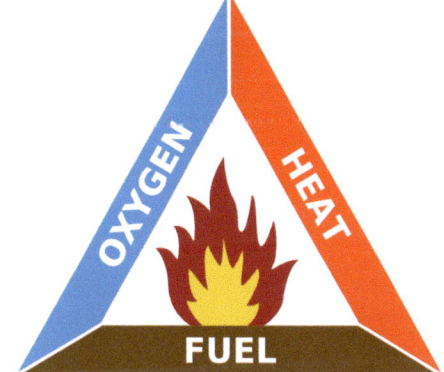

Figure 5.5 The fire triangle
Source: 'Fire triangle'. Licensed under CC BY-SA 3.9 via Wikimedia Commons

burning to occur, oxygen must combine with a fuel. Fuels can be in solid, liquid or gas form to start with, but for flaming combustion to occur, a solid or liquid fuel must be converted into a vapour, which then reacts with oxygen. An oxygen concentration of about 16% is required for combustion to occur and air contains 21%.

4.3 Fire prevention

Prevention is better than cure and there are a number of things you can do to prevent fires from starting:

- Do not smoke in the workplace. The NHS has prohibited smoking in all areas other than those dedicated as smoking zones. Take care with cigarettes and matches: always discard in a suitable place and ensure they are fully extinguished.
- Do not allow the build-up of rubbish or other combustible materials in your work area, corridors or stair enclosures as this is fuel and may create an obstruction to escape routes.
- Do not have fabric, paper or other readily combustible material near electric fires or portable gas heaters.
- Do not leave hotplates or containers, e.g. frying pans, unattended when in use.
- Flammable gases and liquids should be stored in the designated location, e.g. the medical gases stores.
- Defective electrical wiring or equipment must be turned off immediately, marked as defective and reported to the estates department. If possible, also remove from general access.
- Switch off all electrical and gas appliances when they are not in use.
- Check your working area before you leave for the day.
- Ensure that manual fire-fighting equipment is accessible, undamaged and maintained.

4.4 What to do in case of fire

If you discover a fire [DoH, 2013]:
1. **Stay safe:** Never compromise your own safety.
2. **Raise the alarm:** Press your thumb against the glass of the nearest and safest fire call point (fire break glass). Alternatively, repeatedly shout 'FIRE' to warn others.
3. **Phone 999 (or 9 999 from some phones) and request the fire service:** Activation of a building fire alarm does not mean the fire and rescue service is automatically alerted; you should make the emergency call every time.
4. **Get out and close the door:** Go to the designated fire assembly point immediately.

If you hear the fire alarm you should [DoH, 2013]:
1. **Leave your place of work:** Close windows and doors behind you if this can be done quickly.
2. **Calmly exit:** Make your way to the nearest and safest fire exit. Do not run or stop to collect personal belongings.
3. **Encourage others to exit:** Attempt to offer assistance to anyone who appears to be confused or having difficulties, especially people with disabilities. If your usual exit route is blocked by smoke or flames, stop, change direction and find an alternative escape route. You should still meet at the normal assembly point for your workplace.
4. **Do not use lifts:** Their movement assists fire travel and they may stop suddenly if there is a power failure. They may also take you to the scene of the fire. Use the stairs at all times.
5. **Move to your designated assembly point:** Make yourself known to the fire marshal or person who is co-ordinating the evacuation. Note that fire marshals are typically only appointed in larger premises (i.e. not ambulance stations) and are identified by a yellow tabard.
6. **Form an orderly group:** Remain together until a head count is established and until further instructions are given.

4.4.1 Vehicle fires

If a fire breaks out in a vehicle, take the following actions [DSFRS, 2024]:
1. Stop in a safe location.
2. Switch on hazard lights.

3. Switch off the ignition and press the battery isolator button (if the vehicle has one).
4. Release the bonnet, but DO NOT open or touch the bonnet.
5. Get everyone out of the vehicle.
6. Remove medical gas cylinders if possible.
7. Move yourself and any other people away from the burning vehicle.
8. Warn oncoming traffic (if safe to do so).
9. Summon help by dialling 999 and requesting the fire and rescue service and the police.
10. If you believe it is safe to do so, attempt to put out the fire with a dry-powder extinguisher if you are able to. If the fire is in the engine compartment, do not open the bonnet; use the extinguisher through the grill or under the edge of the bonnet. Use with caution and if in doubt, do not attempt to tackle the fire.

5 Stress

5.1 Learning objectives

By the end of this section, you will be able to:
- describe common signs and indicators of stress
- compare strategies for managing stress.

5.2 Introduction

Stress is the adverse reaction people have to excessive pressures or other types of demand placed on them [HSE, 2024d]. There is a clear distinction between pressure, which can create a 'buzz' and be a motivating factor, and stress, which can occur when this pressure becomes excessive.

Six broad areas have been highlighted as being the primary sources of stress at work [HSE, 2024d]:
- **Demands:** This includes issues such as workload, work patterns and the work environment.
- **Control:** How much say the person has in the way they do their work.
- **Support:** This includes the encouragement and resources provided by the organisation, line management and colleagues.
- **Relationships:** This includes promoting positive working relationships to avoid conflict and dealing with unacceptable behaviour.
- **Role:** Whether people understand their role within the organisation and whether the organisation ensures they do not have conflicting roles.
- **Change:** How organisational change (large or small) is managed and communicated in the organisation.

5.3 Signs of stress

Stress can cause changes in those experiencing it, making it important for everyone to look out for changes in a person's or a group's behaviour, particularly in NHS ambulance services, where half of the employees experience work-related stress [PIE, 2014]. However, in many cases only you will notice the changes that occur because of the stress you experience.

Stress can show itself in many ways and people will exhibit different signs and symptoms. Some of the well-known signs and symptoms of stress include:
- behaviour change:
  - difficulty sleeping
  - altered eating habits
  - smoking and/or drinking more
  - avoiding friends and family
  - sexual problems
- physical:
  - tiredness
  - indigestion and nausea
  - headaches
  - aching muscles
  - palpitations
- mental:
  - increased indecision
  - difficulty in concentrating
  - poor memory
  - feeling inadequate
  - low self-esteem
- emotional:
  - mood swings, becoming irritable or angry
  - increased anxiety

- feeling numb
- hypersensitivity
- feeling drained and listless.

5.4 Managing stress

Although stress is not an illness, it can cause serious illness, both mental and physical, if not identified and managed early. The success of coping strategies to help reduce the effects of stress will vary from person to person. Consider some of the strategies that have been recommended [NHS Choices, 2021b]:

- **Be active:** Physical activity can help remove some of the emotional intensity of stress.
- **Eat and drink healthily:** Eat a balanced diet and avoid excessive amounts of caffeine and alcohol.
- **Take control:** This can be easier said than done but identify problems and think about possible solutions. Having a suggestion adopted by an organisation to help in your daily work, particularly when it is benefiting patients, is very satisfying.
- **Connect with people:** A good support network of colleagues, friends and family can ease your work troubles and help you see things in a different way. Talking things through with a friend may also help you find solutions to your problems.
- **Make time for yourself:** Make time to do the things you enjoy. Make time for socialising, relaxing or exercise.
- **Challenge yourself:** Setting yourself goals and challenges, inside or outside of work, such as learning a new language or a new sport can help build confidence, which may help you to deal with stress.
- **Help other people:** Evidence shows that those who help other people, through activities such as volunteering or community work, often become more resilient themselves.

If you believe your stress is serious and having a detrimental impact on your mental health, you may need further support. Your GP, occupational health or employer well-being team can be a good place to start. See the section 'Caring for yourself and colleagues' at the end of Chapter 2, 'The Ambulance Service', for more information.

Chapter 6 Safeguarding Adults and Children

1 Safeguarding adults and children

1.1 Learning objectives

By the end of this section you will be able to:
- define the various types of abuse
- identify the signs and/or symptoms associated with each type of abuse
- describe factors that may contribute to an individual being more vulnerable to abuse
- explain the actions to take if there are suspicions that an individual is being abused
- explain the actions to take if an individual alleges that they are being abused
- identify ways to ensure that evidence of abuse is preserved
- identify national policies and local systems that relate to safeguarding and protection from abuse
- explain the roles of different agencies in safeguarding and protecting individuals from abuse
- identify reports into serious failures to protect individuals from abuse
- identify sources of information and advice about your own role in safeguarding and protecting individuals from abuse
- explain how the likelihood of abuse may be reduced
- describe unsafe practices that may affect the well-being of individuals
- explain the actions to take if unsafe practices have been identified
- describe the action to take if suspected abuse or unsafe practices have been reported but nothing has been done in response.

1.2 Introduction

As a responder, you hold a trusted and privileged position and one from which you can potentially identify and assist victims of abuse or neglect. In order to do this, you will need to have a good understanding of the forms abuse can take, the signs and symptoms of those suffering, what increases a person's risk of being a victim of abuse, and also how to get help and support for victims.

Before going further, consider some of the key phrases associated with safeguarding:
- **Safeguarding:** The process of promoting the welfare of individuals and groups and protecting them from harm, often putting controls and measures in place to do so.
- **Protection:** To keep safe from harm.
- **Abuse:** Any action that causes significant harm to an individual.
- **Harm:** Physical or psychological damage or injury.
- **Maltreatment:** Includes all forms of physical and emotional ill-treatment or abuse.

1.3 Learning from previous cases

The vast majority of abuse and neglect happens behind closed doors and rarely reaches the attention of the public. However, over recent years there have been a number of notable cases, including:
- **Winterbourne View:** In 2011 a BBC *Panorama* programme showed staff at Winterbourne View, a private hospital caring for patients with disabilities, abusing their patients in a range of both physical and psychological manners. A national outcry followed. As a result of the subsequent investigation, 11 members of staff were convicted of criminal offences and the hospital was shut. The investigation also identified that serious warning signs, which had not been properly looked into, had been evident at the hospital for a long time prior to the discovery of abuse [DoH, 2013b].

- **Daniel Pelka:** Daniel died aged 4 years and 8 months following a period of sustained abuse and neglect by his mother and her partner. His death was caused by a serious head injury, but he had been physically beaten and starved for a prolonged period prior to his death. In the serious case review following his death, it was identified that, although the family and Daniel were well known to police, social services, healthcare services and his school, the warning signs had not been correctly picked up on or appropriate action taken. The report said that Daniel was 'invisible against the backdrop of his mother's controlling behaviour' and that professionals involved in his case had failed to 'think the unthinkable' [CSCB, 2014].

Sadly, this failure to notice warning signs is not unique and other equally tragic cases, such as the murders of Victoria Climbié and baby Peter Connelly (Baby P), had very similar findings in their investigations.

Abusers can be skilled at explaining away injuries or unusual behaviour and reassuring professionals about the situation they find. In your front-line role, you may be the only individual that comes into contact with a vulnerable person over a prolonged period of time, so you must be prepared to identify and raise concerns where necessary in order to help prevent further similar cases. You must be prepared to 'think the unthinkable'.

1.4 *Vulnerability*

People are considered to be vulnerable when they are at a greater than normal risk of abuse. For vulnerable adults, this can include, but is not limited to [NHS England, 2024d]:
- those with learning difficulties
- older people who are isolated
- those with memory problems
- those who are dependent on others for support
- those whose carer is addicted to alcohol or drugs
- those who live with a carer.

1.4.1 Abusers of vulnerable adults

Vulnerable adults may be abused by a wide range of people, including relatives and family, professional staff, paid care workers, volunteers, other service users, neighbours, friends and those who deliberately target and exploit the vulnerable [DoH, 2000].

1.4.2 Risk factors for child abuse

All children are vulnerable to abuse, but those who may be more so include those in the following situations [NICE, 2017]:
- parental or carer drug or alcohol misuse
- parental or carer mental health problems
- intrafamilial violence or history of violent offending
- previous child maltreatment in members of the family
- known maltreatment of an animal by the carer or parent
- vulnerable and unsupported parents or carers
- pre-existing disability in the child.

What is common to most of these scenarios for both adults and children is that the abused tend to have reduced support networks or social contacts around them who they can turn to for help and support. The victim tends to have a degree of reliance on the abuser and this gives the abuser a position of power with which to control and manipulate the victim.

1.4.3 Cultural influences

Culture is well recognised as influencing abuse in vulnerable groups and can have a major impact on a person's ability to seek help. Examples where cultural beliefs or difference can worsen abuse situations include [NSPCC, 2014]:
- **Fear of cultural isolation:** Family members who do not abide by cultural practices may be cast out and isolated, making it very difficult for them to seek help and therefore making them increasingly vulnerable. In the most extreme cases, so-called honour violence may even be inflicted on these family members.
- **Cultural beliefs overriding self-interests:** An abuser may make a vulnerable person believe

that abuse is part of a cultural practice, warning their victims they will be socially isolated if they reveal the abuse.

1.5 Forms of abuse

There are four types of abuse common to both adults and children [JRCALC, 2023]:
- physical abuse
- psychological/emotional abuse
- sexual abuse
- neglect.

For vulnerable adults there is also financial abuse.

Additionally, you should also be aware of female genital mutilation (FGM), a form of child abuse.

1.5.1 Physical abuse

Physical abuse, also known as non-accidental injury (NAI), involves contact intended to cause, or result in, pain, injury or other physical harm. It may include striking someone (with or without an object), kicking, grabbing, biting or inappropriate restraint. For older patients in particular, it may also include being handled roughly, or moved in a way that causes pain without the appropriate lifting or moving aids [JRCALC, 2023; Age UK, 2023].

Physical harm can also be caused when a carer or parent fabricates illness, or induces symptoms of an illness, in an adult or child (Munchausen's syndrome by proxy).

Signs may include:
- bruising at multiple stages of repair
- bruises on children who are not yet crawling
- injuries inconsistent with the age of the patient
- frequent attendance at hospital
- inappropriate history for injury demonstrated
- specific injuries, such as cigarette burns and 'hand-grip' bruises
- fear of those around them
- fear of making mistakes
- being very withdrawn and quiet
- delays in seeking help for illness or injury.

You should be particularly mindful of injuries to non-mobile babies. Those aged under a year old are the most vulnerable as they cannot speak for themselves and are totally dependent on others for all of their care. Any injury in a non-mobile baby needs to be reviewed by a suitably qualified clinician, normally a paediatrician at the local hospital.

1.5.2 Psychological/emotional abuse

Psychological, also known as emotional, abuse is a form of abuse characterised by damaging a person's psychological well-being. This is often seen in situations of power imbalance, such as abusive relationships. It may include conveying a feeling of unworthiness, unimportance or being unvalued. It may also include making a person feel ashamed or humiliated through the words or actions of another person.

Over a prolonged period, this form of abuse can allow the abuser to mentally control the abused person and seriously damage emotional and psychological development. All forms of abuse usually contain an element of psychological abuse, as abusers will try to control the actions and behaviour of their victim [JRCALC, 2023; Age UK, 2023].

Signs may include:
- lack of social skills
- low self-worth
- depression
- self-harm
- poor relationships with others
- helplessness
- excessive fear or anxiety.

1.5.3 Sexual abuse

Sexual abuse involves forcing or enticing a person to take part in sexual activity against their wishes, or for which they are not able to consent. Activities may involve physical assault, including penetration (for example, rape or oral sex), or they can be non-penetrative, such as kissing, masturbation or touching the outside of clothing. Sexual abuse can also include non-contact activities, such as indecent exposure, or forcing a person to watch, or to be involved in the production of, explicit sexual material. Grooming a person in preparation for abuse is also a form of sexual abuse [JRCALC, 2023; Age UK, 2023].

Signs may include:
- physical signs such as anal or vaginal soreness
- sexually transmitted infection
- unusual discharge
- inappropriate use of sexual language for age
- child being sexually active at a young age
- guilt or shame
- appearing frightened by or avoiding being near to certain people.

Sexual abuse is increasingly occurring online. Young people in particular are vulnerable to abusers over the internet befriending them and then asking or demanding sexual favours in return [NSPCC, 2020].

Child sexual exploitation is a particular form of sexual abuse where a child receives something (such as food, accommodation, drugs or alcohol) as a result of performing sexual acts on others and/or others performing sexual acts on them.

1.5.4 Neglect

Neglect is the persistent failure to meet a person's physical and/or psychological needs. A carer or parent should take reasonable steps to prevent harm from occurring to a dependant, and failure to do so may be neglect. Neglect can be deliberate or accidental, due to not fully understanding the needs of a dependent person.

Neglect may include:
- failure to provide adequate food, warmth or shelter for a dependant
- failure to ensure adequate access to appropriate medical care.

Signs of neglect include:
- poor appearance and hygiene
- untreated injuries or dental issues
- poor physical development for age
- poor language or communication skills for age
- pressure sores
- signs of malnourishment or dehydration
- dirt, urine or faecal smell in a person's environment.

1.5.5 Financial abuse

This is the unlawful use of a person's property, money or other valuables. It may include an individual being pressured into lending or giving money or other belongings to another person. A carer could start to take control of an individual's personal finances and then use that control to gain profitably without consent. It may also include charging excessive amounts of money for simple services or goods. Relatives are often perpetrators of this kind of abuse and may move into a patient's house in order to be able to exert the influence required to take financial control [Age UK, 2023].

Signs of financial abuse can include:
- unexplained loss of money
- unusual bank account activity
- rapid deterioration in a person's standard of living as they can no longer afford essential goods and services
- a relative or carer moving into the home and taking control.

1.5.6 FGM

FGM is the partial or complete removal of the female genitalia, also known as female circumcision or cutting. It is a practice most commonly observed in certain African countries and also the Middle East [UNICEF, 2023].

FGM is a deeply rooted tradition that acts as a complex form of control over women's reproductive and sexual rights, and although it can be performed at any age from birth through to marriage or first pregnancy, it is most commonly carried out on young girls between infancy and 15 years of age. Being subject to FGM can have long-term physical and mental health impacts on well-being.

FGM is a criminal offence in the UK, and it is also an offence for anyone to take a child in order for FGM to be performed abroad. You are legally required by the Female Genital Mutilation Act 2003 to report to the police [HMG, 2017] if you:
- are informed by a girl under 18 years of age that she has undergone an act of FGM

- observe physical signs that an act of FGM may have been carried out on a girl under 18 years of age.

1.6 Managing abuse or disclosures of abuse

The primary goal in the management of a patient who has suffered abuse should be their long-term safety. The situation may be highly emotionally charged, not least for you as a responder, but your actions in the immediate moments on scene may influence the entire course of protecting a vulnerable person. You should remain calm and professional, and not judge those around you. Situations are rarely as simple as they may initially appear, and in the amount of time you will be in contact with a person it is unlikely that you will discover the full truth.

As a responder, it is likely you will pass your concerns on to a crew or other health professional responding to the same incident as you and they will take on responsibility for making appropriate referrals; however, this may change between organisations and you should be aware of these key principles in managing a safeguarding concern [JRCALC, 2023]:

- Consider not just the patient, but also others present. For example, you may be called to manage an adult with chest pain initially, but if you are concerned about the welfare of a child living in the same house, you have the same duty to report and raise concerns as if that child was the original patient.
- Your first priority should be to manage the presenting condition and ensure medical well-being, i.e. provide the usual clinical management for the presenting complaint.
- Limit your questioning to that which is relevant: stop questioning if your suspicions are confirmed, as unnecessary questioning or probing may affect the credibility of subsequent evidence.
- Accept any given explanation. Even if you do not believe the answer, do not make suggestions to the patient on how an incident may have occurred.
- Do not directly accuse parents or carers of abuse, as to do so may result in refusal of further care or transport, thereby increasing the risk a patient faces.
- Wherever possible you should work in partnership with the parents or carers, and inform them of your concerns and the need to share these with other agencies. The only exemption to this rule is when you believe that doing so may put the patient at greater risk of harm. You will have to exercise judgement on this point and should record in detail your justification for not informing, if that is the option you choose.
- Take any and all accusations seriously: it is not your role to decide on their validity or to investigate further; instead you should refer your concerns to the other health professionals who also attend the incident.
- If a person makes a disclosure, make sure you treat them with respect and dignity, and act in a manner which suggests you believe them. Body language and your words can have a massive influence on a patient's behaviour and confidence in you, and if they feel you do not believe them, they may not disclose what they were going to.
- Complete full and accurate records of events. Where possible try to record word for word what the patient has disclosed.

1.6.1 Reporting an urgent concern

An urgent concern exists where you believe a person may be at immediate risk of further harm. In those circumstances all at scene should ensure the immediate safety of the patient. This can often be best achieved by transporting the patient to hospital where they can be monitored and assessed while awaiting the support of other services.

In the most serious circumstances it may be necessary to contact the police via the EOC with your concerns to ensure immediate patient safety. Remember that in certain circumstances, including the prevention or detection of a serious crime, such disclosures can be made to the police without the patient's consent. It would normally be the decision of the most senior clinician on scene to do this.

Chapter 6 – *Safeguarding Adults and Children*

1.7 Safeguarding referrals

Whenever you believe a person is being abused or neglected, or is at risk of either, a safeguarding referral should be completed. Your organisation will likely have a policy on how this should be achieved, and as a responder it is likely that one of your clinical health professional colleagues will take on the responsibility for making a referral, including any concerns you may have raised.

You should be aware of your local policies for making such referrals but should also have a general understanding of these guidelines for making a referral:

- **Report all concerns for children:** Any concern, however small, should be reported through safeguarding referral pathways. Experienced and qualified safeguarding professionals can judge for themselves whether further investigation or action is required. They will also know whether the patient, place of care or family is known for previous safeguarding concerns, information that may not be available to you.
- **Additional sources of help:** All services should have safeguarding teams including named professionals responsible for safeguarding. These teams are experienced in the management of safeguarding issues and have established relationships with the multidisciplinary teams that work around those issues.
- **Role of social services:** In most areas social services are the main organisation around which safeguarding concerns articulate. Social workers are experienced in dealing with vulnerable people and with cases of abuse and neglect, and can be a great source of support and advice.
- **Escalating concerns:** All care organisations should be well prepared for managing safeguarding concerns, but in the unlikely event that you do not believe that your concerns are being managed in an appropriate manner, you have a duty to escalate your concern. To do this you should speak to a senior manager or a named professional. Ensure you make records of all concerns that you pass on.
- **Preserve evidence:** If you suspect abuse, you may need to consider how to preserve evidence. This could take many forms depending on the form of abuse and might include not touching items you believe have been used to assault a victim, or encouraging a person not to wash or change their clothes if they have been subject to physical or sexual abuse in order to retain evidence [JRCALC, 2023].

1.8 Summary

Safeguarding can be a highly emotive topic for all concerned, and this should be at the front of your mind when managing a situation where safeguarding is a concern. Try to remain calm, impartial and factual and keep the immediate safety of patients as your primary goal. Remember the cases of Winterbourne View and Daniel Pelka, where key signs were missed and professionals failed to 'think the unthinkable'.

Be aware of the signs of abuse or neglect and immediately raise any concerns you have through local policy for doing so. Also be mindful that dealing with safeguarding incidents can be emotionally traumatic for responders. Following such incidents, you may need to make use of your organisation's counselling or support services.

7 Manual Handling

1 Principles of manual handling

1.1 Learning objectives

By the end of this section you will be able to:
- define manual handling
- explain principles for safe moving and handling
- describe what action should be taken if an individual's wishes conflict with their plan of care in relation to health and safety and their risk assessment.

1.2 Introduction

Within your role as a responder, moving and handling will be unavoidable. From carrying your kit bags through to helping to reposition patients, you will be engaged in moving and handling activities constantly. These activities happen in the relatively uncontrolled environment of pre-hospital care while dealing with emergency situations, and it is therefore not surprising that musculoskeletal injuries are one of the highest causes of sickness for all emergency service staff, including those working for ambulance services [Hignett, 2015].

Knowing the basics of moving and handling principles and following the techniques contained within this chapter will help to reduce, though not eliminate, the risk of you sustaining a musculoskeletal injury, which as we will discuss can range from minor through to life-changing debilitating injuries.

As a responder, it is unlikely you should need to frequently move patients, and you should only undertake any movement which your organisation has trained you to do, but occasionally it may be unavoidable, such as moving a patient from a chair to the floor to perform CPR.

1.2.1 Definitions

The Health and Safety Executive (HSE) [2016] defines manual handling operations as the transporting or supporting of loads, including lifting, lowering, pushing, carrying or moving loads. A load may be either inanimate, for example a box or a trolley, or animate, for example a person or animal.

1.3 Consequences of poor manual handling

Responding for an ambulance service, it is inevitable that occasionally you will need to perform some moving and handling tasks. It is well known that poor moving and handling techniques, as well as repetitive tasks, significantly increase the risk of musculoskeletal injuries, particularly in the back. Musculoskeletal injuries are a significant cause of sickness and the leading cause of back injury for ambulance service staff.

One of the most common injuries is a 'slipped disc', also known as a herniated disc (Figure 7.1).

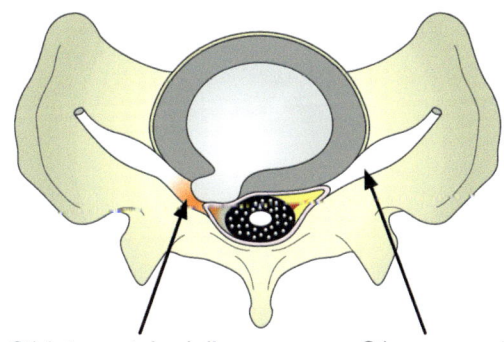

Figure 7.1 Herniated disc

1.3.1 Herniated disc

The spinal column is constructed of vertebrae, with intervertebral discs in between. These discs, which are designed to help take the load through the spine and to cushion the vertebrae, can be damaged by repetitive action or sudden movements, causing the outer layer (the annulus fibrosis) to rupture and protrude beyond the normal diameter of the vertebrae.

When this happens, it pinches on the nerves, causing significant pain and even potential nerve damage (Figure 7.2) [Nellist, 2013]. Most commonly, due to the natural curvature and the increased weight in this area, this occurs in the lumbar region, meaning that the nerves involved often include the sciatic nerve and lead to sciatic leg and back pain, which is very uncomfortable.

1.3.2 Consequences to others

You should also consider that it would not be just you who can be injured by poor or inappropriate moving and handling techniques. It is likely that any inappropriate technique will also lead to injury of your colleagues and even potentially your patient.

It is an unavoidable issue that sometimes you will need to undertake moving and handling procedures in high-pressure emergency environments, but even then you should continue to apply good principles of moving and handling to ensure that nobody is injured by such actions.

1.4 Risk assessment

In Chapter 5, 'Health and Safety', you learnt about risk assessment; manual handling is a perfect example of a set of actions for which you need to undertake a risk assessment before taking action. The difficulty in emergency situations is that the time available to make this risk assessment may be short.

There are five steps to take [HSE, 2024e]:
1. Identify the hazards.
2. Assess the risk by deciding:
   - who might be harmed and how
   - what you're already doing to control the risks
   - what further action you need to take to control the risks
   - who needs to carry out the action
   - when the action is needed by.

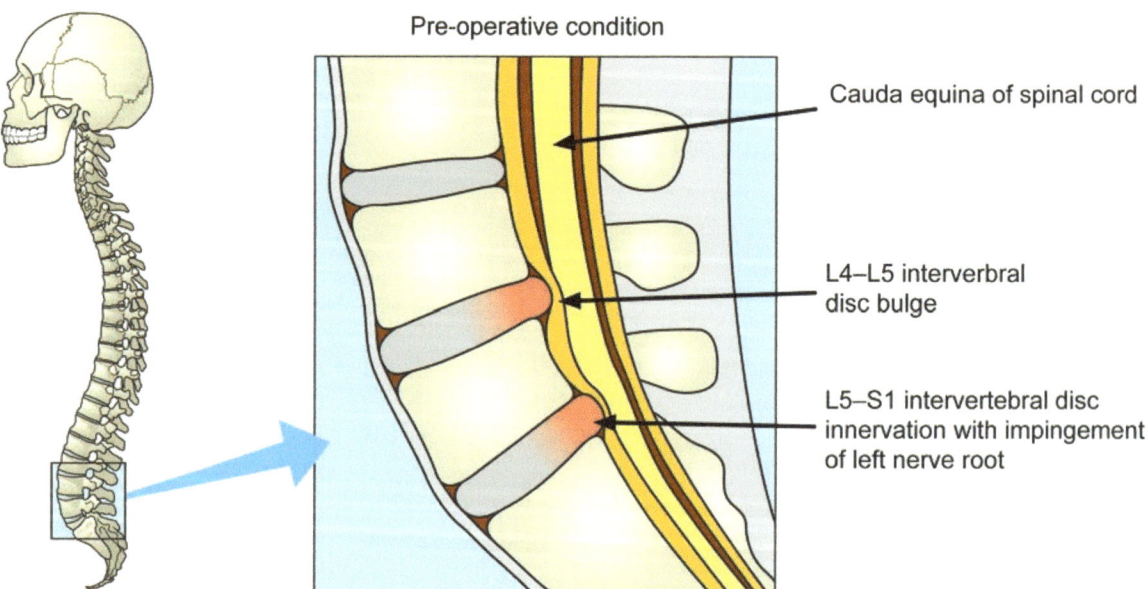

Figure 7.2   Lumbar spine

Principles of manual handling

3. Control the risk by asking yourself:
   - Can I get rid of the hazard altogether?
   - If not, how can I control the risk so that harm is unlikely?
4. Record your findings and implement them.
5. Review your assessment and update if necessary.

This is not very user-friendly or specific to manual handling, and so these steps can be encapsulated in the TILEE acronym [HSE, 2024f]:

- **Task:** Consider whether the lift:
  - involves holding the load away from the body
  - involves long distances
  - requires strenuous effort or twisting.
- **Individual:** Consider whether the lift:
  - requires specialist training
  - presents a hazard
  - is something you and your colleagues are capable of performing (including differences in height and weight)
  - should be undertaken if either you or one of your colleagues is pregnant.
- **Load:** Consider whether the load is:
  - heavy or bulky
  - difficult to get hold of
  - unstable
  - unpredictable
  - harmful
  - likely to grab out when alarmed at being carried down the stairs.
- **Environment:** Determine the presence of:
  - constraints on posture, e.g. low ceiling, confined spaces
  - poor, uneven flooring
  - hot/cold/wet weather
  - poor lighting
  - noise.
- **Equipment:** Consider what equipment:
  - is available
  - will reduce risk to you and the patient
  - is safe to use
  - you are trained and competent to use.

1.4.1 Reducing risk

Legal responsibility

The Manual Handling Operations Regulations 1992, as amended in 2002, bring together European Directive 90/269/EEC on the manual handling of loads, general duties placed on employers by the Health and Safety at Work etc. Act 1974, and the requirements of the Management of Health and Safety at Work Regulations 1999 to detail how employers should reduce or remove the risk from moving and handling injury so far as is reasonably practicable [HSE, 2016].

This should be done by assessing the risk, reducing it so far as is practicable and then regularly reviewing the risk to see if further controls are required.

An example of this is ambulance stretchers. Stretchers used to have to be lifted manually by two people and this led to a large number of injuries. To help reduce the risk, a new generation of ambulance stretchers was introduced that included hydraulic foot pumps, thus reducing the manual handling load. More recently, mechanically powered stretchers have been introduced (Figure 7.3). This further reduces the load and therefore the risk of injury.

Reducing the load in practice

Once you have identified a risk relating to manual handling, you will need to determine how best to

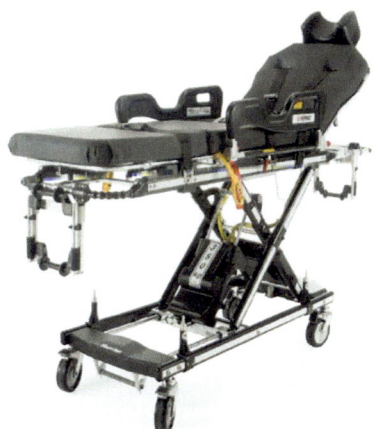

Figure 7.3 A Ferno mechanically powered ambulance stretcher

manage this. Strategies for managing risk are best considered in advance, for example during your training, or by consulting manuals or guidance provided by your service and the HSE. When you are at the patient's side, however, these approaches are not suitable. You will seldom work alone, so ask colleagues for advice and don't be afraid to request additional help if your risk assessment suggests this would be beneficial. This is especially true for larger patients or where manoeuvres will be difficult due to limited access.

You should not use equipment you are not familiar with, but some equipment does come with a manual or simple diagrams printed on its surface, which you can use to remind yourself about the correct way round it should be used, or the sequence of actions required. Don't forget that other manual handling equipment may be available in your location, such as hoists, which can help reduce the risk to you and the patient. However, this will usually rely on a trained member of staff being available to help you.

Patients who refuse manual handling aids

It is unlikely during the course of your work that you will encounter patients who refuse to be transferred or lifted using manual handling aids. However, some policies are unlawful in relation to a patient's human rights, such as blanket no-lifting policies, no lifting unless life or limb are at risk, and no lifting if equipment could physically affect the transfer [*A & Ors v East Sussex CC*].

This does not mean, however, that patients have a right to be manually handled without aids, just that consideration needs to be given to alternatives on a case-by-case basis. For example, a patient who refuses to be hoisted up off the floor does not have a right to be lifted by the ambulance crew, but an alternative, such as a lifting cushion, could be utilised instead. In the event that a compromise cannot be reached, contact your line manager while on scene to assist with decision-making.

1.5 *Biomechanics*

Biomechanics is the application of the physical laws of mechanics to the human body. In order to reduce the risk of injury and facilitate manual handling, it is important to be aware of the following mechanical principles [Smith, 2011]:

- force
- gravity
- friction
- stress and strain
- pressure
- levers
- moment of force or turning force
- stability and equilibrium.

1.6 *General principles*

The next section covers specific moving and handling equipment and techniques, but it is helpful to know the basic principles to adopt when approaching a manual handling task [Skills for Health, 2020].

There is no such thing as a completely 'safe' lift, but try to keep the weights for lifting and lowering in the zones shown in Figure 7.4. If you are twisting, reduce weights by 10% if you are required to twist beyond 45°, and by 20% if you must twist beyond 90° [HSE, 2020].

1.6.1 Procedure

Take the following steps to safely lift or handle a load:

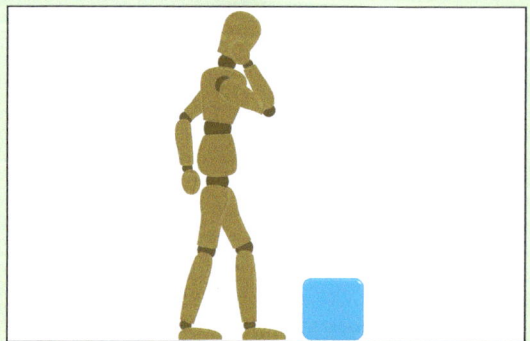

1. **Think before handling.** Plan the lift. Can handling aids be used? Where is the load going to be placed? Will help be needed with the load? Remove obstructions such as discarded wrapping materials. Can you reduce the moving and handling manoeuvre? For a long lift, consider resting

Principles of manual handling

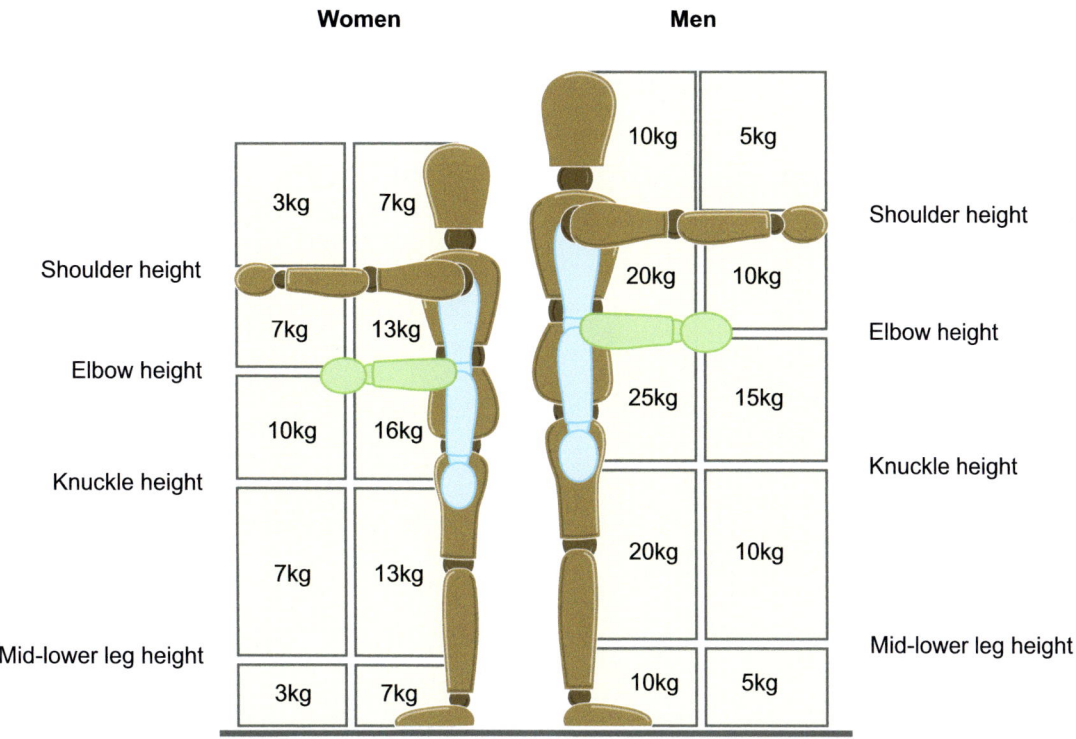

Figure 7.4 Guideline weights for lifting and lowering

Procedure – *cont*

the load midway on a table or bench to change grip.

2. **Prepare the load.** Whatever your load may be, prepare it so that it is as safe as possible to move. This may include securing items if carrying a load of medical stores, or warning a patient what is going to happen and instructing them not to grab out with their hands when on a chair.

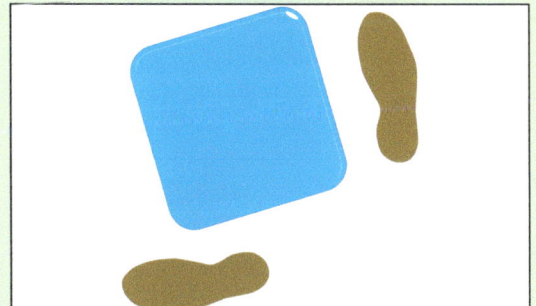

3. **Adopt a stable position.** The feet should be apart with one leg slightly forward to maintain balance (alongside the load if it

Procedure – *cont*

is on the ground). The worker should be prepared to move their feet during the lift to maintain their stability. Avoid tight clothing or unsuitable footwear, which may make this difficult.

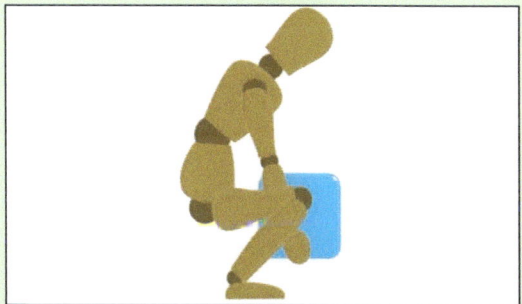

4. **Start in a good posture.** At the start of the lift, slight bending of the back, hips and knees is preferable to fully flexing the back (stooping) or fully flexing the hips and knees (squatting). Don't flex the back any further while lifting. This can happen if the legs begin to straighten before starting to raise the load.

Chapter 7 – Manual Handling

Procedure – *cont*

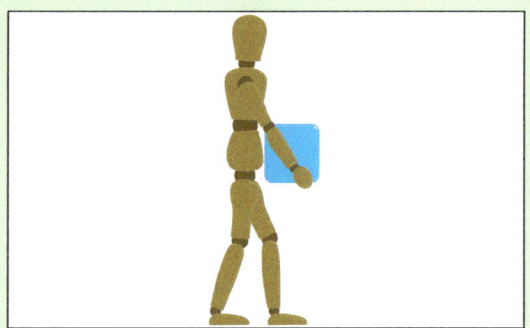

5. **Keep the load close to the waist.** Keep the load close to the body for as long as possible while lifting. Keep the heaviest side of the load next to the body. If a close approach to the load is not possible, try to slide it towards the body before attempting to lift it.

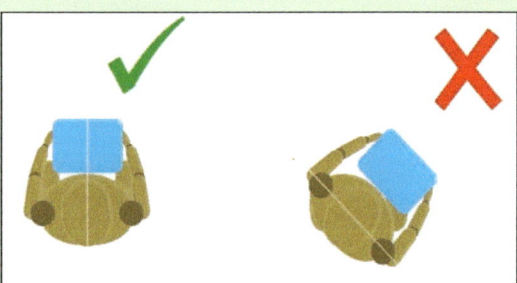

6. **Avoid twisting the back or leaning sideways, especially while the back is bent.** Shoulders should be kept level and facing in the same direction as the hips. Turning by moving the feet is better than twisting and lifting at the same time.

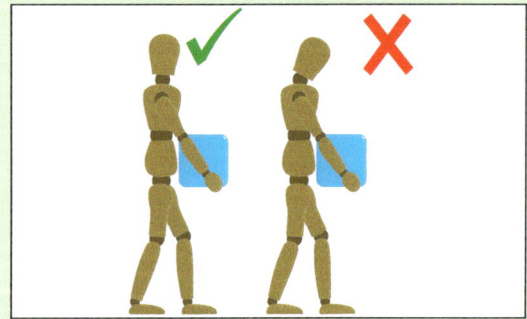

7. **Keep the head up when handling.** Look ahead, not down at the load, once it is held securely. Move smoothly. The load should not be jerked or snatched as this can make

Procedure – *cont*

it harder to keep control and can increase the risk of injury. Don't lift or handle more than can be easily managed. There is a difference between what people can lift and what they can safely lift. If in doubt, seek advice or get help.

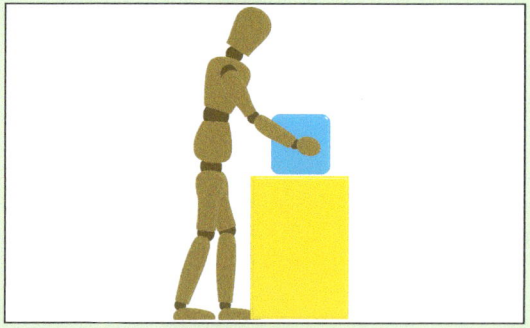

8. **Put down, then adjust.** If precise positioning of the load is necessary, put it down first, then slide it into the desired position.

1.7 Handling aids

Your organisation should provide aids to assist in manual handling. In the ambulance service, this may include:
- handling belts
- slide sheets
- transfer (banana) boards
- turntables
- lifting cushions/chair
- powered ambulance stretcher
- a carry chair
- tail lifts on the back of the ambulance.

As a responder, it is unlikely that you will have many of these available to you all the time and you should limit your moving and handling to only that which is immediately required, and that you can perform safely. The ambulance staff that will be backing you up will have been trained extensively in moving and handling and will have aids for reducing the risk, so you should wait for this wherever possible.

While the above remains the case for the majority of responders, there are an increasing number of services that are providing some responders with additional training and equipment to help patients get up off the floor when they have had a fall and are otherwise not obviously injured. This is in response to the severe delays which patients have experienced in recent years wating for ambulances, where lying on the floor for a prolonged period can worsen their condition. In these circumstances your service will provide you with specific training on the equipment and techniques that should be used, and you should follow these for your own safety and that of the patient.

2 Moving and handling equipment and techniques

2.1 Learning objectives

By the end of this section you will be able to:
- describe the aids and equipment that may be used for moving and positioning
- describe the impact of specific conditions on the correct movement and positioning of an individual.

2.2 Introduction

This section provides guidance on different techniques that can be utilised for moving and handling patients. As has already been mentioned, as a responder you may not be trained in all of these techniques by your service and should only perform those that you have been trained in, can safely undertake on your own and which cannot wait until additional help arrives.

2.3 Patients on the floor

The usual advice from a call handler in response to a 999 call is to advise the caller not to move the patient. Usually this will be the case for you as a responder as well, and the patient should not be moved until an ambulance crew has assessed them as being uninjured.

There are a number of techniques for helping a patient to get from the floor to seated in a chair by themselves and these have been included below; however, these have been included for information in case you should ever need to assist an ambulance crew in performing them, as it is unlikely you would ever utilise these techniques yourself without an ambulance crew being present.

For patients who are unable to get themselves up from the floor, it is likely a lifting device, such as a lifting cushion or lifting chair, will be required. You should be aware of such equipment being carried by your service, and in some circumstances it can be helpful if you let the EOC know this while you are awaiting backup as they can ensure they send the appropriate resource.

2.3.1 Instructing a patient to get off the floor – one-chair method

In order to undertake this procedure, the patient needs to be able to roll on to their side and be able to kneel, so it may not be suitable for patients with knee and hip problems.

Procedure

Take the following steps to instruct a patient to get off the floor using a single chair [Smith, 2011b]:

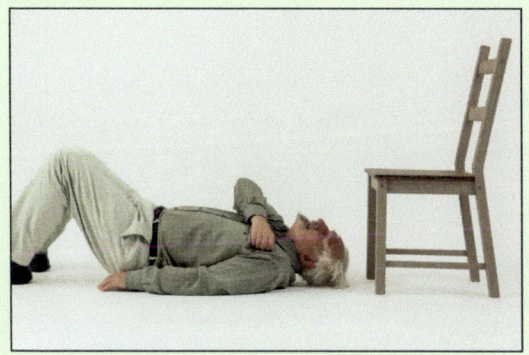

1. Position a chair at the head end of the fallen patient. Instruct them to bend their knees up and to bring one arm across their chest.

Chapter 7 – Manual Handling

Procedure – *cont*

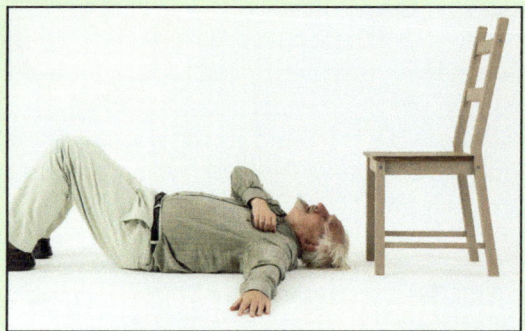

2. Instruct the patient to move their other arm away from the body.

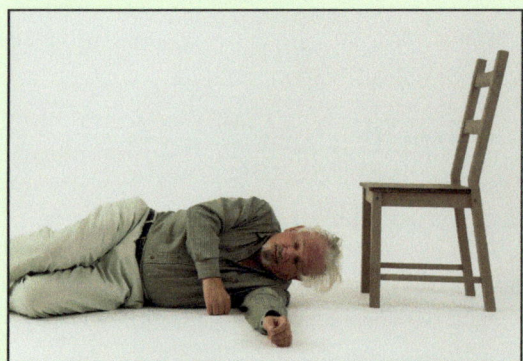

3. Instruct the patient to roll on to their side, and to bring their arm over their body so that it is flat on the floor.

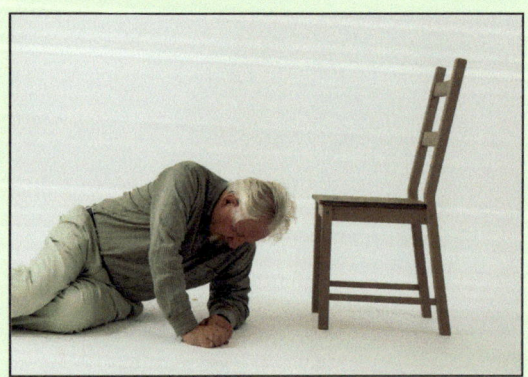

4. Instruct the patient to push up on their hand and at the same time push up on their forearm that is resting on the floor, until they are half-sitting.

Procedure – *cont*

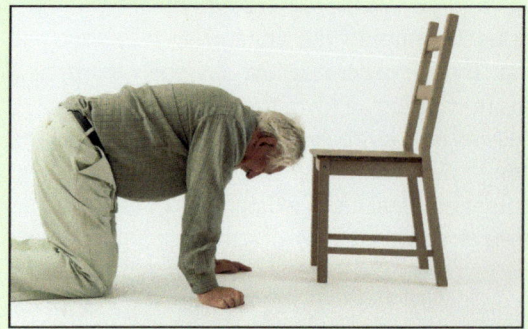

5. Continue to verbally support the patient as they continue to push upwards, until they end up on all fours facing the chair.

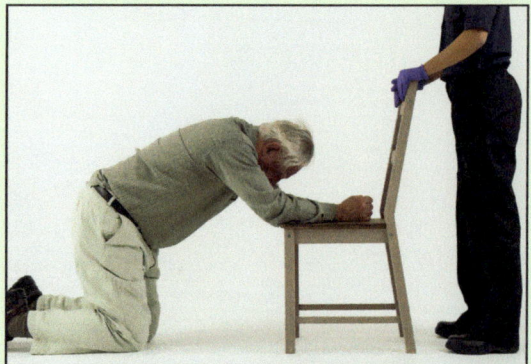

6. While holding the chair steady, instruct the patient to lower their arms on to the chair and ask them to lean on to the seat of the chair.

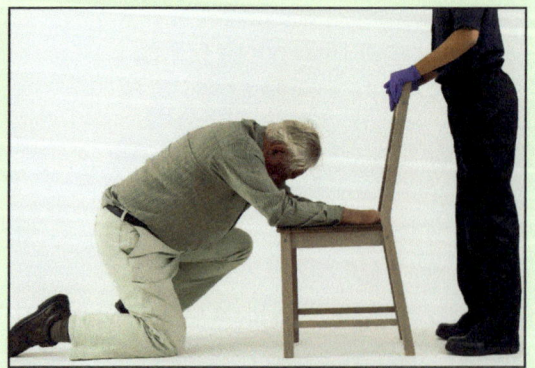

7. Instruct the patient to raise their stronger leg and place the foot of that leg on the floor.

Moving and handling equipment and techniques

Procedure – *cont*

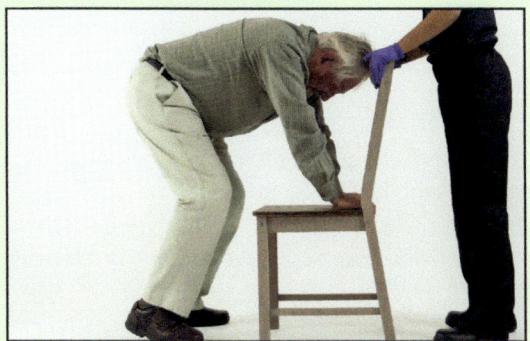

8. Instruct the patient to push up and straighten their legs.

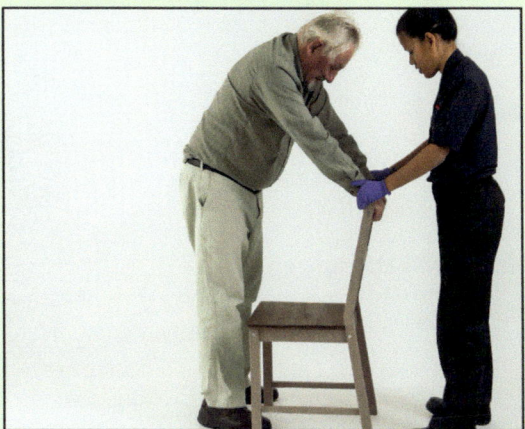

9. Allow the patient time to stabilise themselves and stand up straight, placing their hands on the chair.

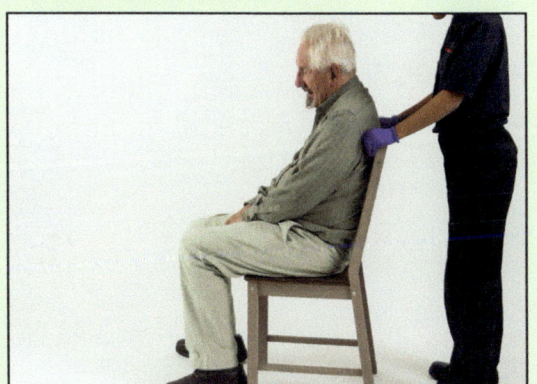

10. Instruct the patient to carefully turn and sit on the chair.

2.3.2 Instructing a patient to get off the floor – two-chair method

Procedure

Take the following steps to instruct a patient to get off the floor using two chairs [Smith, 2011b]:

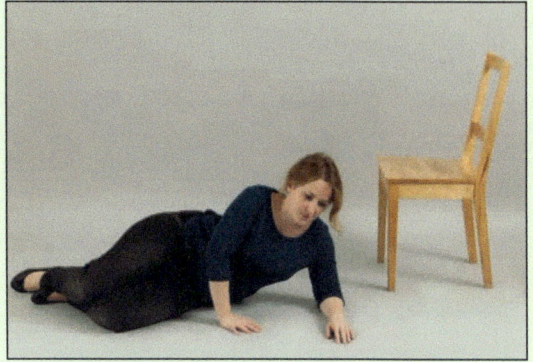

1. Position a chair at the head end of the fallen patient. Instruct them to bend their knees up and roll into side-lying. They should then bring one arm over the chest until their hand is flat on the floor. Instruct them to push up with one hand and lower arm into a side-sitting position as in the one-chair method.

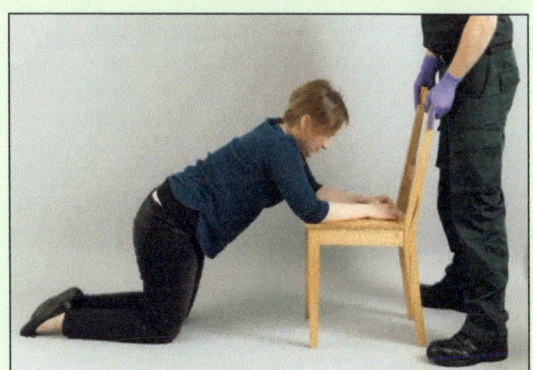

2. Instruct the patient to face the chair and place their forearms on the chair.

Chapter 7 – Manual Handling

Procedure – *cont*

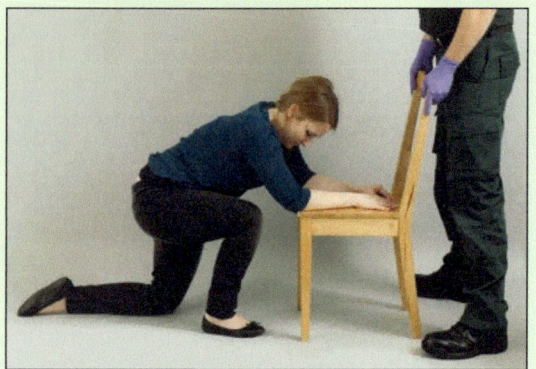

3. Instruct the patient to bend one knee and place the foot of that leg on to the floor while at the same time pushing up on their forearms and hands.

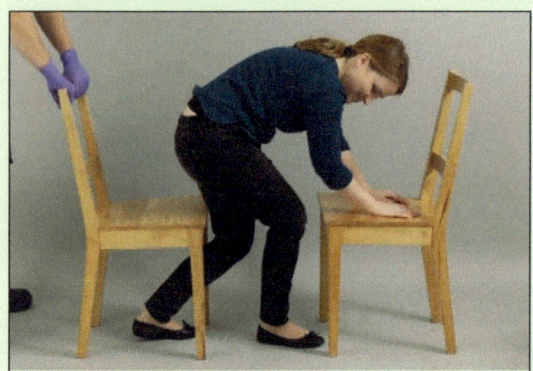

4. Place a second chair behind the patient, ensuring it is under their hips.

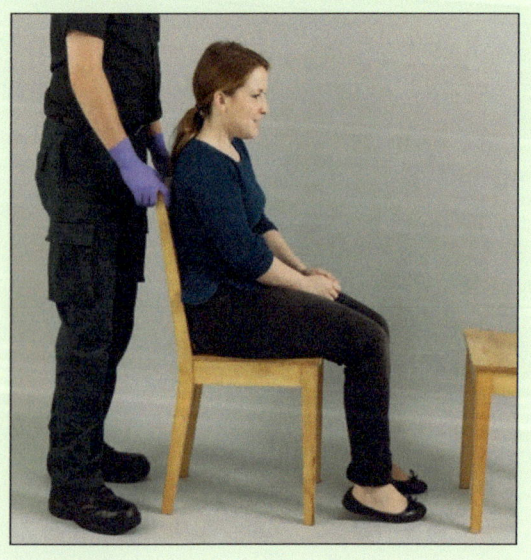

Procedure – *cont*

5. Instruct the patient to sit backwards on to the chair.

2.3.3 Lifting chairs

Lifting chairs are devices that can be used to lift a patient who has fallen, sustained no significant injuries but is unable to get themselves back up from the floor. Prior to a patient being lifted from the floor, they must be assessed for injuries. You should follow your local service guidelines for how this assessment should be conducted. One example is the use of the 'Help Fall' post-fall decision-making tool (Figure 7.5), but you should use whichever tool or process your local organisation has adopted.

Indications
- Patients who have fallen and are unable to get back up without assistance and have suffered no significant injury.

Contra-indications
- Patients who have suffered an injury or where the patient is unable to reliably communicate if they are injured.
- Patients who are not fully conscious so unable to follow commands or provide reliable feedback during the lift.
- Patients weighing over 150 kg.

Advantages
- Can be used by a single person to help get someone off the floor.

Disadvantages
- Can be unstable if patient moves too much once raised.

Moving and handling equipment and techniques

In association with:

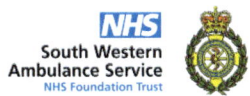

Post Falls Decision Making Tool for Care Homes

When a person has a fall, or has been found on the floor, use this tool to check for any injury or new symptoms prior to moving them. Please then follow the appropriate course of action.

MAJOR INJURY OR SYMPTOMS
- Loss of, or reduced level of, consciousness
- Airway or breathing problems
- Severe or uncontrollable bleeding
- New central neck or back pain
- Swelling or bruising around eyes or behind an ear
- Blood or clear fluid coming from inside an ear
- New onset of chest pain
- FAST test positive
- Repeated vomiting since the fall (not before)
- New lower limb deformity or swelling
- Any seizure activity
- Fallen from height of more than 1 metre and hit head

Actions for carer:
1. Do not lift the person
2. Call 999 for an ambulance
3. Give first aid as needed
4. Document all findings

MINOR INJURY OR SYMPTOMS
- New bruising or wounds
- Mild discomfort
- Isolated injury to an arm
- New loss of memory leading up to or after the fall
- Dizziness or an episode of vomiting since the fall (not before)
- No apparent injuries but person taking anti-coagulants
- Any other concerns by carer

Actions for carer:
1. Give first aid as needed
2. Safely lift or assist the person from the floor
3. Contact GP, NHS 111 or local community provider for advice and follow up
4. Observe the person for at least 24 hours for any new symptoms
5. Document all findings

NO INJURY OR SYMPTOMS
- Conscious and responding as usual
- No apparent injury, bruising or wounds
- No head injury
- No new pain or discomfort (verbal or non-verbal)
- Able to move limbs on command or spontaneously
- No sign of limb deformity, shortening or rotation

Actions for carer:
1. Safely lift or assist the person from the floor
2. Observe the person for at least 24 hours for any new symptoms
3. Document all findings

If there are any changes in the person's condition causing concern, you should contact the GP, NHS 111 or local community provider, for advice. Contact 999 should any symptoms in the red section arise.

Get the HelpFall Web App:

This guidance covers most situations care staff are likely to encounter when a person falls, but it cannot foresee every possible scenario. It must be used together with clinical judgement (in nursing homes), common sense and in line with the duty of care.

© Copyright Felgains Ltd 2022   Version 1.2   felgains.com/helpfall

Figure 7.5 Help Fall checklist

Chapter 7 – Manual Handling

Procedure

Take the following steps to use the Raizer 2 Lifting Chair [DHG, 2023]:

1. Ensure the patient is comfortable, has been assessed for injuries following local protocol and is suitable to be assisted with the Raizer chair.
2. Ensure you have all the required components and the chair is charged and ready to be used.
3. With the patient lying on their back, bend their knees and slide the seat of the chair under their thighs.
4. Ensure the seatbelt is fitted to the backrest tube prior to connecting the backrest to the seat.
5. By supporting the patient's elbow, gently roll them so one shoulder comes off the ground. Insert the corresponding backrest piece under the elevated shoulder, sliding it down into place. A confirmatory tone will sound from the seat once the backrest is in place.
6. Repeat the process on the other side so that both backrests are in place.
7. Ensure the seatbelt is securely fastened to the patient at this point.
8. Fit the four legs so that they are slotted into the relevant positions. They can be fitted in any order and all legs can be fitted in any position. A tone will sound after each leg has been correctly fitted, and once all four legs are fitted a double confirmation tone will sound.
9. Check that the LED signal on the side of the device has changed from yellow to green. This indicates the device is ready to lift the patient.
10. If supplied, fit the headrest now. If this is not supplied, the operator may need to support the head/neck of the patient as the chair lifts them. Brief the patient as to what is going to happen.
11. Position the patient so their shoulders are on the chair and their arms are crossed. Make sure the path of travel for the chair legs is not obstructed and that they will not crush limbs as they operate.

Procedure – *cont*

12. Using the remote control (if supplied) or the control panel on the side of the chair, push the up arrow and maintain pressure on the button as the patient is lifted. The chair will stop automatically once it reaches the upright position.
13. If at any point you need to stop, release the button and, if required, push the down arrow to lower the patient again. There is also an emergency stop should it be required.
14. Once in the upright position, the patient can be assisted to step away from the chair. Note: Never use the Raizer chair as a wheelchair. The fitted wheels are for assisting the legs to raise, not to facilitate pushing a patient in the chair.

2.4 Patients who need to be transferred to the floor

On occasion it may be necessary to move a patient from a seated position to the floor; this is most likely when the patient has collapsed and is unresponsive, so you can assess them and place them in the recovery position or perform CPR if necessary.

This procedure is best performed with three rescuers. When this is not possible, it can be performed with two or one; however, the fewer the rescuers the greater the risk to those performing the manoeuvre.

As a responder, it is likely you will need to perform this procedure on your own so you should be aware of the risks and only perform it when required and waiting would be detrimental to the patient.

2.4.1 Procedure

Take the following steps to move a patient from a seated position to the floor when they are unresponsive [RCUK, 2015]:

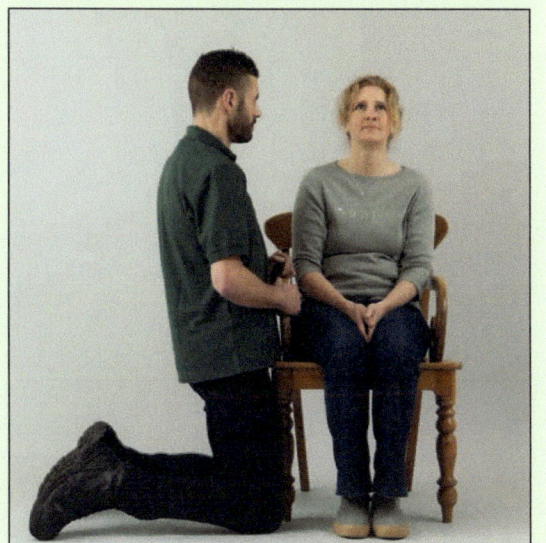

1. Kneel on the floor, to one side of the patient.

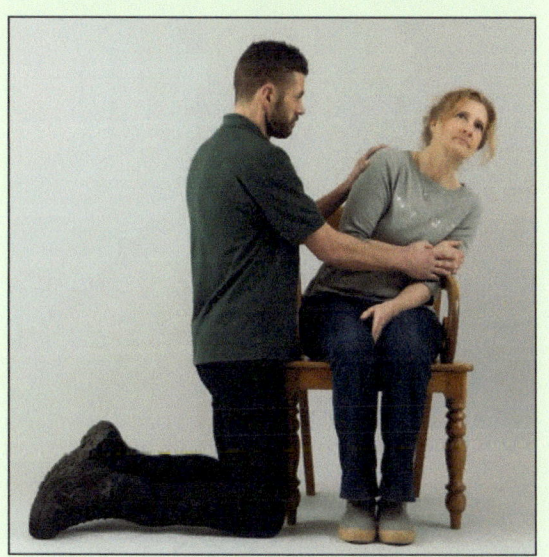

2. Position the patient's arm that is closer to you across their chest and push their trunk away from you.

Procedure – *cont*

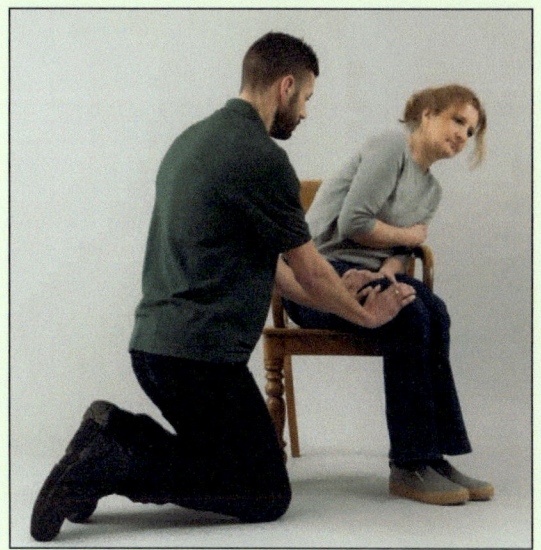

3. Push against the patient's lower thigh which is nearer to you with both hands to position the patient's hip towards the front of the chair.

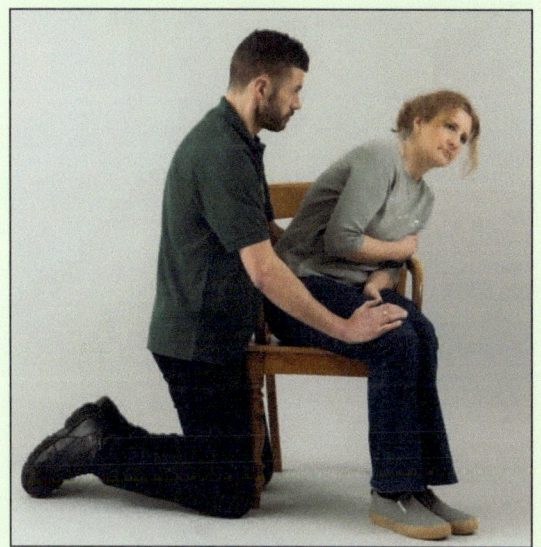

4. Place one hand behind the patient and around their further hip. Place your other hand on the patient's thigh closer to you.

Chapter 7 – Manual Handling

Procedure – *cont*

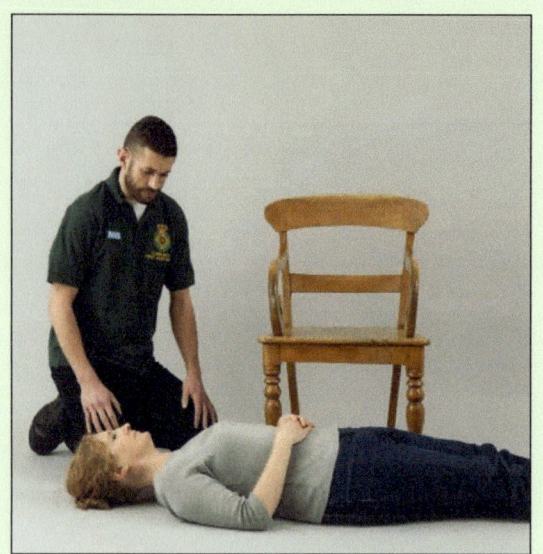

5. Pull with the hand that is on the hip and push with the hand that is on the thigh to move the patient down to the floor.

8 Scene Assessment

1 Scene assessment and safety

1.1 Learning objectives

By the end of this section you will be able to:
- outline and explain the parts of an initial scene assessment
- explain the importance of ensuring scene safety prior to approaching any incident for:
  - patients
  - yourself
  - your colleagues
  - bystanders
- describe the components of a dynamic risk assessment model.

1.2 Introduction

Despite the name, scene assessment begins before you physically arrive at the patient's location. You will be passed details of the incident, with further details provided as you respond if the EOC obtains new information about the incident. Your service will have agreed criteria for incidents that are appropriate for you (as a responder) to attend. This will vary, but typically would not include incidents on motorways or where patients and/or bystanders are known to be intoxicated with alcohol, for example.

To help you cover the essential aspects of a scene assessment, consider using the SCENE mnemonic [JRCALC, 2023]:
- **S:** Safety
- **C:** Cause including the nature of illness (NOI) or mechanism of injury (MOI)
- **E:** Environment
- **N:** Number of patients
- **E:** Extra resources needed.

1.3 Safety

Maximising the safety of everyone on scene requires risk assessment. The ambulance service has many formal, written risk assessments, but these cannot legislate for all eventualities. In order to reduce the risk to you as a responder, patients and bystanders, it is necessary to undertake a more fluid and mental (i.e. in your head as opposed to a written-down) risk assessment. This is known as a dynamic risk assessment (DRA) and relates to the fact that the environment or situation is dynamic, rather than the risk itself. DRA underpins subsequent decision-making and is focused on thinking BEFORE you act, and not the other way around [Asbury, 2014]. The National Ambulance Resilience Unit (NARU) has published a DRA model to assist with risk assessments while on scene (Figure 8.1).

1.4 Cause

Although you are likely to have been passed details about the incident or call you are attending, you should not be completely led by this. Establishing the presenting complaint from the patient's perspective will come later on in the assessment process, but you may be able to determine what has happened from the scene, particularly in trauma cases. However, it is important to keep an open mind even at this stage. For example, a medical-sounding call, such as a patient with low blood sugar, may also have a traumatic component if, for example, they fell and injured themselves as a result. In addition, while it is unlikely that you would be sent to an incident that was known to involve hazardous substances, their presence may not be known until after you arrive on scene, so it is important that you can recognise their presence and know what initial actions you should take. This is explained in the 'Hazardous materials' section of this chapter.

Chapter 8 – Scene Assessment

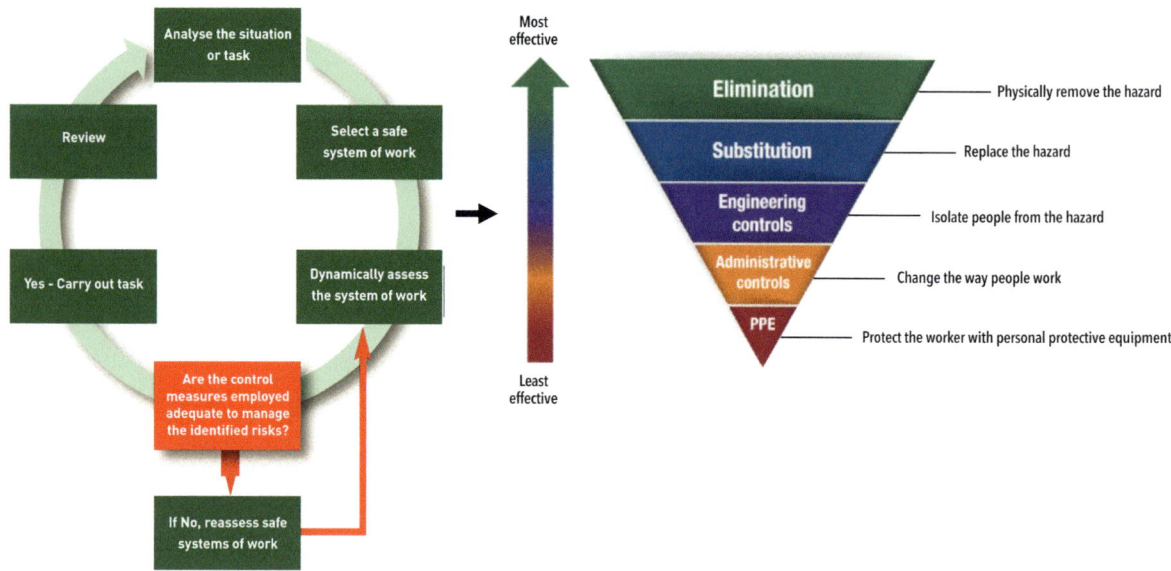

Figure 8.1 DRA model

Source: National Ambulance Resilience Unit, National Ambulance Service Command and Control Guidance (July 2019). Source for artwork on right-hand side (hierarchy of control measures) – HSE: L25 – PPE at Work – Guidance on Regulations (4th Ed., 2022), p.10, Figure 1).

If it turns out that your patient has been injured, find out about the MOI, which you will cover in Chapter 16, 'Trauma'. Knowledge of the MOI can assist in determining what injuries may have been sustained. Equally, for medical patients, establishing the NOI can assist with the diagnosis, particularly in cases where bystander and/or patient information is limited (for example if the patient was discovered unresponsive). Clues from the scene, for example medical equipment such as home oxygen or hoists, medication and/or care notes, may provide clues as to the underlying problem [Bledsoe, 2014].

1.5 Environment

Consider whether there are any environmental factors that need to be taken into account, for example, the risk of harm to the patient due to the development of hypothermia. The terrain may be an issue, particularly if the patient is located well away from roads that are suitable for a vehicle. In these cases helicopters and/or mountain rescue teams can prove useful.

Other risky environments include confined spaces, where there may be a risk of low levels of oxygen and/or the presence of toxic/explosive substances (such as carbon monoxide). These require specialist equipment and rescue knowledge that is typically provided by HARTs or the fire and rescue service [Bledsoe, 2014; NARU, 2022].

1.6 Number of patients

Usually, you will only be called to incidents where there is a single patient. However, it is important to clarify the number of patients early on in your assessment to help identify patients who may have wandered off from the scene or are currently hidden from view.

1.7 Extra resources

You will normally have at least one member of ambulance staff backing you up on scene. However, depending on your assessment, it may be clear that you require additional help and/or equipment from other emergency services. For example, you may require the police to keep a scene safe, or additional ambulances, including the air ambulance, for patient transport. Pass your assessment on to the EOC as early as possible so additional help can be organised.

2 Major incidents

2.1 Learning objectives

By the end of this section you will be able to:
- define the term 'major incident'
- state the ambulance service's responsibilities with regard to a major incident
- describe the mnemonic METHANE
- describe how to use the ten second triage tool.

2.2 Introduction

According to the Civil Contingencies Act 2004, an emergency is defined as:
- an event or situation which threatens serious damage to human welfare in a place in the UK
- an event or situation which threatens serious damage to the environment of a place in the UK
- war, or terrorism, which threatens serious damage to the security of the UK.

To distinguish this definition of emergency from the regular emergency work of the ambulance service, the term used most often is 'major incident'.

NHS ambulance services are classed as category 1 (primary) responders under the Civil Contingencies Act 2004. As such, these organisations are expected to have plans in place to prevent emergencies, and to reduce, control and mitigate emergencies once they occur [NARU, 2019]. In addition, business continuity arrangements need to be in place to ensure services are maintained to patients even in the event of disruptions, such as severe weather or an IT failure, for example. Collectively, all these activities fall under the umbrella term 'emergency preparedness, resilience and response' (EPRR) [NHS England, 2022].

You are very unlikely to be called to attend a major incident as a responder. However, it is important for you to have an awareness since by their nature major incidents typically have a significant impact on an ambulance service's ability to maintain a 'normal' response to routine emergency calls.

2.3 Classification of incidents

NHS organisations are required to develop emergency preparedness arrangements for three levels of incident [NHS England, 2022]:
- **Business continuity incident:** An event or occurrence that disrupts, or might disrupt, an organisation's normal service delivery to below acceptable pre-defined levels. This might be due to a sudden, temporary surge in 999 calls, or a failure of the computerised dispatch system used in the EOC, for example.
- **Critical incident:** Any localised incident where the level of disruption results in an organisation temporarily or permanently losing its ability to deliver critical services, or where patients and staff may be at risk of harm. Sustained high volumes of 999 calls together with long turn-around times at local EDs have led to ambulance services declaring critical incidents.
- **Major incident:** Any occurrence that presents a serious threat to the health of the community or causes such numbers or types of casualties as to require special arrangements to be implemented.

2.4 Types of major incident

Major incidents can arise from a number of causes, including [NHS England, 2022]:
- **Rapid onset (sometimes called 'big bang'):** Develops quickly, and usually with immediate effect, thereby limiting the time available to consider response options. Examples include serious transport accidents, an explosion or series of smaller incidents.
- **Rising tide:** A developing infectious disease epidemic, or a capacity/staffing crisis.
- **Cloud on the horizon:** A serious threat such as a major chemical or nuclear release developing elsewhere and needing preparatory action.
- **Headline news:** Public or media alarm about a personal threat.

- **Chemical, biological, radiological, nuclear and explosives (CBRNe):** Actual or threatened dispersal of CBRNe materials (one or several, or in combination with explosives), with deliberate criminal, malicious or murderous intent.
- **Hazardous materials (HAZMAT):** Accidental incident involving hazardous materials.
- **Cyber security incident:** A breach of a system's security policy to disrupt its integrity or availability, or the unauthorised access or attempted access to a system.
- **Mass casualty:** An incident (or series of incidents) causing casualties on a scale that is beyond the normal resources of the emergency and healthcare services' ability to manage.
- **Marauding terrorist attack (MTA):** An act of terrorism, utilising firearms and/or explosives (known as a marauding terrorist firearms attack, MTFA), although less sophisticated weapons such as knives and vehicles can also be used. As the name implies, the location of the incident can change over time as the terrorists are often mobile, sometimes striking multiple locations simultaneously [Chauhan, 2018].

2.5 Role of the ambulance service

NHS ambulance trusts have the responsibility for alerting, mobilising and co-ordinating the NHS response to short-notice or sudden-impact emergencies. This includes [NARU, 2019]:
- initiating and maintaining a command and control system to provide appropriate support and guidance to all NHS responders and other agencies
- co-ordinating all NHS communications on scene
- managing the health, safety and welfare of all NHS responders
- providing casualty triage, treatment and transport, including the selection of appropriate receiving hospitals
- provision of specialist incident response capabilities, including hazardous area working, decontamination of casualties and response to terrorist incidents.

During a major incident, the response of the ambulance service revolves around seven key principles [Mackway-Jones, 2012]:
- **Command and control:** Each emergency service on scene has an incident commander, but the police usually take overall command.
- **Safety:** Personal safety is paramount and the appropriate PPE must be worn. This does not always happen when crews are faced with a major incident. Of particular concern are hazardous materials or CBRNe incidents.
- **Communication:** This is the most common failing at major incidents [Mackway-Jones, 2012]. Modern radio networks used by the ambulance service should in theory alleviate some of the problems that have occurred in the past, but the use of runners should be considered if required.
- **Assessment:** A rapid initial assessment of the scene can provide an estimate of the number of those injured and the severity of their injuries. This can be refined as the incident unfolds.
- **Triage:** This is the dynamic process by which casualties are sorted into priorities for treatment. It needs to be repeated frequently.
- **Treatment:** 'Do the most for the most' is the standard mantra. This depends on the skills of the providers, severity of injuries and time on scene. The nature of the environment and casualty load may restrict the ability of the providers to give 'gold standard' care.
- **Transport:** Most patients will probably be transported to hospital by ambulance, but alternative methods of transport can be used. The aim is to get the right patient to the right place at the right time.

2.6 M/ETHANE model

The M/ETHANE model is an established reporting framework which provides a common structure for responders to share incident information with the EOC. It is recommended that this format is used for all incidents and is updated as the incident develops. For incidents falling below the major incident threshold, M/ETHANE becomes an 'ETHANE' message (Figure 8.2) [JESIP, 2023a].

Major incidents

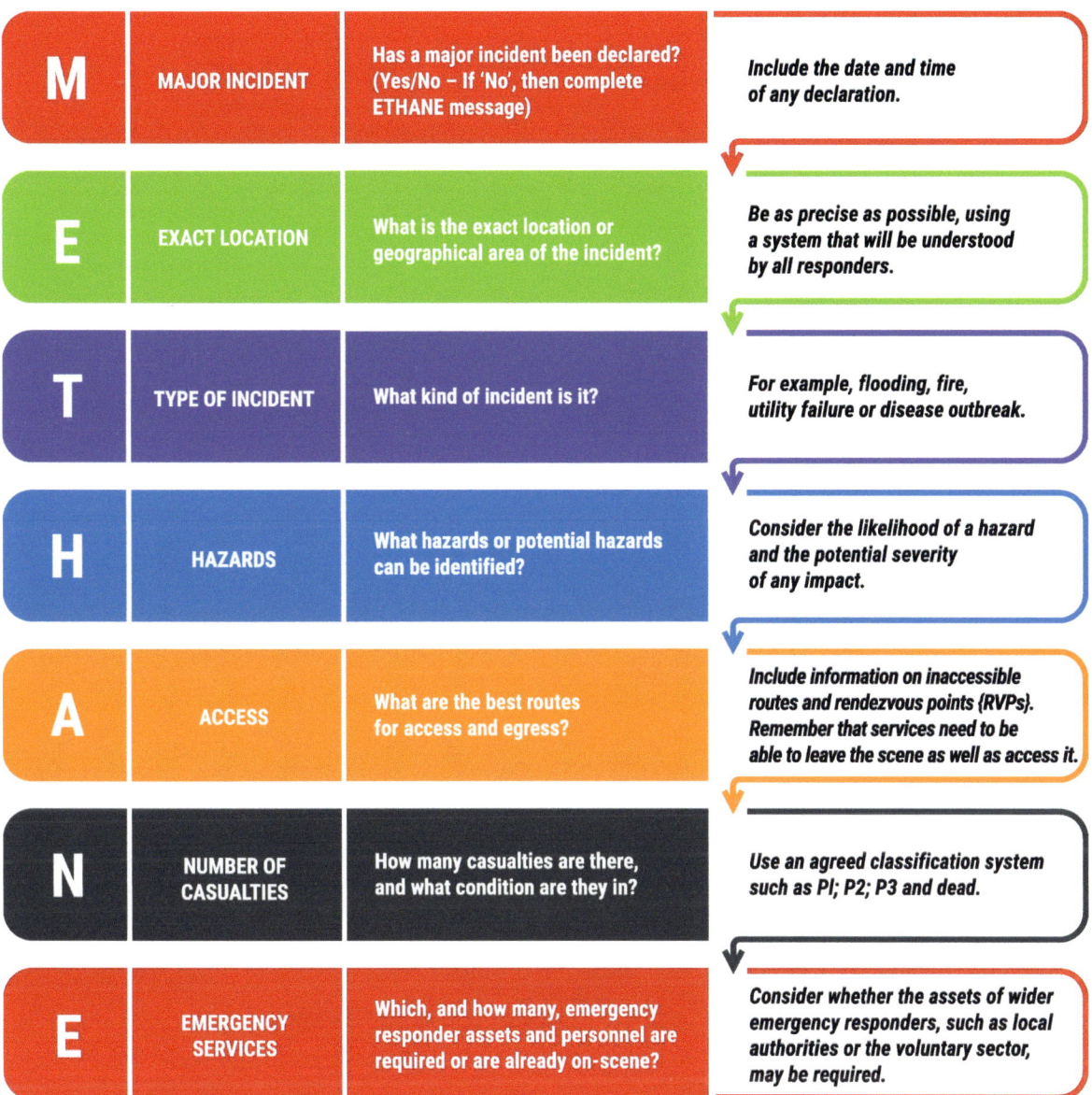

Figure 8.2   M/ETHANE model

2.7 Ten second triage

The aim of triage is to do the most for the most, and it should be used any time that the number of casualties exceeds the number of skilled rescuers. It is a dynamic process and therefore needs to be repeated multiple times during the care of each casualty. In the event that you are a responder at a major incident, you may be asked to undertake the initial triage of casualties using the ten second triage model (TST) [Vassallo, 2024]. This has advantages over other tools (such as the NHS major incident triage tool, MITT) in that it does not involve measuring any physiological parameters, such as breathing or heart rate, making it quick to perform and reducing the cognitive load that comes with responding to major incidents (Figure 8.3). Casualties are allocated to one of four

Chapter 8 – *Scene Assessment*

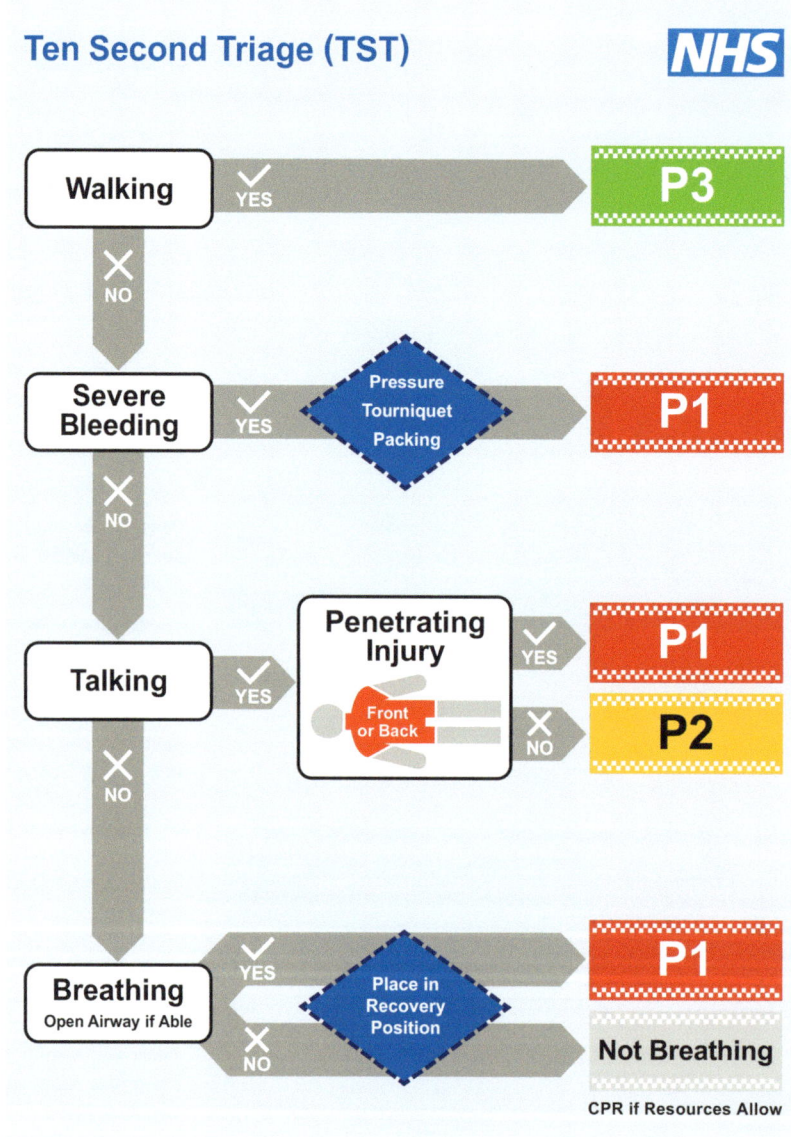

Figure 8.3   Ten Second Triage

categories, with the placement of a coloured band. These are:
- white on red: P1 priority one
- black on yellow: P2 priority two
- white on green: P3 priority three
- black on silver: not breathing.

3 Hazardous materials

3.1 *Learning objectives*

By the end of this section you will be able to:
- describe the systems for labelling hazardous substances

Hazardous materials

- describe how to find out information about a hazardous substance
- describe the risks when attending a hazardous substance incident
- describe actions which need to be undertaken when attending a hazardous substance or CBRNe incident.

3.2 Introduction

There is a good chance if you have a look in the cupboard under your kitchen sink or in your shed/garage that you will find a hazardous/dangerous substance. Since the key component of scene assessment is safety for yourself, patients and bystanders, it is important that you appreciate how readily available hazardous substances are. Patients who are contaminated with a hazardous substance can easily contaminate others. On a grander scale are incidents involving transport vehicles, most commonly on the road, but also by rail, sea and air. You will not be tasked to these types of incidents, as you will not have the training or equipment to be able to safely attend. These are incidents for the fire and rescue service and HART to deal with. However, if you can identify the hazardous substance early, this can assist commanders in determining what resources are required.

Information about the hazardous material can be obtained from a number of sources [HSE, 2017]:
- the packaging and associated warning labels
- emergency telephone advice from services such as Chemsafe or TOXBASE (typically accessed through the ambulance EOC)
- the driver and the documentation being carried in the case of vehicular incidents.

3.3 Labelling of hazardous substances

The classification, labelling and packaging (CLP) of hazardous substances is specified under the Great Britain CLP Regulations (GB CLP). Part of these regulations defines what information must be provided on the label of a hazardous substance or mixture (Figure 8.4) [HSE, 2023].

3.3.1 CLP pictograms

The CLP outlines nine pictograms (Table 8.1) and two signal words that accompany the pictograms [HSE, 2022a; HSE 2022b]:
- **Danger:** Substances and mixtures with the most severe hazards.
- **Warning:** Substances and mixtures with less serious hazards.

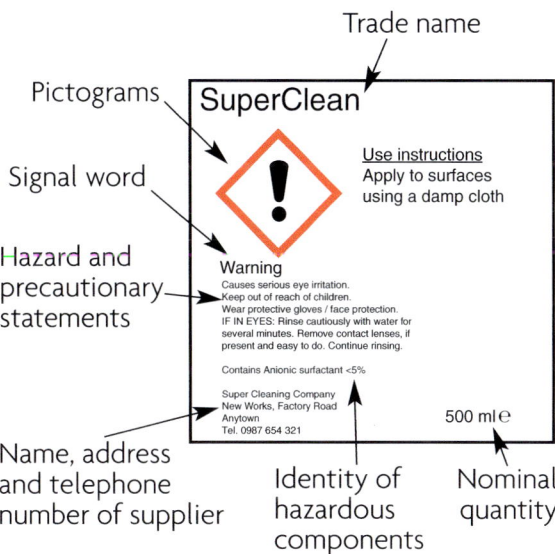

Figure 8.4 An example label for a hazardous mixture [EC, 2013]

Chapter 8 – Scene Assessment

Table 8.1   CLP pictograms and sample hazard statements

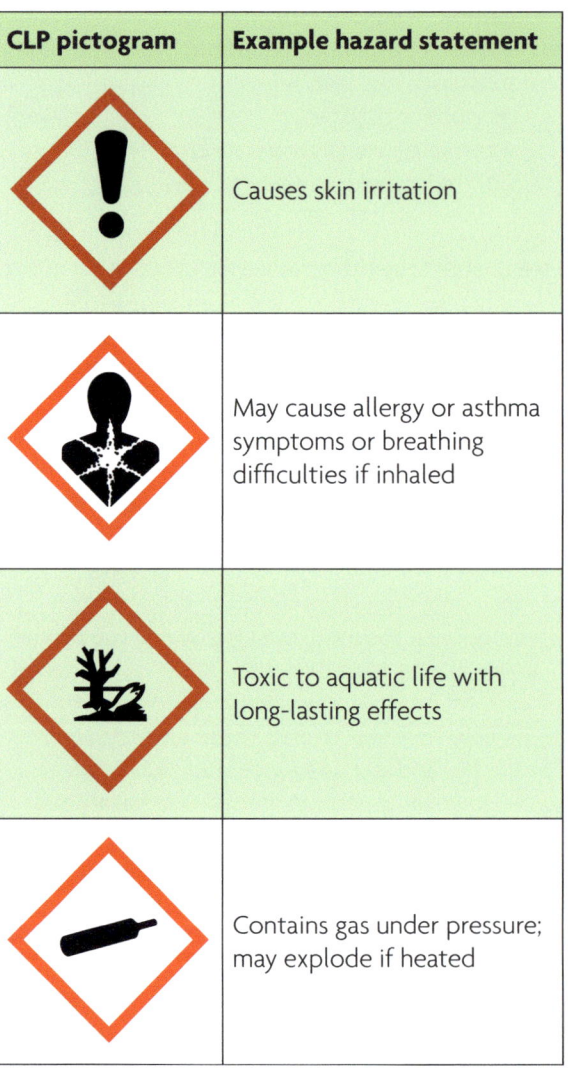

CLP pictogram	Example hazard statement
	Explosive; mass explosion hazard
	Extremely flammable gas/aerosol/liquid/solid
	May cause or intensify fire; oxidiser
	Fatal if swallowed
	Causes severe skin burns and eye damage

CLP pictogram	Example hazard statement
	Causes skin irritation
	May cause allergy or asthma symptoms or breathing difficulties if inhaled
	Toxic to aquatic life with long-lasting effects
	Contains gas under pressure; may explode if heated

3.4   Responder actions at scene

In the event that an 'ordinary' emergency call turns out to involve hazardous substances, or you come across an incident that appears to involve hazardous substances, withdraw and await specialist teams, such as the HART. Inform the EOC as soon as possible that the incident involves hazardous substances.

Chapter 9 Patient Assessment

1 Patient assessment process

1.1 Learning objectives

By the end of this section you will be able to:
- state the components of the patient assessment process
- describe the ‹C›ABCDE approach to initial patient assessment, including:
  - catastrophic haemorrhage
  - airway
  - breathing
  - circulation
  - disability
  - exposure
- state the components of the tool AVPU to assess level of consciousness
- outline how to obtain a patient history using the acronyms SAMPLE and SOCRATES
- describe the steps in a 'head-to-toe' assessment.

1.2 Introduction

Once you have completed your scene assessment, the next step is to conduct a patient assessment. This chapter will break down the patient assessment process into its separate parts so you can explore them further. Figure 9.1 shows the patient assessment process from start to finish. This chapter and some of the subsequent chapters are going to cover this in some detail, so just concentrate on the order of the assessment process, rather than on what it is you are expected to do during each stage [RCUK, 2021a; JRCALC, 2023].

1.3 Primary survey

The primary survey (Figure 9.2) is a swift patient assessment and management process, which can be completed within 60–90 seconds [JRCALC, 2023]. It is designed to be a step-wise approach, meaning that any abnormalities identified in one step should be addressed before moving on to the next. Patients who have suffered traumatic injuries should have a check for life-threatening (or catastrophic) haemorrhage, before you check the patient's airway. In addition, in this group of patients you should give consideration to the

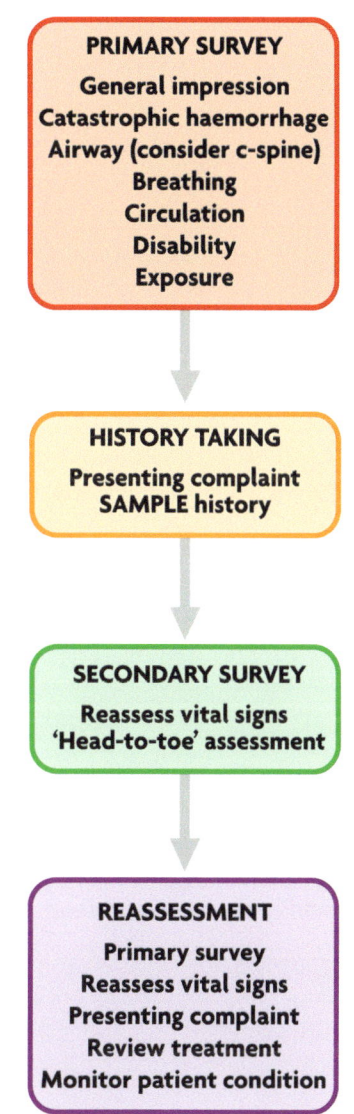

Figure 9.1 The patient assessment process

Chapter 9 – Patient Assessment

PRIMARY SURVEY
General impression
Catastrophic haemorrhage
Airway (consider c-spine)
Breathing
Circulation
Disability
Exposure

Figure 9.2   The primary survey

patient's cervical spine and avoid unnecessary movement of the head and neck. This is covered in more detail in Chapter 16, 'Trauma'.

1.3.1 General impression

The general impression is your first and immediate assessment of the patient and their current location, which will give you an early indication as to how sick and/or injured your patient is. Some of this information you will have already gathered from your scene assessment. As you approach a patient ensure that you are wearing appropriate PPE. Note the patient's approximate age, and signs of obvious frailty, injury or disability, as your management and expectations of what the patient can do will vary. For example, a 1-year-old child will not present in the same way as an adult. In addition, patient positioning can give you early clues. Is the patient sitting up and smiling (Figure 9.3a) or are they lying apparently lifeless on the floor (Figure 9.3b)? This step relies heavily on experience and intuition and can be challenging [NAEMT, 2019].

This is also your chance to assess how responsive the patient is. If the patient is awake, introduce yourself with 'Hello, my name is…' and identify yourself as being from the ambulance service. Ask how they would prefer to be addressed.

If the patient appears not to be awake or is unconscious, check for responsiveness by asking them if they are all right, or try giving them a command such as 'Open your eyes'. If they do not respond, gently shake the patient's shoulders. Patients who fail to respond are critically ill until proven otherwise [RCUK, 2021a].

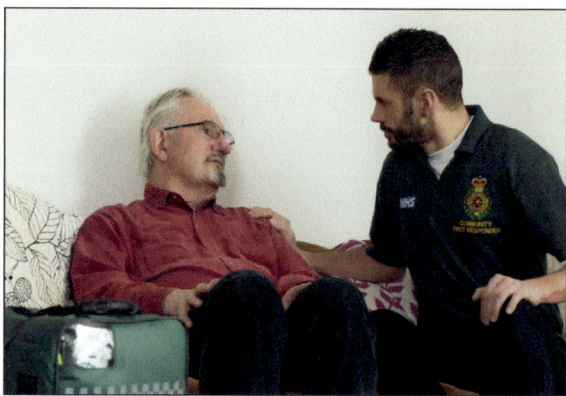

Figure 9.3a   General impression. Patient sitting up and smiling

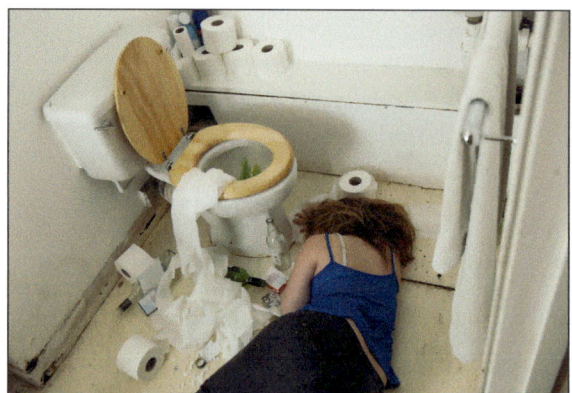

Figure 9.3b   General impression. Patient lying apparently lifeless on the floor

1.3.2 Catastrophic haemorrhage

Bleeding that is likely to cause death in minutes is referred to as a catastrophic haemorrhage. This bleeding needs to be stopped, even before assessing the airway, to prevent the patient from bleeding to death. This is covered in Chapter 16, 'Trauma'.

1.3.3 Airway

Assessment of the airway involves three steps:
- **Look** for signs of airway obstruction.
- **Listen** for noisy or absent breathing.
- **Feel** for air movement as the patient breathes.

Remember, the primary assessment proceeds in a step-wise manner. Any signs of obstruction such as snoring or gurgling sounds need to be addressed now, before moving on to breathing. You will learn how to deal with airway problems in Chapter 10, 'Airway'.

1.3.4 Breathing

Once you have a patent (open) airway, you are ready to move on to breathing. As with the airway, you will adopt a look, listen, feel approach.

A victim who is barely breathing or is taking infrequent, slow and noisy gasps is not breathing normally [Olasveengen, 2021]. If this is accompanied by no signs of life (not moving, no normal breathing or coughing), you should commence basic life support (see Chapter 20, 'Cardiac Arrest').

If they are breathing, you will need to decide whether it is adequate. You can start with the respiratory rate and depth of breathing (indicated by chest movement).

1.3.5 Circulation

You can obtain a good idea of the patient's circulation by looking at the colour of their limbs (usually the hands as they are the most accessible and normally visible). Feeling for a pulse is a skill that you will cover in Chapter 12, 'Circulation'. The pulse can tell you the heart rate and adequacy of the cardiac output, particularly if distal pulses such as the wrist are absent when a central pulse (such as found in the neck) is palpable. Clearly, a patient who does not have a pulse needs CPR immediately. This is covered in Chapter 20, 'Cardiac Arrest'.

1.3.6 Disability

Disability in the primary assessment refers to the patient's level of consciousness, or how awake they are. There are many causes of unconsciousness and these are covered in Chapter 13, 'Disability'. During the primary assessment, you will need to check three things to assess the patient's disability [JRCALC, 2023]:
- level of consciousness
- pupils
- blood sugar.

Level of conciousness
A rapid assessment of the patient's level of consciousness (LOC) can be undertaken using the acronym AVPU:
- **A:** Alert
- **V:** Responds to verbal stimulus
- **P:** Responds to pain
- **U:** Unresponsive.

Pupils
When looking at a patient's pupils, you are interested in whether they are of equal size and react to light. There are a number of reasons why this may not be the case and you'll find out about these in Chapter 13, 'Disability'.

Blood sugar
Hypoglycaemia, or low blood sugar, is a cause of reduced level of consciousness, which can usually be corrected by the administration of glucose, either orally (by mouth) or intravenously. In addition, there are drugs which can mobilise the body's own glucose stores and you'll be learning about these in Chapter 15, 'Medical and Surgical Emergencies'.

1.3.7 Exposure

You will undertake a full 'head-to-toe' assessment later in the patient assessment process, but a quick look early on will provide you with clues to obvious illness/injury that needs to be managed quickly. For example, some types of rashes (e.g. non-blanching) signal serious illness such as sepsis. It also provides a chance to identify sites of hidden bleeding that you did not pick up on earlier on in your assessment.

Working out of hospital, however, you do need to be mindful about maintenance of patient privacy by not unnecessarily exposing them and ensuring that they do not lose body heat.

1.4 *History taking*

1.4.1 Presenting complaint

The presenting complaint is usually the reason you have been called to the patient (Figure 9.4). The majority of presenting complaints fall into the

> **HISTORY TAKING**
> Presenting complaint
> SAMPLE history

Figure 9.4 History taking

categories of pain, discomfort and/or abnormal body function. Sometimes this is explicit ('I have terrible chest pain') but can be vague, particularly in the elderly ('I just don't feel right today'). Avoid using words like 'problem' or 'complaint' when finding out the reason for the emergency call (despite the fact that it is referred to as the 'presenting complaint' within medical circles!) [Innes, 2018].

1.4.2 SAMPLE history

Once you know the presenting complaint, you will need to ask further questions. At the bare minimum, this should include the parts of the SAMPLE acronym:
- **S:** Signs and symptoms of the presenting complaint
- **A:** Allergies (particularly to medication or food)
- **M:** Medications
- **P:** Past medical history
- **L:** Last oral intake
- **E:** Events that led to the current illness or injury.

Signs and symptoms of the presenting complaint
To help you organise the signs and symptoms of the presenting complaint, you can use the SOCRATES acronym. This was originally designed with assessment of pain in mind, but can be helpful for other presenting complaints.
- **S:** Site
- **O:** Onset
- **C:** Character (how does the patient describe their symptom, particularly pain? Is it sharp or dull, for example?)
- **R:** Radiation
- **A:** Association (are there any other signs and symptoms associated with the presenting complaint?)
- **T:** Timing
- **E:** Exacerbating/relieving factors
- **S:** Severity.

1.4.3 Allergies and medication

Allergies
The range of drugs that you can administer is limited, but there is still scope for patient harm if administered inappropriately. You should always ask the patient about any allergic reactions to medication they have received in the past. It is also a good idea to ask about other allergies, such as those caused by food, animals, pollen or metal [Innes, 2018].

Medication
Ask if the patient's medication can be made available for the ambulance crew when they arrive. It is also a good idea to ask about any over-the-counter medicines (i.e. those not prescribed by a doctor, but obtained from a pharmacist or supermarket), as well as herbal and homeopathic remedies. Don't forget to consider whether illicit drugs have been taken by patients. In addition, there are cases where patients take medication prescribed for other family members or friends.

1.4.4 Past medical history

You will probably cover some of the patient's medical history while obtaining the history of the presenting complaint, but the following questions will help you uncover other medical illnesses or surgery that may prove helpful [Innes, 2018; Gregory, 2010]:
- Have you had any illnesses that you saw your GP about?
- Have you had to take any time off work because of ill health?
- Have you had any operations?
- Have you been admitted to hospital, and if so, why?
- Have you suffered any injuries?

1.4.5 Last oral intake and events leading to illness/injury

Last oral intake
Find out when the patient last had anything to eat or drink. This information is useful for patients who are unconscious or who may require surgery, as patients with a full stomach are at risk of aspiration.

Also, you may be able to identify the onset of food poisoning and/or food allergies [Gregory, 2010].

Events leading to the illness or injury

This is also known as the history of the presenting complaint and if you have used the SOCRATES acronym, you will have already obtained most of the information required.

Additional information that is useful to obtain includes [Gregory, 2010]:
- **Associated symptoms:** For example, does the patient have shortness of breath and nausea with their chest pain?
- **Previous episodes:** Find out what happened last time, including any diagnoses made or hospital admissions.
- **Effect on daily living:** Does the presenting complaint interfere with getting to the toilet or making a cup of tea, for example?

1.5 Secondary survey

The secondary survey is often tailored to your findings from the primary survey and history (Figure 9.5). For example, if the presenting complaint is shortness of breath, then you are going to ensure that you obtain a respiratory rate and oxygen saturations.

1.5.1 Reassess vital signs

Your ambulance service may have a specified minimum set of observations to obtain, but this will generally include:
- respiratory rate
- oxygen saturations
- pulse rate
- blood pressure
- LOC (AVPU)
- pain score
- blood sugar
- temperature.

SECONDARY SURVEY
Reassess vital signs
'Head-to-toe' assessment

Figure 9.5 The secondary survey

Being able to record vital signs accurately is a fundamental skill and these will be explored in depth in the relevant chapters later in the book.

1.5.2 'Head-to-toe' assessment

It is not always appropriate to perform a 'head-to-toe' or full-body examination for every patient, but in cases of multiple injury, or in cases when the patient is found collapsed and the history is limited or non-existent, it can be helpful to identify signs of injury, or illness. The assessment outlined here is a rapid full-body assessment. Clinicians that you work with are likely to perform more thorough assessments on specific areas of the body depending on the presenting complaint.

Procedure

Take the following steps to perform a 'head-to-toe' assessment [JRCALC, 2023]:
1. Look at the face for obvious injuries such as lacerations, bruising, fluid and deformities.
2. Inspect the area around the eyes and eyelids.
3. Check the eyes for redness and the presence of contact lenses.
4. Assess the pupils with a pen torch to ensure that they react to light.
5. Look behind the ears for bruising and in the ears for signs of fluid or blood leaking out.
6. Look for bruising, lacerations and deformity around the head and then gently feel for tenderness and depressions of the skull.
7. Feel the cheekbones for tenderness, symmetry and instability.
8. Feel the maxilla (the bone just below the nose).
9. Check the nose for blood and fluid leaking out.
10. Feel the jaw.
11. Assess the mouth and nose for cyanosis (blue-tinged skin), foreign bodies (including loose teeth and/or dentures), bleeding, lacerations and deformities.
12. Smell the patient's breath for specific odours (such as pear-drops, which can be present in some diabetic patients).

Chapter 9 – Patient Assessment

Procedure – *cont*

13. Look at the neck and note any obvious lacerations, bruises and/or deformity. Look for bulging veins in the neck and feel the trachea to ensure it is centrally located.
14. Feel the back of the neck for tenderness and deformity.
15. Look at the chest for any obvious injury and watch the chest rise and fall as the patient breathes.
16. Gently feel the ribs to ensure they are intact and to identify if they are tender. Don't press over any obvious bruising or fractures.
17. Check the abdomen and pelvis for obvious injury and gently feel the abdomen, which should be soft and non-tender.
18. Look at the pelvis for signs of injury, then gently feel the iliac crests for signs of instability, tenderness or crepitus. Do not compress the pelvis (sometimes called 'springing').
19. Check the extremities (arms and legs) for lacerations, bruises, swelling, deformities and the presence of medical bracelets. Feel for distal pulses and check motor and sensory functions. Compare the right and left sides.

REASSESSMENT
Primary survey
Reassess vital signs
Presenting complaint
Review treatment
Monitor patient condition

Figure 9.6 Reassessment

1.6 Reassessment

The first thing you'll probably notice about the reassessment section is that it contains many of the things you have already undertaken as part of the patient assessment process (Figure 9.6). As with scene safety, a patient's clinical condition is dynamic and frequently changes, either due to the illness and/or injury they have acquired or as a result of an intervention you have performed, such as defibrillation. Frequent reassessment will mean that you will not miss these changes.

Chapter

10 Airway

1 Airway anatomy

1.1 Learning objective

By the end of this section you will be able to:
- identify and describe the structures of the upper and lower airway.

1.2 Introduction

The respiratory system is made up of a number of structures (Figure 10.1):
- nose
- mouth
- pharynx (throat)
- larynx (voicebox)
- trachea (windpipe)
- bronchi
- lungs.

Structurally, the respiratory system is split into two halves: the upper and lower respiratory systems. The upper consists of everything above the vocal folds (also referred to as cords), and the lower, the cricoid cartilage and lower structures.

1.3 Upper airway

1.3.1 Nose

This is mostly constructed from cartilage, and is external to the skull. Its orifices (nostrils, or nares) open into the nasal cavity of the skull, which is divided by the nasal septum. The nasal cavity contains the superior, middle and inferior turbinates (Figure 10.2), which increase the internal surface area of the nasal cavity, which in turn increases the temperature and humidity of air that passes through during breathing [Drake, 2019].

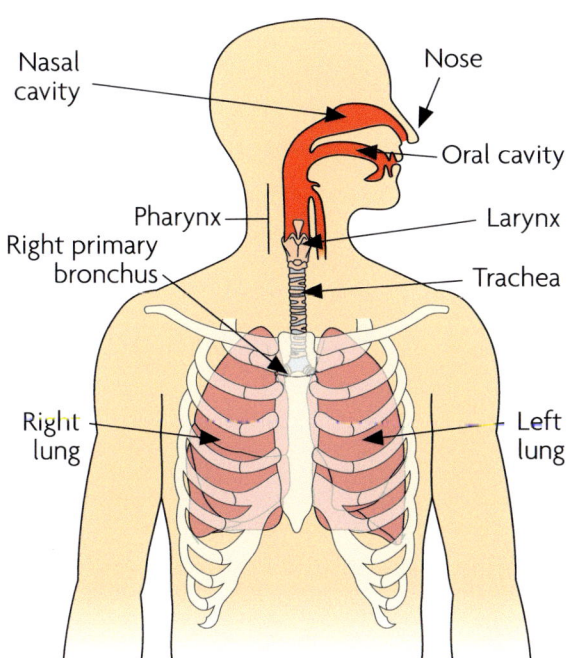

Figure 10.1 The structures of the respiratory system

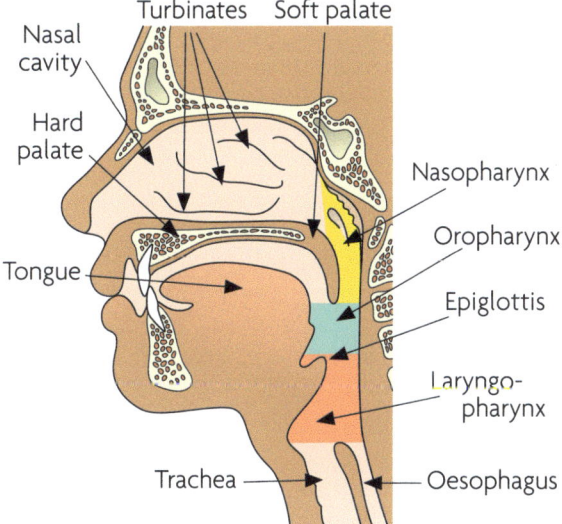

Figure 10.2 The upper airway

Chapter 10 – Airway

1.3.2 Mouth

The mouth (or oral cavity) starts at the lips and is continuous with the oropharynx posteriorly. The roof of the mouth is made up of the hard and soft palates, with the floor made up of mostly soft tissue, including the tongue (Figure 10.3). The tongue is a muscular, non-compressible tissue that attaches to the mandible, stylohyoid process and hyoid bone. The tongue, in the past, was accused of being the most common cause of obstruction. However, research conducted on adult anaesthetised patients has demonstrated that it is usually the soft palate and epiglottis that cause obstruction of the airway, not the tongue [Shorten, 1994].

1.3.3 Pharynx

The pharynx is a funnel-shaped tube extending from the back of the nasal cavity to the top of the oesophagus. Although a continuous structure, it is typically divided into three sections anatomically (Figure 10.2):
- nasopharynx
- oropharynx
- laryngopharynx.

Nasopharynx
This is the area at the back of the nasal cavity, above the level of the soft palate. It is bordered by the sloping base of the skull above and mostly skeletal muscle on either side, forming a domed vault at the top of the pharyngeal cavity.

Elevation of the soft palate during swallowing helps to ensure that food does not rise up into the nasal cavity. The tissues that cover the top of the nasopharynx contain the pharyngeal tonsils. In severe cases, enlargement of these can block the nasopharynx.

Oropharynx
This is the area posterior to the oral cavity, below the level of the soft palate but continuous with the nasopharynx, and above the margin of the epiglottis (which marks the start of the laryngopharynx). Anteriorly, the palatoglossal folds mark the boundary between the oral cavity and oropharynx.

Laryngopharynx
This is continuous with the oropharynx, running from the superior margins of the epiglottis to the top of the oesophagus around the level of the sixth cervical vertebra (spinal bone) in adults.

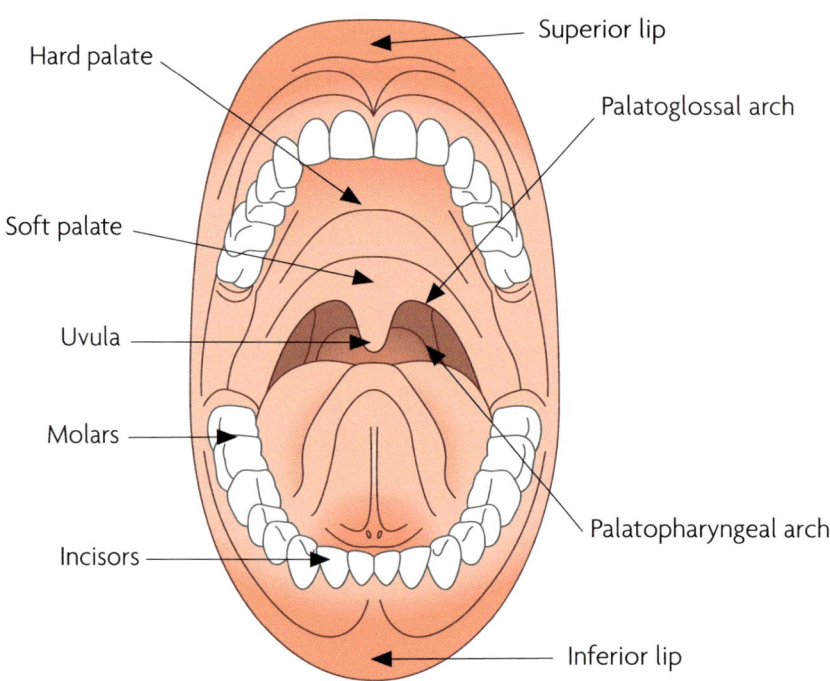

Figure 10.3   The oral cavity

Airway anatomy

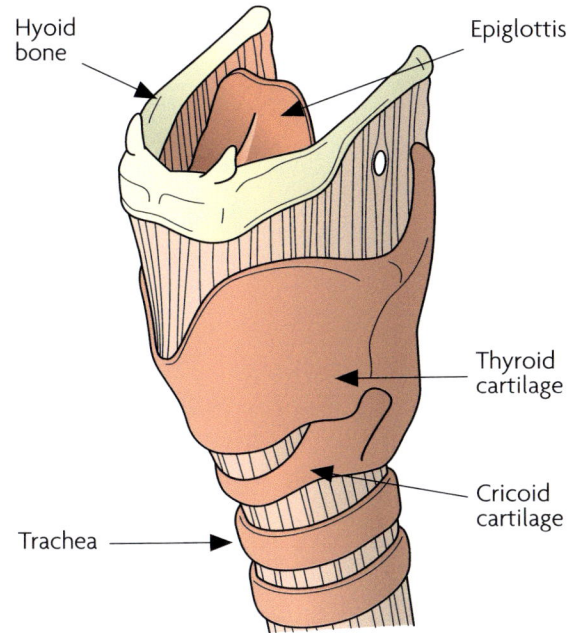

Figure 10.4 The larynx

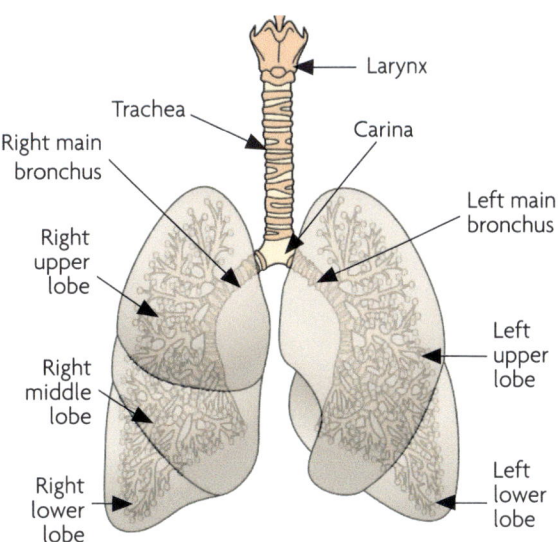

Figure 10.5 The lower airway

1.3.4 Larynx

The larynx is a hollow structure made up of muscles and ligaments. In adults it is cylindrical in shape, with the narrowest part of the airway at the level of the vocal cords. It is continuous with the trachea below and opens into the laryngopharynx posteriorly.

The larynx is suspended from the hyoid bone above, and trachea below, by a series of membranes and ligaments, which makes it very mobile within the neck (Figure 10.4). During swallowing it moves upwards and forwards, causing the epiglottis to swing downwards, effectively closing the laryngeal inlet while at the same time opening the oesophagus.

As well as acting as a valve to close off the respiratory tract during swallowing, the larynx also produces sound for speech, singing, etc.

1.4 Lower Airway

1.4.1 Trachea

The trachea extends from the cricoid cartilage to approximately the level of the sixth thoracic vertebra where it splits into the left main bronchus and right main bronchus (together, the bronchi) at the carina (Figure 10.5). In an adult the trachea is approximately 12–15 cm long and consists of C-shaped cartilages, which are completed posteriorly by the trachealis muscle [Kovacs, 2011].

1.4.2 Bronchi

The left main bronchus and right main bronchus split into secondary bronchi, tertiary bronchi, the bronchioles and finally the terminal bronchioles. The right main bronchus is more vertical, wider and shorter than the left, which explains why objects that are inhaled (foreign bodies) tend to end up here. In a similar design to the trachea, the main bronchi are incomplete rings of cartilage.

1.4.3 Lungs

The lungs are a pair of spongy, cone-shaped organs located in the thoracic (chest) cavity. They are separated by the mediastinum, a region in the thoracic cavity that contains the heart, major vessels, oesophagus and trachea, among others. This means that in the event that one lung collapses, due to air entering the thoracic cavity after a traumatic injury, for example, the other lung may remain inflated.

The lungs are covered by the pleura, which consists of two layers: the parietal pleura, which covers the wall of the thoracic cavity, and the visceral pleura, which covers and adheres to the surface of the lungs. In between is the pleural cavity, a potential space filled with fluid to prevent friction and allow the pleurae to slide over each other during breathing. It also helps the membranes stick together due to the surface tension of the fluid in a similar way that a glass with a wet bottom lifts the coaster it is sitting on.

The lungs extend from the diaphragm to just above the clavicles. The left lung is smaller than the right due to the space taken up by the heart. It also has only two lobes, the upper and lower, whereas the right lung has three, the upper, lower and middle lobes [Tortora, 2017].

2 Assessing and managing the airway

2.1 Learning objectives

By the end of this section you will be able to:
- identify clinical signs that indicate a need to manage the airway
- explain factors that affect airway patency and the step-wise approach to airway management
- explain how to perform a range of manual airway manoeuvres
- describe how to appropriately size and insert oro- and nasopharyngeal airways
- describe the equipment required for suction and how to use it safely.

2.2 Introduction

More often than not, your patient will be conscious and able to talk, scream or cry, indicating that they have a patent airway. In some cases, however, you will need to assist them in opening and maintaining their airway. Basic manoeuvres with nothing more than your hands are often enough to open and keep open a patient's airway, but things can change and it is important that you frequently reassess airway patency, i.e. perform a dynamic airway assessment.

In this section, the following manoeuvres will be described:
- recovery position
- head tilt–chin lift
- jaw thrust
- jaw thrust with head tilt.

Once the manual manoeuvres have been covered, the following more advanced procedures will be described:
- suction
- insertion of an oropharyngeal airway (OPA)
- insertion of a nasopharyngeal airway (NPA).

2.3 Assessing the airway

In Chapter 9, 'Patient Assessment', you were introduced to the three-step approach to airway assessment:
- **Look:** As you approach the patient, note their position as it can give you an indication of the patency of the airway. Conscious patients who have adopted a tripod position (Figure 10.6) or

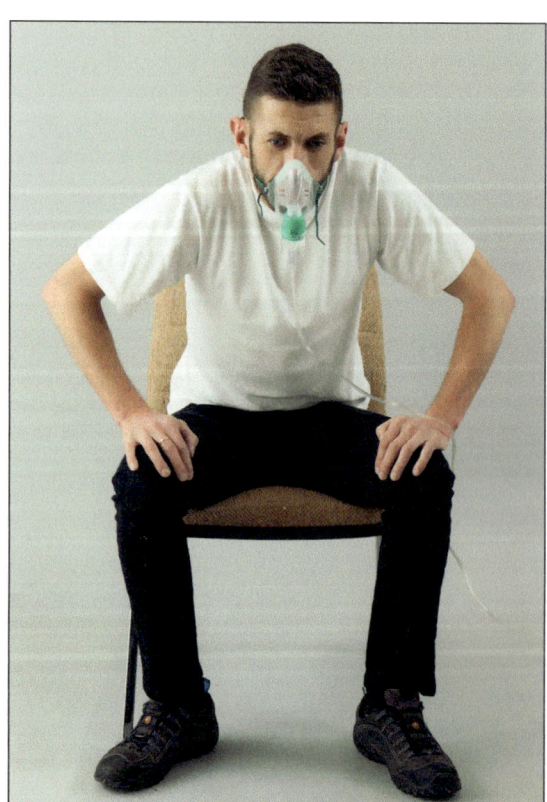

Figure 10.6 A patient in the tripod position

who are showing other signs of increased work of breathing may have a partially obstructed airway.

- **Listen:** When assessing the airway, listen for the presence of additional sounds (which can often be heard without the need for a stethoscope). High-pitched inspiratory (although sometimes can be expiratory too) sounds can be a sign of upper airway narrowing (known as stridor). Lower-pitch sounds usually heard on expiration (wheeze) are a sign of partial lower airway obstruction, particularly in acute exacerbations of conditions such as asthma or chronic obstructive pulmonary disease (COPD). Other sounds include snoring, typically due to the soft tissues of the pharynx relaxing, and gurgling, due to fluid, secretions and vomit, etc. Snoring can usually be remedied with manual airway manoeuvres or an adjunct such as an oropharyngeal airway, whereas gurgling is an indication that the patient's airway requires suction.
- **Feel:** You will not always need to place your ear close enough to your patients to feel their breath on your cheek! However, in unresponsive patients it is important to determine if there is airflow and not just rely on chest movement. The chest can move even in complete airway obstruction, and is sometimes associated with a see-saw, paradoxical movement of the abdomen and the chest. So, as the chest expands, the abdomen sinks and vice versa.

2.4 *Step-wise approach to the airway*

In general, you will start with basic manoeuvres, such as the head tilt–chin lift or recovery position for patients who have an obstructed airway. Depending on the patient's condition and potential threats to their airway, you may elect to escalate their management to include an airway adjunct, such as an OPA or NPA. It is important to provide an early update to the EOC if your patient requires airway manoeuvres or adjuncts to maintain airway patency, or if you cannot obtain a patent airway despite attempting the manoeuvres and using the adjuncts you have been trained to use.

To help guide your decision-making when deciding on which airway manoeuvre to use, or when to escalate your airway management to include the use of an airway adjunct, a step-wise approach to airway management has been published in the UK Ambulance Clinical Practice Guidelines [JRCALC, 2023]. We have provided a modified version in Figure 10.7 which is appropriate for responders but, as always, consult your local guidance and procedures.

2.5 *Manual airway manoeuvres*

Manual airway manoeuvres can be achieved with just your (or a colleague's) hands. They are great for the initial management of the airway, and in some cases may be all that is required.

2.5.1 Recovery position

Indications
- A spontaneously breathing but unconscious patient who does not have a spinal injury.

Contra-indications
- Patients with spinal injuries.
- Patients who require assisted ventilation or insertion of an advanced airway.

Advantages
- Simple and quick to perform, even for a single rescuer.
- Does not require equipment.
- Encourages postural drainage of secretions or vomit from the patient's mouth.

Disadvantages
- Not a definitive airway (does not guarantee that the patient will not aspirate).
- Sometimes difficult to assess patient's breathing and undertake other examinations or monitoring.

Chapter 10 – *Airway*

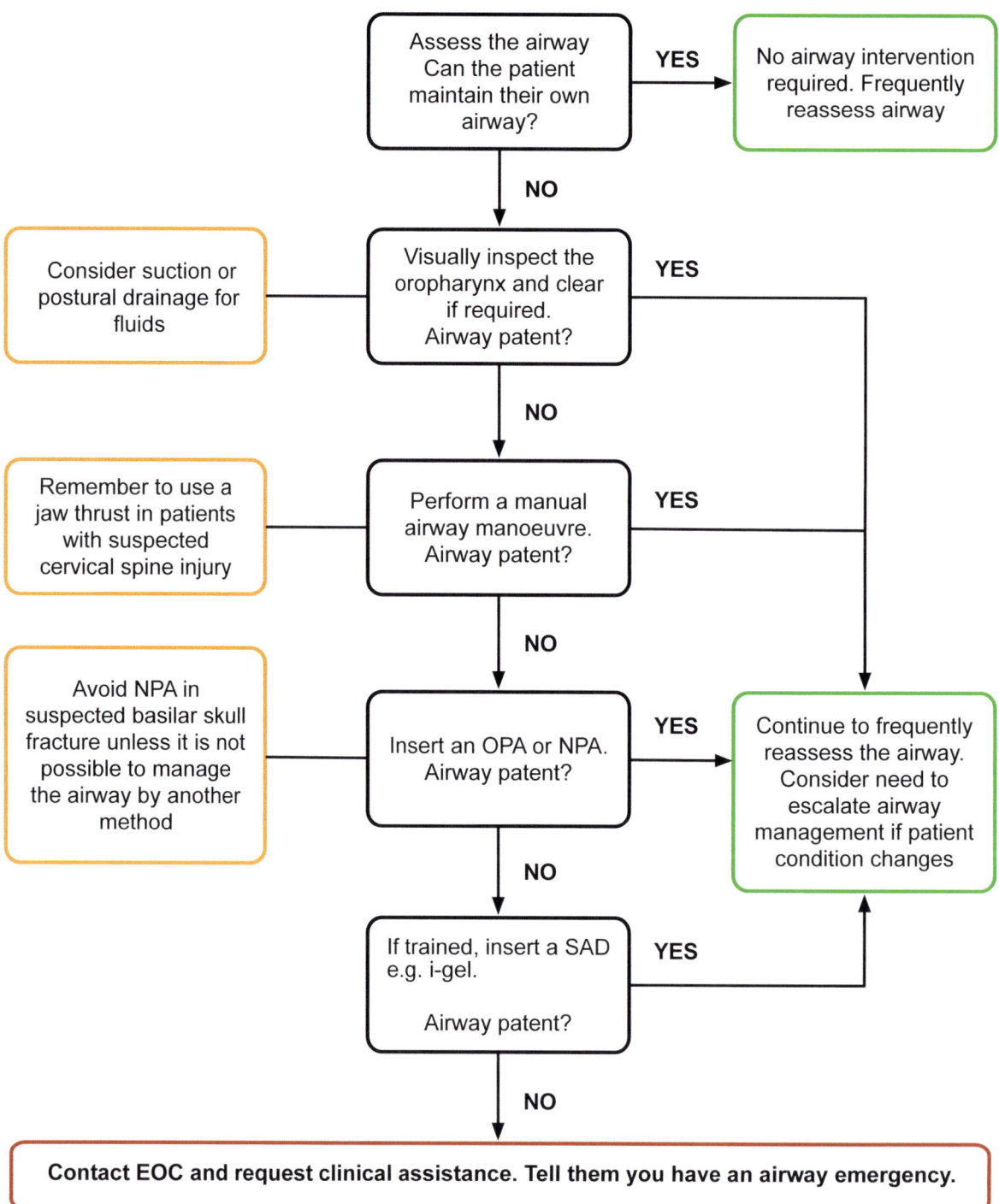

Figure 10.7 Step-wise approach to airway assessment and management

Assessing and managing the airway

Procedure

Take the following steps to place a patient in the recovery position [Pilbery & Lethbridge, 2022]:
1. Don appropriate PPE, and undertake appropriate hand hygiene.
2. With the patient lying supine, kneel beside them and straighten both of their legs. Quickly check if they have any items in their pockets that should be removed before rolling the patient.

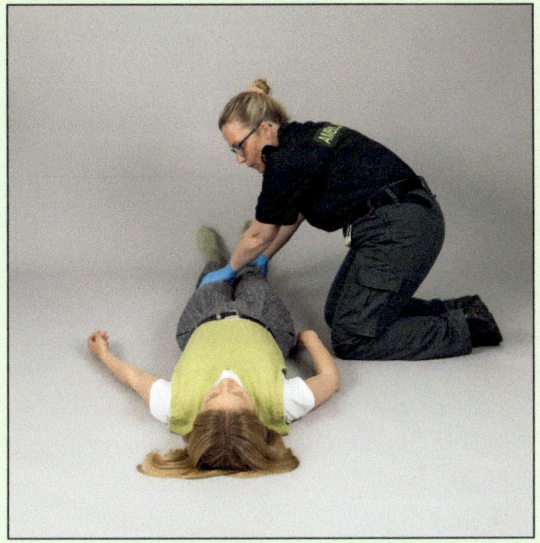

3. Place the arm nearer to you at right angles to their body, with the arm bent at the elbow and palm of the hand facing upwards.

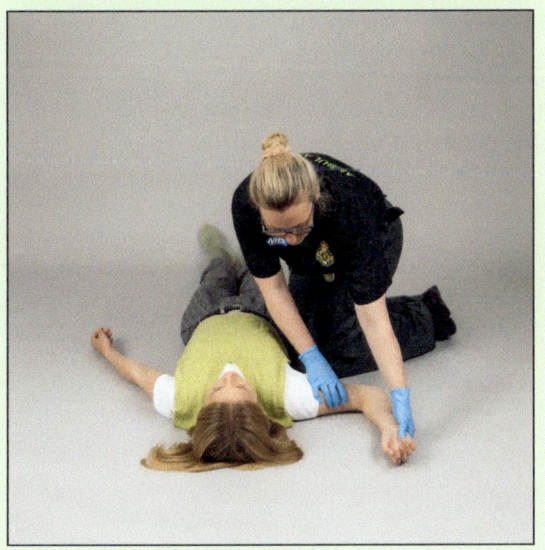

Procedure – *cont*

4. Bring the other arm across the chest and hold the back of their hand against the cheek that is nearer to you. Don't let go.

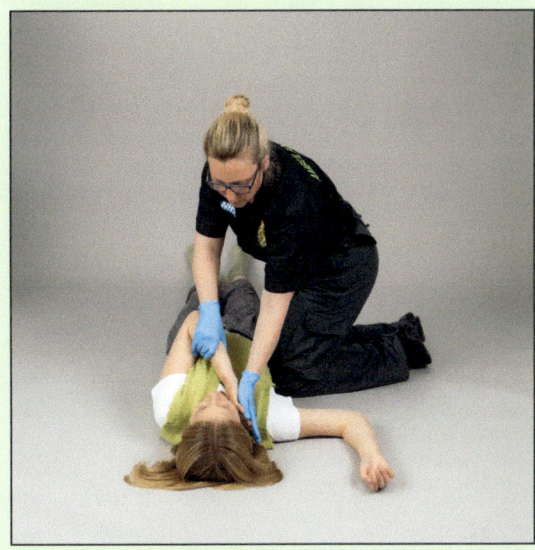

5. With your other hand, grasp the leg further away from you just above the knee and lift upwards so the leg flexes. Keep the foot on the ground.

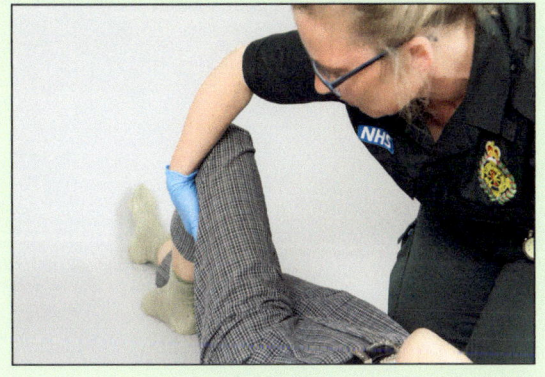

Chapter 10 – Airway

Procedure – *cont*

6. While supporting the head, pull the leg towards you, so that the patient rolls to face you.

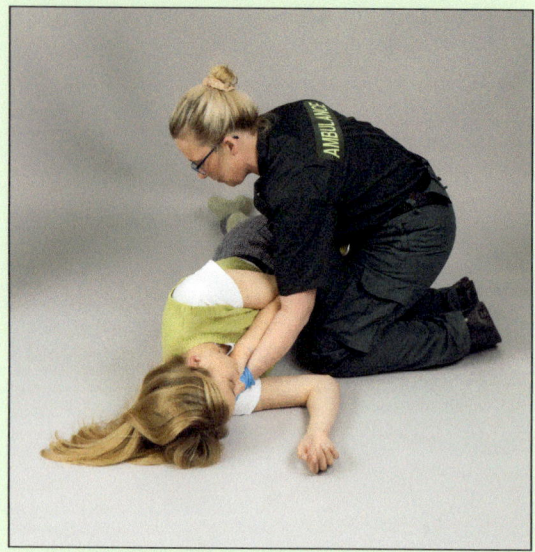

7. Adjust the upper leg so that the patient's hip and knee are bent at right angles.

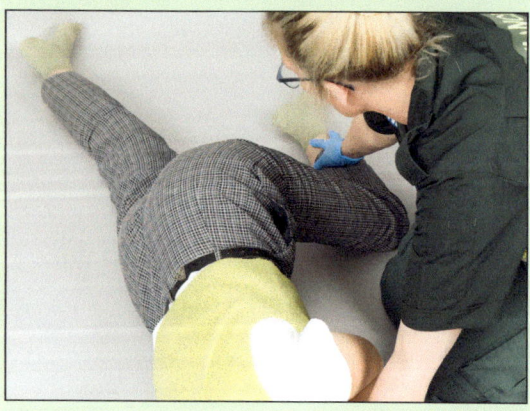

Procedure – *cont*

8. Tilt the head back to ensure the airway remains open. Adjust the patient's hand that is under their cheek if required, to maintain head tilt and keep the patient facing slightly downwards. Reassess frequently.

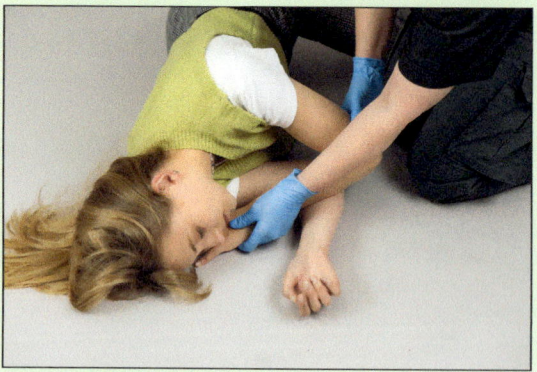

9. Document the procedure.

2.5.2 Head tilt–chin lift

Indications
- Unresponsive patients who have an airway obstruction caused by loss of pharyngeal muscle tone.

Contra-indications
- Suspected cervical spinal injury.

Advantages
- No equipment is required.
- Technique is simple and non-invasive.

Disadvantages
- Does not protect the airway from aspiration.
- Not suitable for patients with a suspected cervical spinal injury.
- Requires practice and experience to perform effectively, especially with more challenging airways, for example in obese patients.

Procedure

Take the following steps to perform a head tilt–chin lift [Pilbery & Lethbridge, 2022]:
1. Don appropriate PPE, and undertake appropriate hand hygiene.

Procedure – *cont*

2. With your patient lying on their back (supine), position yourself at the patient's side. Place the hand closer to the patient's head on their forehead and gently tilt the head backwards.

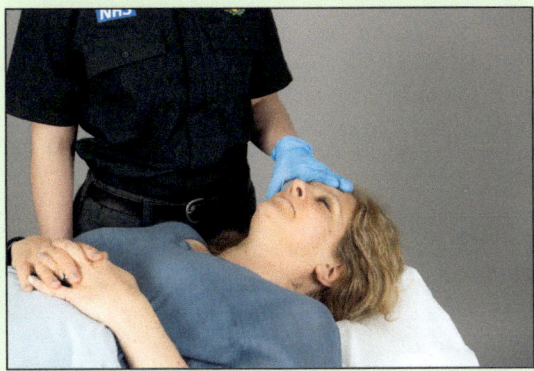

3. Place two fingers on the bony part of the chin and gently lift upwards.
   Take care not to overextend the neck.

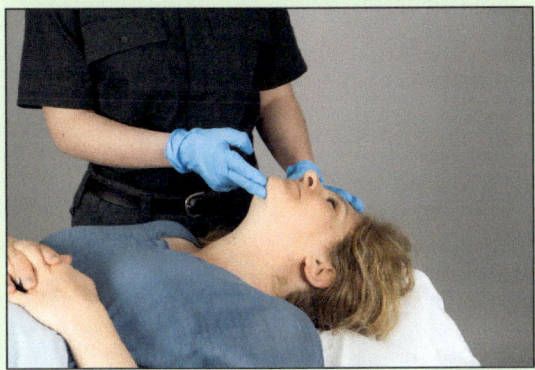

4. Check for procedure success by adopting a look, listen, feel approach.

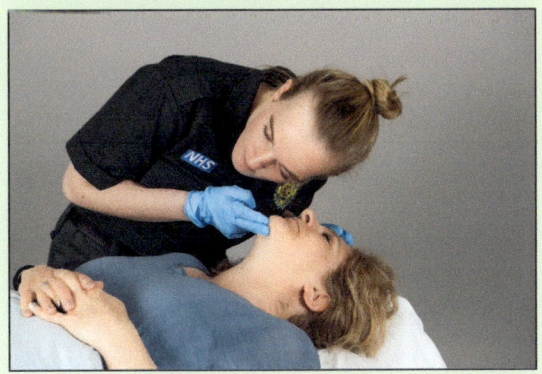

5. Document the procedure.

2.5.3 Jaw thrust

Indications
- Unresponsive patients who have an airway obstruction caused by loss of pharyngeal muscle tone.
- Alternative technique when head tilt–chin lift has been unsuccessful.

Contra-indications
- Responsive patients.

Advantages
- No equipment is required.
- Technique is simple and non-invasive.
- Maintains neutral alignment of the head when cervical spine injury is suspected.

Disadvantages
- Does not protect the airway from aspiration.
- Difficult to maintain for long periods.
- Requires an assistant to provide ventilations, if required.

Procedure

Take the following steps to perform a jaw thrust [Pilbery & Lethbridge, 2022]:
1. Don appropriate PPE, and undertake appropriate hand hygiene.
2. With your patient lying on their back (supine), identify the angle of the mandible.

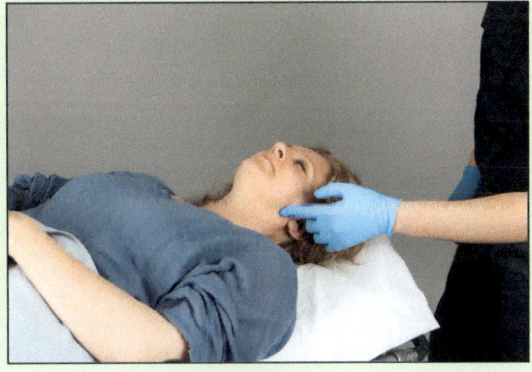

Chapter 10 – Airway

Procedure – *cont*

3. Place your fingers behind the mandible and lift in an upwards and forwards direction.

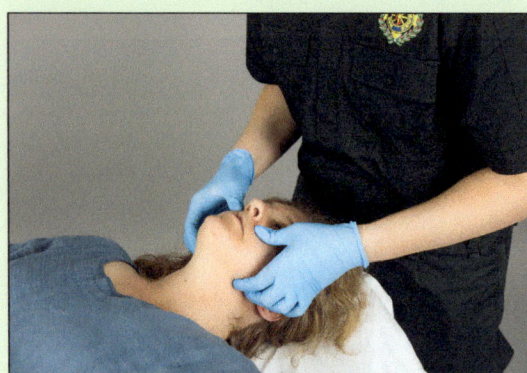

4. Using your thumbs, open the patient's mouth.

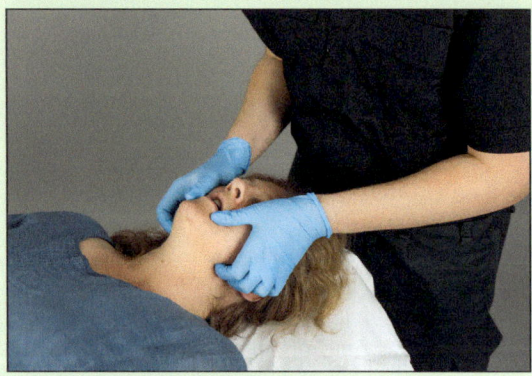

5. Document the procedure.

2.5.4 Triple airway manoeuvre

Indications
- Unresponsive patients who have an airway obstruction caused by loss of pharyngeal muscle tone.
- Head tilt–chin lift and jaw thrust have been unsuccessful.

Contra-indications
- Responsive patients.
- Suspected spinal injury.

Advantages
- No equipment is required.
- Technique is simple and non-invasive.

Disadvantages
- Does not protect the airway from aspiration.
- Not suitable for patients with a suspected cervical spinal injury.
- Difficult to maintain for long periods.
- Requires an assistant to provide ventilations, if required.

Procedure

Take the following steps to perform the triple airway manoeuvre [Pilbery & Lethbridge, 2022]:

1. Don appropriate PPE, and undertake appropriate hand hygiene.
2. With your patient lying on their back (supine), identify the angle of the mandible.

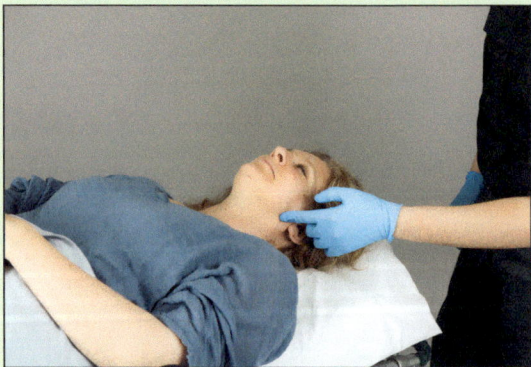

3. Place your fingers behind the mandible and lift in an upwards and forwards direction.

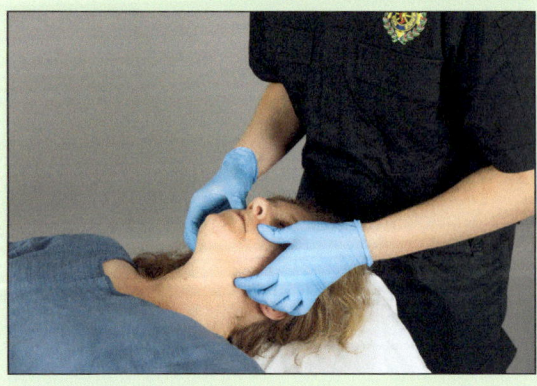

Assessing and managing the airway

Procedure – cont

4. Using your thumbs, open the patient's mouth.

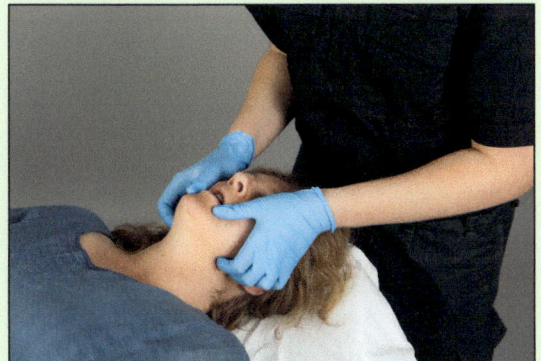

5. Tilt the head backwards.

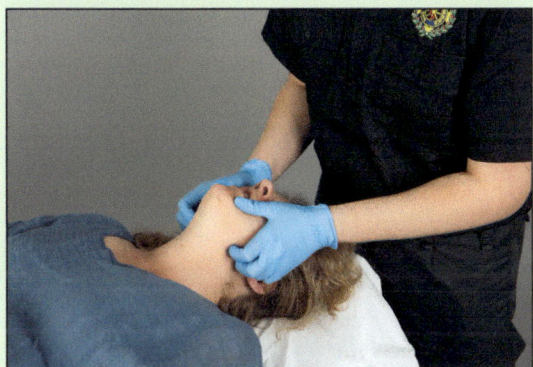

6. Document the procedure.

2.6 Suction

If you can hear gurgling in the airway, then you should think suction. Suctioning an airway involves removing vomit, blood and secretions with suctioning equipment. If you have suction available, it is likely to be a hand-operated device (Figure 10.8). Make sure you are familiar with the operating instructions for the devices you carry.

Indications
- Patients who cannot maintain and clear their own airway and in whom vomit, blood or secretions are at risk of entering the lower respiratory tract.

Contra-indications
- Patients who can maintain and clear their own airway.

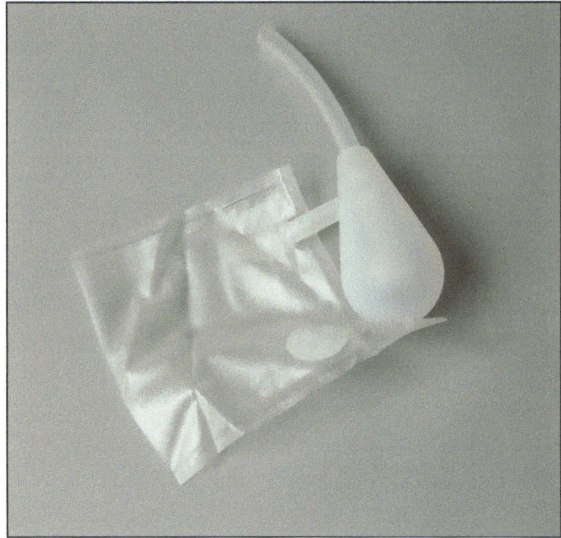

Figure 10.8 Hand-operated suction device

Advantages
- Reduces risk of aspiration of vomit, blood and secretions.
- Supports maintenance of a clear airway.

Disadvantages
- Suctioning removes air as well as secretions.
- Might not be possible to use with patients who have limited mouth opening.
- May not be sufficient to overcome continuous emesis (vomiting) or haemorrhage.

Procedure

Take the following steps to perform suction using a handheld suction device [Randle, 2009; Roberts, 2014]:

1. Don appropriate PPE, and undertake appropriate hand hygiene.
2. Prepare your equipment. You will need:
   - suction device assembled, with catheter attached, if provided separately
   - oxygen.
3. Consider adjusting the patient's position to allow for postural drainage and pre-oxygenate the patient, if you have time.
4. Open the patient's mouth and insert the catheter into their mouth without suctioning. Make sure you can always visualise the end of the suction catheter.

Chapter 10 – Airway

> **Procedure – cont**
> 5. Apply suction by squeezing the bulb or trigger (depending on suction device type) while gently withdrawing the suction device from the patient's mouth. Suction for no more than 10 seconds.
> 6. Re-oxygenate the patient and reassess the airway. Further suction attempts may be required.
> 7. Document the procedure.

Notes

In cases of severe bleeding or active vomiting, positioning the patient to allow for postural drainage is more important: for example, turning a patient on to their side when they are immobilised on an orthopaedic stretcher [Nutbeam, 2013].

Although prolonged suctioning will cause hypoxia (which is why suctioning for no more than 10 seconds is suggested), an airway obstructed by blood or vomit will not allow any air exchange and is likely to result in aspiration. In this case, patient positioning and aggressive suction will be required until the airway is at least partially clear. Re-oxygenation can then be performed and suction repeated as required [NAEMT, 2020].

2.7 Airway adjuncts

Airway adjuncts are devices that assist in airway management. Probably the most commonly used airway adjunct is the oropharyngeal airway, also known as a Guedel airway (Figure 10.9), but there are others, including the nasopharyngeal airway.

2.7.1 Insertion of an OPA

Indications
- An unresponsive patient with an absent gag reflex.
- Patient requires bag-valve-mask (BVM) ventilation.

Contra-indications
- Patient has a gag reflex.

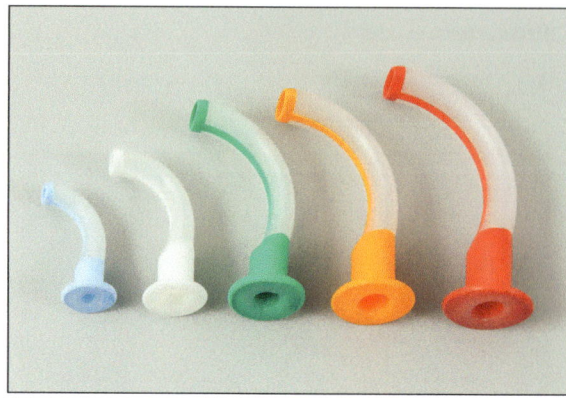

Figure 10.9 A collection of oropharyngeal airways

Advantages
- Easy to place.
- Technique is simple and minimally invasive.

Disadvantages
- Tongue can be pushed back during insertion, making obstruction worse.
- Does not protect against vomiting or aspiration.

> **Procedure**
>
> Take the following steps to insert an OPA [Pilbery & Lethbridge, 2022]:
> 1. Don appropriate PPE, and undertake appropriate hand hygiene.
> 2. Select the correctly sized OPA by measuring the vertical distance between the patient's incisors and the angle of the jaw.

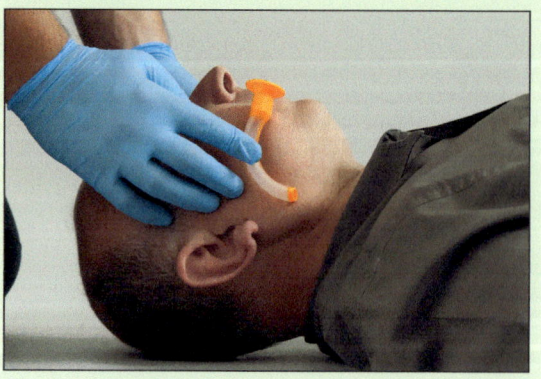

Assessing and managing the airway

Procedure – *cont*

3. Open the patient's mouth and check it is clear of foreign bodies, vomit, blood or secretions. Suction if required.

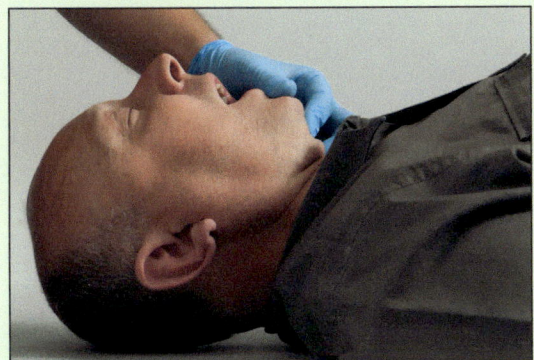

4. Insert the airway 'upside down' along the roof of the mouth until it reaches the soft palate.

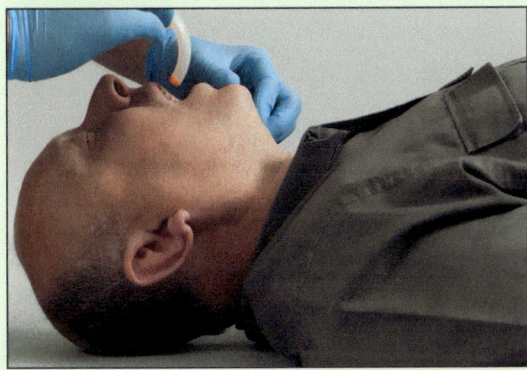

5. Rotate the OPA through 180°.

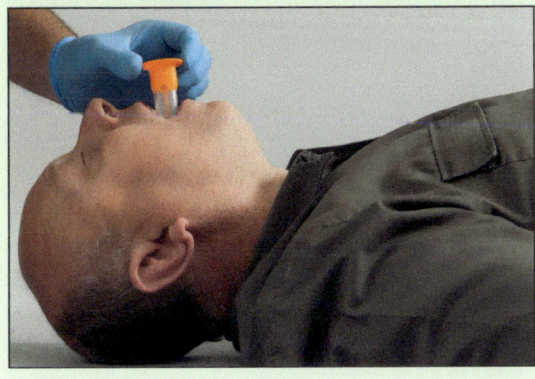

Procedure – *cont*

6. Advance the OPA until it rests in the pharynx. Consider using a jaw thrust to assist with final seating of the OPA. Remove immediately if the patient gags.

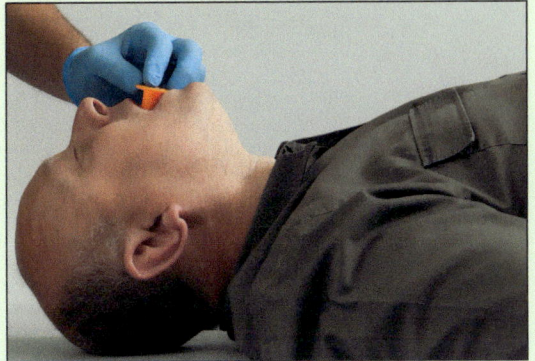

7. Continue to provide manual manoeuvres such as head tilt–chin lift or jaw thrust as appropriate.
8. Document the procedure.

2.7.2 Insertion of a NPA

Indications
- An unresponsive patient, or a patient with a reduced LOC who has an intact gag reflex.

Contra-indications
- Patients who do not tolerate the procedure.

Cautions
- Patients who have a suspected basal skull fracture or other serious head injury (oropharyngeal airways are preferred, unless these are not possible to insert because of trismus [involuntary spasm of the jaw muscles which keeps the mouth tightly closed], for example).
- Patients with nasal polyps.

Advantages
- Can be suctioned through.
- Can be tolerated by patients who are not unconscious.
- Does not require the mouth to open.

Disadvantages
- Can cause bleeding.
- Does not protect against aspiration.

Chapter 10 – Airway

Procedure

Take the following steps to insert a NPA [Pilbery & Lethbridge, 2022]:
1. Don appropriate PPE, and undertake appropriate hand hygiene.
2. Prepare the following:
   - an appropriately sized NPA, which is generally considered to be a 7 for an average adult male and 6 for an average adult female
   - water-soluble gel
   - suction.

   If the NPA you are using comes with a safety pin, insert it through the non-bevelled end.

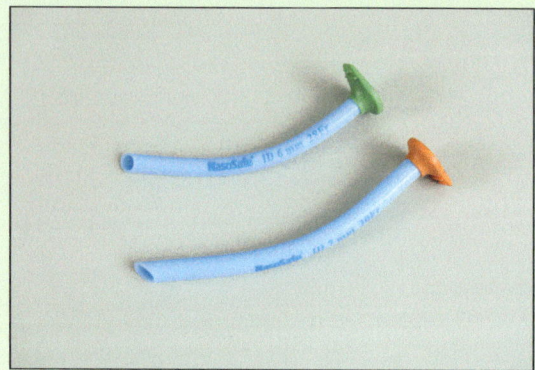

3. Lubricate the NPA, ensuring that the gel does not go over the open ends of the airway.

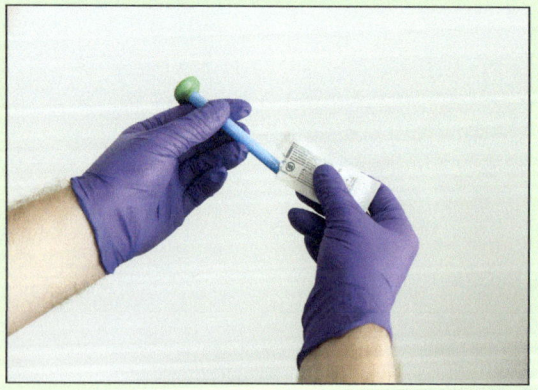

Procedure – cont

4. Insert the NPA posteriorly and with the bevel facing the nasal septum. This means that the right nostril is usually used, although if the left is clearly larger, then this can be used.

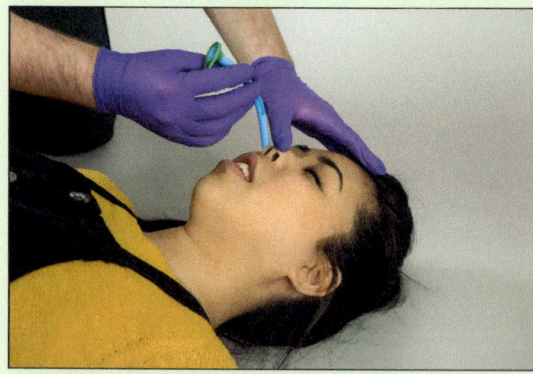

5. If resistance is felt when inserting the NPA, twist the device a little; if it still cannot be advanced, consider changing nostril or using a smaller-size NPA. Check for blanching of the patient's nostrils. If this occurs, the NPA should be removed and a smaller-diameter NPA inserted instead.

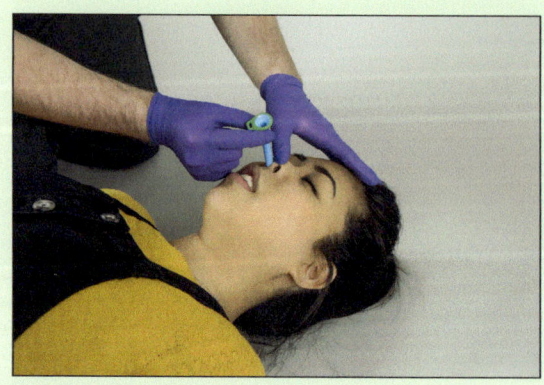

Tracheostomies

Procedure – *cont*

6. Confirm position by listening for breath sounds and ensuring the chest rises and falls.

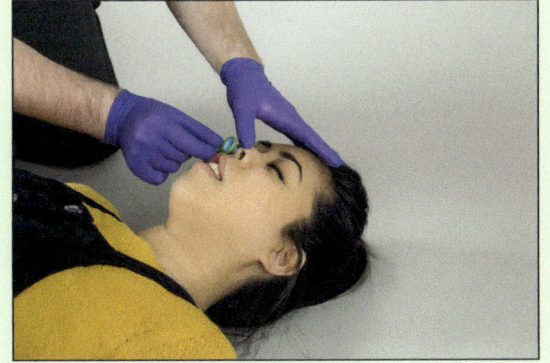

7. Document the procedure.

3 Tracheostomies

3.1 Learning objectives

By the end of this section you will be able to:
- explain the difference between laryngectomy and tracheostomy
- describe how to manage the airway of a patient with a laryngectomy or a tracheostomy.

3.2 Introduction

A tracheostomy is an artificial opening made into the trachea through the neck (Figure 10.10). Patients have them inserted for a number of reasons, including [Feber, 2006; Bowers, 2007]:

- following trauma or surgery to the head and neck, which leads to an airway obstruction
- bypassing a tumour which obstructs the upper airway
- for prolonged ventilation
- for some types of chronic disease where minimising the anatomical dead space is beneficial
- to provide access to chest secretions in the event of respiratory insufficiency
- to protect from aspiration in the event of impaired swallow reflex (for example, neuromuscular disorders).

As the name suggests, a laryngectomy is the removal of the larynx. This is typically due to involvement of the larynx in oral, pharyngeal and laryngeal cancers. If the patient requires a total laryngectomy, the larynx is removed and the trachea cut and stitched to the front of the neck [NTSP, 2014]. This is important for subsequent management, because these patients cannot be ventilated from the mouth and/or nose.

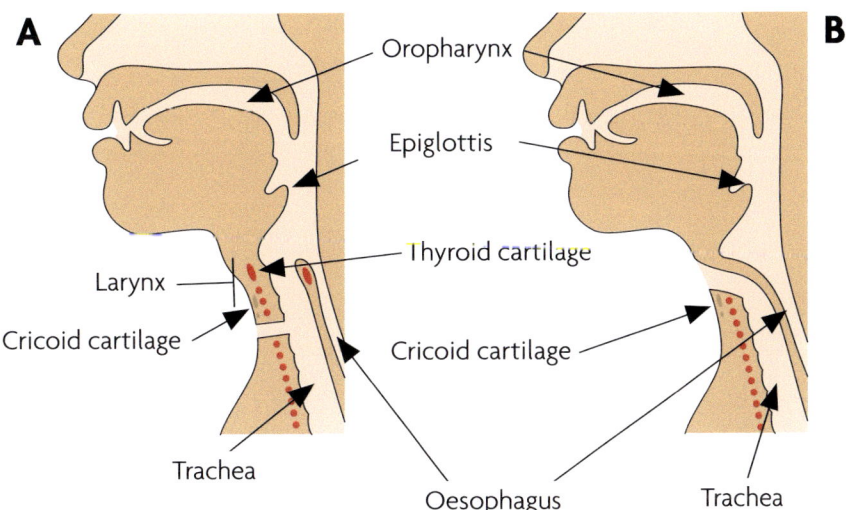

Figure 10.10 The anatomical differences between A) tracheostomy and B) laryngectomy

3.3 Tracheostomy tubes

There is a wide variety of tracheostomy tubes, which can seem rather overwhelming. However, tubes are broadly classified into the following categories [NTSP, 2014]:
- cuffed/uncuffed
- with/without inner cannula
- fenestrated/unfenestrated.

3.3.1 Cuffed/uncuffed tubes

As with adult endotracheal tubes, a cuffed tracheostomy tube has a soft balloon around the distal end, which is inflated by injecting air into the pilot balloon via the injection port (Figure 10.11). These are used when patients require positive-pressure ventilation (PPV) and/or when the patient cannot protect their own airway from secretions. Note that if the cuffed tube is inflated and the lumen becomes blocked or occluded, the patient will not be able to breathe!

Uncuffed tubes tend to be used in longer-term patients, but since they lack the cuff, it is important that these patients have an effective cough and gag reflex to minimise the chance of aspiration. These tubes are not suitable for PPV.

3.3.2 Inner cannulas

Tracheostomy tubes with an inner cannula (sometimes called double-cannula or double-lumen tubes) consist of an outer tube or cannula, which maintains airway patency, and an inner cannula, which can be removed for cleaning and/or disposed of and replaced (Figure 10.12). Uncuffed, double-cannula tracheostomy tubes are the safest type to use in the community [NTSP, 2014].

3.3.3 Fenestrated tubes

These tracheostomy tubes have an opening on the outer cannula which allows air to pass through the patient's oropharynx and nasopharynx. This is helpful because it allows the patient to talk and produce an effective cough. However, fenestrations increase the risk of aspiration and prevent PPV unless a non-fenestrated inner cannula is used. Non-fenestrated inner cannulas should also be used if the patient requires suction (Figure 10.12).

3.4 Management of the tracheostomy patient

Patients with tracheostomies have a potentially patent upper airway, since the upper airway and trachea are anatomically connected. However,

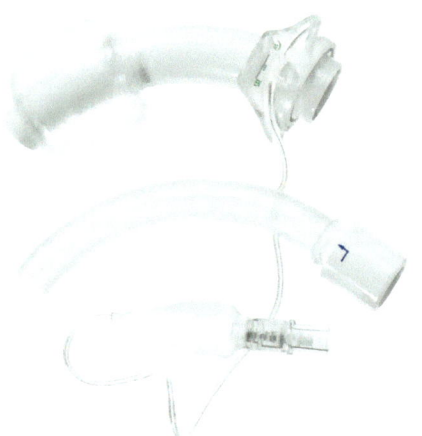

Figure 10.11 A cuffed, unfenestrated tracheostomy tube (top). Inner cannula with no fenestrations (middle). Pilot balloon and inflation valve for tracheostomy cuff (bottom)

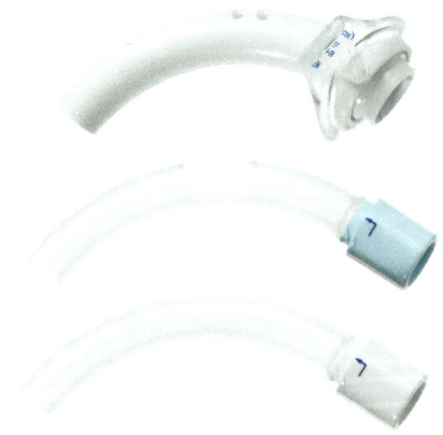

Figure 10.12 An uncuffed, fenestrated tracheostomy tube (top). Inner cannula with opening for fenestrations (middle). Inner cannula with no fenestrations (bottom)

it is quite possible that the reason the patient had a tracheostomy in the first place is that their upper airway is difficult or impossible to manage [McGrath, 2012].

3.4.1 Help and equipment

You will not be able to manage on your own and assistance is vital. If a relative or carer is present, it is quite possible that they know more about tracheostomy management than you do, so listen to their advice and encourage them to help.

Patients may well have equipment to hand, such as replacement tubes, but you can manage with the equipment from your response bag:
- airway adjuncts such as oropharyngeal and nasopharyngeal airways
- BVM.

3.4.2 Airway and breathing

Check and open the upper airway as normal. Look, listen and feel for breathing at the face and tracheostomy site for no more than 10 seconds.

If the patient is breathing, apply high-flow oxygen to both face and tracheostomy. This may require two cylinders, or the addition of a flowmeter into the Schrader valve of the oxygen cylinder. If the patient is not breathing, is making agonal gasps or there are no signs of life, start chest compressions and follow the basic life support (BLS) algorithm while continuing to troubleshoot the tracheostomy, since this may be the cause of the cardiac arrest [Olasveengen, 2021].

3.4.3 Tracheostomy patency

Start by checking for and removing the following:
- decannulation caps (used when removing tracheostomies), which can block the end of the tracheostomy
- obturator (inserted inside the tracheostomy when first inserting a tube into the patient, Figure 10.13)
- speaking valve, which must not be used with an inflated cuffed tube (Figure 10.14)
- blocked humidification device such as Swedish nose.

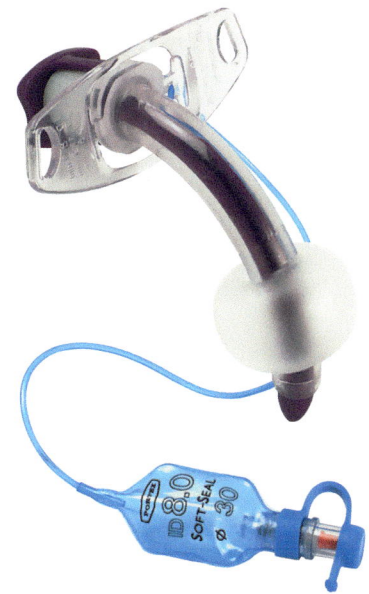

Figure 10.13 A tracheostomy tube with an obturator inside

If the tracheostomy tube is a double-cannula design, remove the inner cannula, but remember that with some types of tubes the connector required for BVM ventilation is mounted on the inner cannula. Pass a suction catheter through the tube and into the trachea to check patency. It should pass easily through the tube. If the suction catheter passes through the tube, suction it and attempt to ventilate the patient. If this fails and the

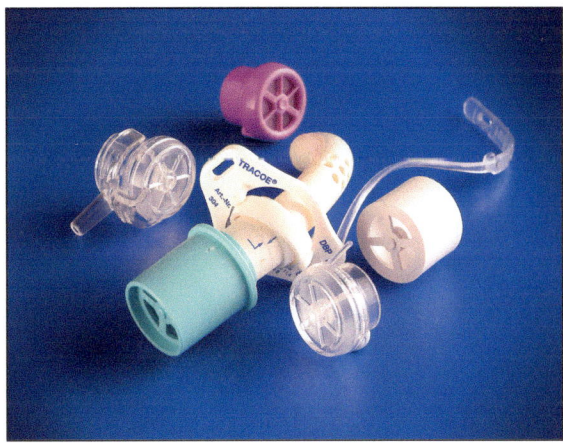

Figure 10.14 A selection of speaking valves. These should be fitted to cuffed tubes

tube has a cuff, deflate it and reassess the patient using the same look, listen and feel technique as before at both the face and the stoma site.

3.4.4 Next steps

If everything attempted thus far has failed to improve the patient's condition, remove the tube. Reassess the patient again and hopefully they will be breathing. If the patient is in cardiac arrest, continue with BLS. Attempt to oxygenate the patient via the oral route, but don't forget to cover the stoma site with swabs or a gloved hand. Use standard airway adjuncts to achieve effective ventilation. Alternatively, a paediatric face mask can be placed over the stoma and the patient ventilated. If there is a large air leak from the mouth and/or nose, occlude them both during PPV.

3.5 Management of the laryngectomy patient

Unlike patients with a tracheostomy, laryngectomy patients do not have any connection between the upper airway and their lungs. Do not attempt to ventilate via the mouth/nose. Laryngectomy patients do not normally have tracheostomy tubes either, but may have a tracheo-oesophageal puncture (TEP) valve fitted to allow for speech. This may be visible inside the stoma, but should not be removed. They are usually fitted with a one-way valve to prevent aspiration [NTSP, 2014].

Since these patients have, in effect, no upper airway, it cannot be obstructed by an inappropriate head position. Due to the reduction in anatomical dead space, chest compressions typically generate sufficient tidal volume to negate the need for PPV if this proves difficult to administer. Instead, just provide a supply of high-flow oxygen to the stoma site.

Tracheostomies are ten times more commonly performed than laryngectomies, so in the event that there is any uncertainty about whether the stoma is a laryngectomy or tracheostomy site, it is better to apply oxygen to both face and stoma.

3.5.1 Help and equipment

As with tracheostomy patients, patients who have had laryngectomies are not patients who you can manage alone, and assistance is vital. If a relative or carer is present, it is quite possible that they know more about laryngectomy management than you do, so listen to their advice and encourage them to help.

Patients may well have equipment such as replacement tubes to hand, but you can manage with the BVM from your response bag.

3.5.2 Airway and breathing

Check and open the upper airway as normal unless you are sure the patient has a laryngectomy. Look, listen and feel for breathing at the stoma site for no more than 10 seconds. If the patient is breathing, apply high-flow oxygen to the stoma site. If the patient is not breathing, is making agonal gasps or there are no signs of life, start chest compressions and follow the BLS algorithm while continuing to troubleshoot the laryngectomy stoma, since this may be the cause of the cardiac arrest.

3.5.3 Laryngectomy stoma patency

Most patients will not have a tube in place, but you should remove any stoma cover (sometimes called a 'button') if in place. If a tracheostomy tube is in place and is of a double-cannula design, remove the inner cannula, but remember that with some types of tubes the connector required for BVM ventilation is mounted on the inner cannula.

Pass a suction catheter through the stoma and into the trachea to check patency. It should pass easily into the trachea. If it does, the stoma is patent, so suction the trachea and attempt to ventilate the patient if they are not breathing. If this fails and there is a cuffed tracheostomy tube in place, deflate it and reassess the patient.

3.5.4 Next steps

If everything attempted thus far has failed to improve the patient's condition, remove any tracheostomy tubes, if present. Reassess the patient again and hopefully they will be breathing. If the patient is in cardiac arrest, continue with BLS.

Attempt to ventilate the patient using a paediatric face mask placed over the stoma. If this fails, a suitably qualified clinician will need to intubate the stoma with either a smaller-diameter tracheostomy or endotracheal tube.

4 Choking in adults

4.1 Learning objectives

By the end of this section you will be able to:
- define foreign body airway obstruction (FBAO) and list some common causes
- state the signs that an adult is choking due to a FBAO
- describe the procedure for managing the choking adult.

4.2 Introduction

A FBAO, as the name implies, is a mechanical obstruction of the airway occurring anywhere between the mouth and carina (where the left and right bronchi split from the trachea). Common causes include [Walls, 2012]:
- foreign bodies
- blood
- secretions
- teeth
- vomit.

It is not known how common FBAO is in adults. Death from FBAO is thankfully rare, mostly because airway obstructions that cause choking are witnessed [Olasveengen, 2021]. In England and Wales, around 270 people die each year as a result of a foreign body (FB) in the respiratory tract. Most of these are over 65 years of age [ONS, 2021].

4.3 Recognition

The signs of choking in an adult depend on the severity of the airway obstruction that has occurred. Typically, the episode will have

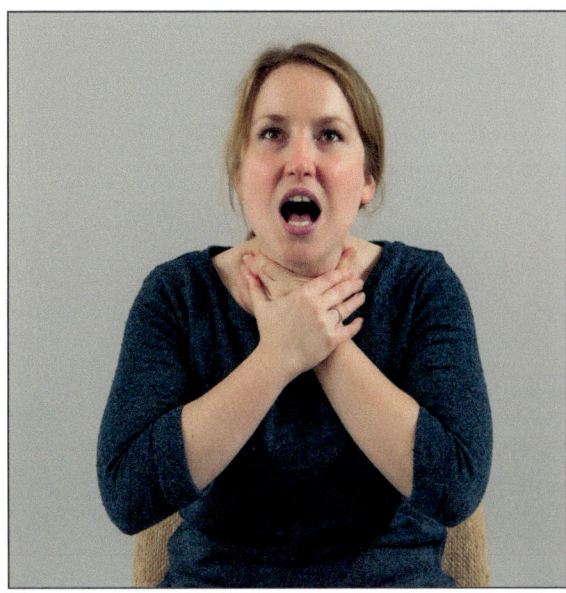

Figure 10.15 A choking victim clutching their neck

occurred while eating, will cause a sudden onset of respiratory distress, is often associated with coughing and gagging, and if the patient is still conscious, they may clutch their neck (Figure 10.15).

In the case of a mild airway obstruction, if you ask the patient if they are choking, they will still be able to speak and confirm that this is the case. They will also be able to breathe and cough.

However, in cases of severe airway obstruction, the patient will be unable to speak, so may only be able to respond to you by nodding their head in response to your question about whether they are choking. Any attempts at coughing will be silent, and if this continues the patient will lose consciousness, possibly before your arrival [RCUK, 2021a].

4.4 Management

Start by determining the severity of the obstruction. In adults, this is typically determined by the patient's response to the question 'Are you choking?' A patient who can reply 'Yes', i.e. can speak, cough and breathe, is classified as mild, whereas the patient who is clutching their throat, is unable to speak and who cannot breathe falls into the severe category.

Chapter 10 – Airway

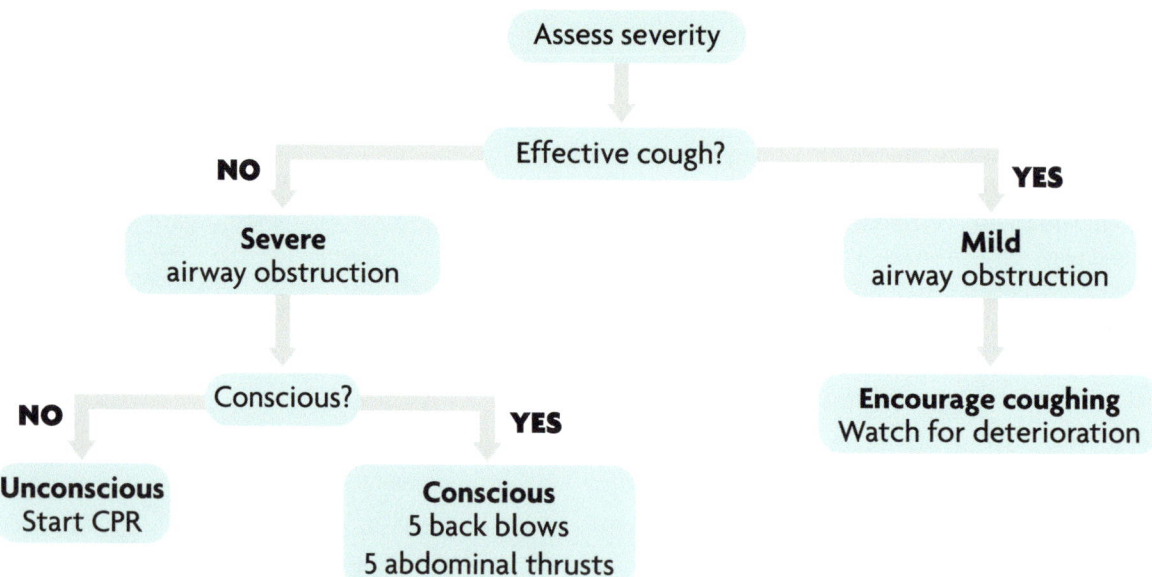

Figure 10.16 The FBAO algorithm for adults

4.4.1 Conscious and choking

If the patient is coughing, do not perform any interventions other than encouraging the patient to continue coughing.

If the obstruction is severe, administer up to five back blows, by standing just to the side and slightly behind the patient, leaning them forward, and then administering sharp blows between the shoulder blades with the heel of one hand.

If this fails, move on to abdominal thrusts. Position yourself behind the patient and place a clenched fist between the umbilicus (belly button) and the ribcage. Grasp the fist with your other hand and pull sharply upwards and inwards up to five times.

Repeat the back blows/abdominal thrusts until the obstruction is relieved, or the patient becomes unconscious [Olasveengen, 2021].

4.4.2 Unconscious and choking

Lay the patient on their back and start chest compressions and ventilations at a rate of 30:2. Do not attempt blind finger sweeps in an attempt to remove unseen solid material as this may make the airway obstruction worse. However, if there is material clearly visible in the mouth, suction or a finger sweep can be used to remove the obstruction [Olasveengen, 2021].

4.4.3 Adult FBAO management algorithm

Figure 10.16 shows the FBAO management algorithm, which summarises the explanation provided in the previous section.

5 Choking in the paediatric patient

5.1 Learning objective

By the end of this section you will be able to:
- demonstrate how to manage a choking paediatric patient with a FBAO.

5.2 Introduction

It is estimated that around 20 children aged 0–14 years of age per 100,000 population will experience at least one food-related choking episode each year. It is more common in boys and children under 1 year of age [Chapin, 2013]. Since most choking episodes involving infants and children are witnessed by an adult, intervention can commence straight away, as long as the adult knows the correct action to take [RCUK, 2021b].

5.3 The paediatric airway

Children's airways more readily obstruct than those of adults, and are particularly sensitive to soft-tissue swelling. With a tracheal diameter of around 4 mm in infants compared with 8 mm in the adult, small amounts of swelling dramatically increase airflow resistance and the work of breathing required to maintain adequate ventilation.

The most dramatic differences are found in infants. By the age of 10–12 years, children have mostly adult anatomy, albeit smaller in size [Walls, 2012; Benger, 2009]. Other differences include the following [AAP, 2018; RCUK, 2021b]:

- Infants have a large, prominent occiput (back of the skull), which results in neck flexion if they are laid supine on a flat surface. Use padding under the torso to maintain a neutral alignment.
- The glottic opening is at the level of the first cervical vertebra (C1) in infants, descending to C3–C4 by the age of 5 years, resulting in a high, anterior larynx.
- The epiglottis is horseshoe (or omega) shaped, floppy and proportionally larger than that of an adult.
- The tongue is proportionally larger than that of adults, occupying more of the mouth.
- The narrowest portion of the airway in children is at the level of the cricoid ring due to their funnel-shaped larynx, compared to the more cylindrical shape of the adult larynx.

5.4 Recognition

Most choking episodes in children and infants usually occur when a FB enters their airway during feeding or playing and are often witnessed by a carer. However, remember to ask about any recent history of playing with or eating small objects and consider choking in any child with a sudden onset of breathing problems.

Choking due to a FBAO will result in a sudden onset of respiratory distress and is often accompanied with coughing, gagging or stridor.

The severity of the obstruction can be determined by the effectiveness of the patient's ability to cough. An effective cough is better than external manoeuvres, so an actively coughing child should be encouraged to continue to do so. Other signs of a mild obstruction include [Voorde, 2021]:

- crying/verbal response to questions
- long cough
- able to take breaths before coughing
- fully alert.

Contrast this with signs of a severe airway obstruction and an ineffective cough:

- unable to verbalise
- quiet/silent cough
- unable to breathe
- cyanosis
- decreasing level of consciousness.

5.5 Management

The management of the choking paediatric patient depends on their ability to effectively cough and on whether they are conscious or unconscious (Figure 10.17) [Voorde, 2021].

5.5.1 Conscious and choking infants

If the infant is conscious but their cough is ineffective or absent, deliver back blows. Sit on a chair or kneel on the floor and place the infant across your lap in a prone (face-down) position. Support their head with the thumb and fingers of one hand at the angle of their jaw, taking care not to compress the soft tissues. Administer up to five sharp blows between their scapulae (shoulder blades) with the heel of your other hand.

If these fail, turn the infant on to their back with their head downwards. Locate the landmarks for chest compression (i.e. one finger-width above the xiphisternum) and administer up to five chest compressions, making them sharper and slower than those administered during cardiac arrest.

Continue to alternate between back blows and chest thrusts until either the obstruction is cleared or the infant becomes unconscious.

Chapter 10 – Airway

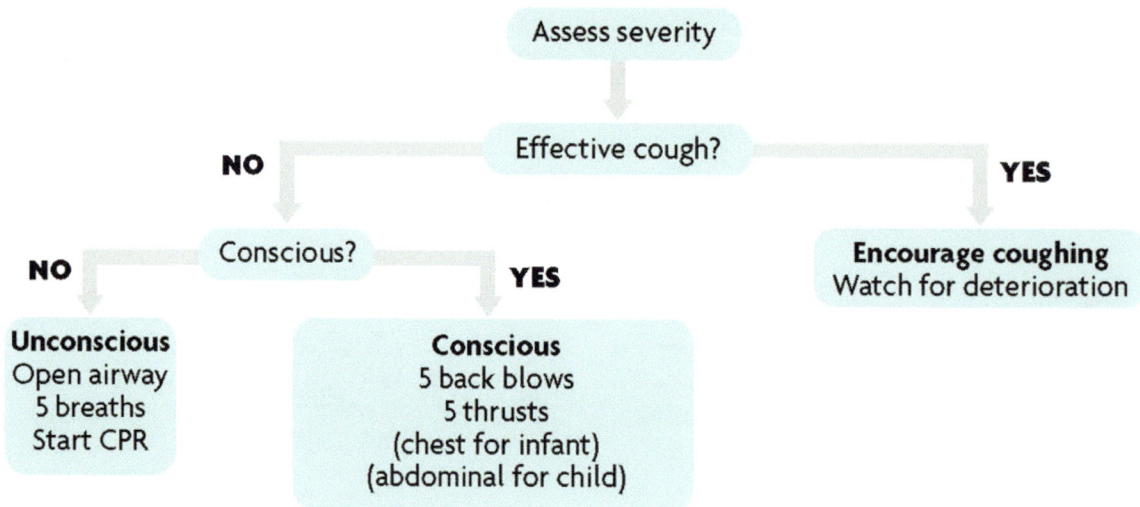

Figure 10.17 Management of FBAO in the paediatric patient

5.5.2 Conscious and choking children

If the child is conscious but their cough is ineffective or absent, deliver back blows. Support them in a head-down position and administer up to five inter-scapular blows.

If this does not clear the obstruction, administer abdominal thrusts by standing behind the child and leaning them forward. Place a clenched fist midway between the xiphisternum and umbilicus (belly button). Grasp the fist with your other hand and pull inwards and upwards, up to five times.

Continue to alternate between back blows and abdominal thrusts until either the obstruction is cleared or the child becomes unconscious.

5.5.3 Unconscious and choking

If a child or infant becomes, or is, unconscious, place them on their back with appropriate padding to maintain an open airway. Check the mouth for a visible obstruction and make a single attempt to remove it if a FB is visible.

Attempt to ventilate, but if this does not cause chest expansion try repositioning the head and try again. If after five attempts you still cannot ventilate the child or infant, move on to chest compressions and alternate with further ventilations using a ratio of 15:2.

11 Breathing

1 Respiratory system physiology

1.1 Learning objective

By the end of this section you will be able to:
- describe and explain the function of the respiratory system.

1.2 Introduction

In Chapter 10, 'Airway', you learnt about the structure (or anatomy) of the respiratory system, but it is also important to understand its function (physiology). Functionally, the respiratory system is split into two portions [Tortora, 2017]:
- **Conducting portion:** This is made up of the interconnecting cavities and tubes starting at the mouth and nose and ending at the terminal bronchioles. These filter, warm and moisten the air and transfer it to the lungs and out again.
- **Respiratory portion:** This is made up of the tissues inside the lungs that exchange the gas. It consists of the respiratory bronchioles, alveolar ducts and sacs, and the alveoli. This is where gas exchange between the air and blood occurs.

These portions combined enable the respiratory system to perform its functions, which are:
- gas exchange, which imports oxygen (O_2), which is taken up into the blood and delivered to the body's cells, and expires the waste gas, carbon dioxide (CO_2)
- assisting in the regulation of blood acidity levels
- removing small amounts of heat and water
- filtering inspired air, producing vocal sounds and containing receptors that provide a sense of smell.

1.3 Respiration

Respiration is the process of gas exchange in the body (mainly of oxygen and carbon dioxide). It consists of three steps [Tortora, 2017]:
- **Pulmonary ventilation:** The process of moving air into and out of the lungs. It is divided into inspiration (inhalation), when air is moved into the lungs, and expiration (exhalation), when air is moved out of the lungs.
- **External respiration:** The exchange of gases between the alveoli of the lungs and the blood inside the pulmonary capillaries.
- **Internal respiration:** The exchange of gases between the blood in capillaries around the body and tissue cells.

1.4 The lungs

In order to understand ventilation and external respiration, we need to cover a little more anatomy. Recall from section 1, 'Anatomy', in Chapter 10, 'Airway', that the lungs extend from the diaphragm to just above the clavicles. The left lung is smaller than the right due to the space taken up by the heart. It also has only two lobes, the upper and lower lobes, whereas the right lung has three: the upper, lower and middle lobes [Tortora, 2017].

The lungs are divided into lobes by deep grooves known as fissures. Both lungs have an oblique fissure, but the right lung also has a horizontal fissure (Figures 11.1, 11.2 and 11.3).

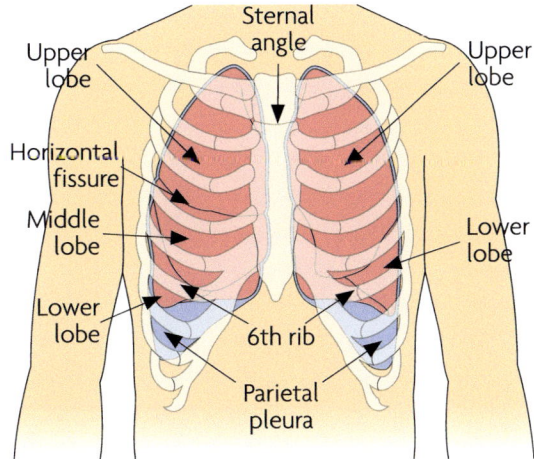

Figure 11.1 Anterior view of the lungs in relation to surface anatomy

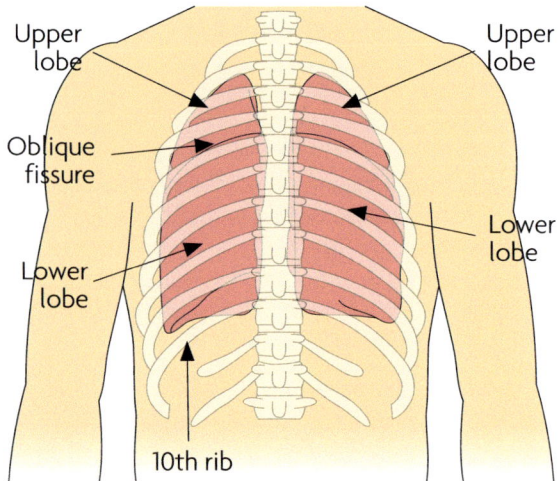

Figure 11.2 Posterior view of the lungs in relation to surface anatomy

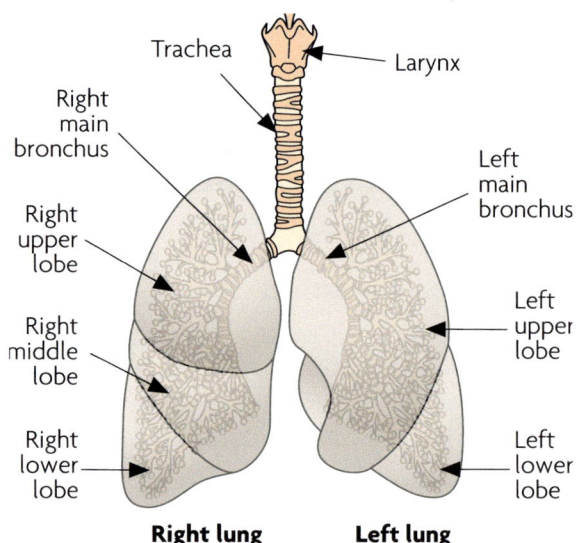

Figure 11.4 The lower respiratory tract showing the left and right bronchi

1.4.1 Lobes, lobules and alveoli

Each lobe of the lungs has its own secondary branch (bronchus), branching from the right and left primary bronchi (Figure 11.4).

These in turn divide into tertiary bronchi, each supplying a segment of lung called a bronchopulmonary segment. Within these are many much smaller components known as lobules, within which are contained three to five respiratory units, which is where the gas exchange occurs. Respiratory units (or acini) emerge from the terminal bronchioles and consist of several respiratory bronchioles, which subdivide into alveolar ducts and, finally, the alveoli [Hickin, 2015].

Alveoli

The alveoli are cup-shaped pouches with very thin walls that enable the exchange of oxygen and carbon dioxide with the pulmonary capillaries that surround them. There are around 150–400 million in each normal lung, creating a surface area for gaseous exchange of approximately 50–100m^2 [Hickin, 2015].

1.5 Mechanics of breathing

1.5.1 Air pressure

Air moves into and out of the lungs because ventilation changes the pressure inside the alveoli. This is achieved by changing the volume of the thoracic cavity (the contents of the body surrounded by the ribs and diaphragm). As the volume inside this cavity increases, the pressure inside decreases (a relationship known as Boyle's Law). This causes the lungs to expand, increasing their volume and so decreasing the alveolar pressure.

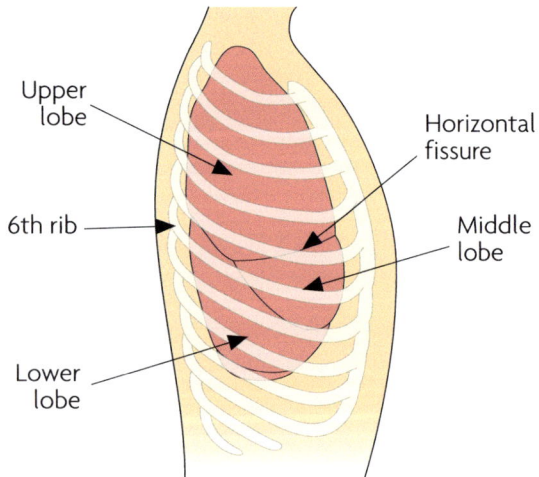

Figure 11.3 Lateral view of the lungs in relation to surface anatomy

Since air moves from areas of high pressure to low pressure, once the pressure inside the alveoli drops below that outside the body, i.e. atmospheric pressure, air enters the lungs. At the end of inspiration, the volume of the thoracic cavity decreases, and the pressure rises; once it becomes higher than that of atmospheric pressure, air leaves the lungs [Hickin, 2015].

1.5.2 Inspiration

During normal, quiet respiration, most of the work of respiration is undertaken by the diaphragm. This is a dome-shaped muscle that seals the thoracic cavity from the abdomen. When it contracts, it flattens and descends, increasing the volume inside the thoracic cavity, and is responsible for about 75% of the air entering the lungs.

The remaining 25% of air entering the lungs is as a result of the external intercostal muscles contracting, which pulls the ribs upwards and outwards like a bucket handle [Tortora, 2017].

1.5.3 Expiration

During normal, quiet respiration, expiration is a passive process as no muscles are involved. This is because of elastic recoil, a property of the thoracic wall and the lungs to 'spring back' to their original position after they are stretched by the muscles of inspiration.

1.5.4 Forceful breathing

When exercising and in other instances when the body requires more oxygen, additional, accessory, muscles can be used to aid inspiration and expiration (Figure 11.5). These can often be seen in use by patients in respiratory distress.

1.6 Gas exchange

You have already read that gas moves from areas of high pressure to low, and it turns out that this is the case even for a mixture of gases. Take room air, which you are breathing in. It is made up of the following (percentages are approximate) [Tortora, 2017]:
- oxygen (O_2): 20.9%
- nitrogen (N_2): 78.6%
- carbon dioxide (CO_2): 0.04%
- other gases/water vapour: 0.46%

The pressure each of the gases exerts to make up the pressure of air is known as the gas's partial pressure. For example, the partial pressure of oxygen (PO_2) in the air is 21 kilopascals (kPa).

Each gas acts independently of the others, so in the alveoli, oxygen moves from an area of higher pressure (the alveoli) to an area of lower oxygen pressure (the pulmonary circulation), by a process known as diffusion.

1.6.1 Diffusion

Diffusion is a process by which molecules (such as oxygen and carbon dioxide) move around. It has two key characteristics [Hickin, 2015]:
- Diffusion occurs from areas of high concentration to areas of low concentration.
- Diffusion continues until both areas have the same concentration of molecules.

Oxygen diffuses from the alveoli into the pulmonary circulation, whereas carbon dioxide has a higher partial pressure inside the pulmonary circulation so moves across into the alveoli, where it can be expired. In this way, oxygen is taken up by the body and the waste gas, carbon dioxide, is removed [Tortora, 2017].

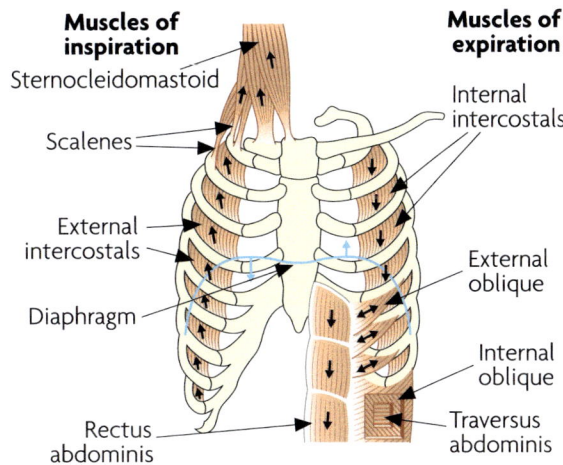

Figure 11.5 Muscles of inspiration and expiration

1.7 Control of breathing

The muscles of respiration are dependent on the nervous system to tell them to contract and relax. This is achieved through two types of nervous system control [Tortora, 2017]:

- **Voluntary (or conscious) control:** This originates in the cerebral cortex and is the way you can control your breathing by holding your breath or controlling the flow of air in order to play a wind instrument, for example. In addition, other centres in the brain, such as the hypothalamus and limbic system, can stimulate respiration, allowing laughing and crying to affect the breathing pattern.
- **Automatic control:** This originates from groups of nerve cells (neurons) in the brain stem (mainly the pons and medulla). The neurons in the medulla are responsible for the basic rhythm of breathing and send impulses to the inspiratory muscles via the phrenic and intercostal nerves. Expiratory neurons generally become active only during forceful breathing, such as when exercising.

The respiratory centres containing these inspiratory and expiratory neurons are influenced by sensory input from nerves around the body. For example, stretch receptors prevent the lungs from being overinflated and others are linked to receptors that can detect movement, stimulating the respiratory centres to increase ventilation during exercise.

Breathing is also regulated by the partial pressures of oxygen (PaO_2) and carbon dioxide ($PaCO_2$), and hydrogen ion concentration (pH) in the blood. $PaCO_2$ is the most important and has the most profound effect on respiration. Special sensory neurons called chemoreceptors are located close to the medulla (central chemoreceptors) and in the walls of the aortic and carotid arteries [Tortora, 2017].

Note: The extra 'a' in PaO_2 and $PaCO_2$ denotes the partial pressure of oxygen and carbon dioxide in arterial blood.

2 Using medical gases safely

2.1 Learning objectives

By the end of this section you will be able to:
- describe dangers of using compressed gas
- outline the safe use, storage and handling of medical gases
- state the guidelines for the use of oxygen therapy, including:
  - indications
  - contra-indications
- outline the safe use of entonox including:
  - the properties of entonox
  - complications of environmental temperature with regard to Entonox
  - the benefits of Entonox therapy
  - indications
  - cautions and contra-indications
- explain the use of facial barriers, the bag-valve-mask and mechanical ventilators.

2.2 Introduction

There are two main medical gases in use by ambulance services: oxygen and Entonox (Figure 11.6). These gases are compressed into cylinders of varying sizes. Typically, you will have a small, portable cylinder for carrying into a patient's house, but there are likely to be larger, heavier cylinders which are fitted to the ambulance and are generally removed only when empty and they need replacing.

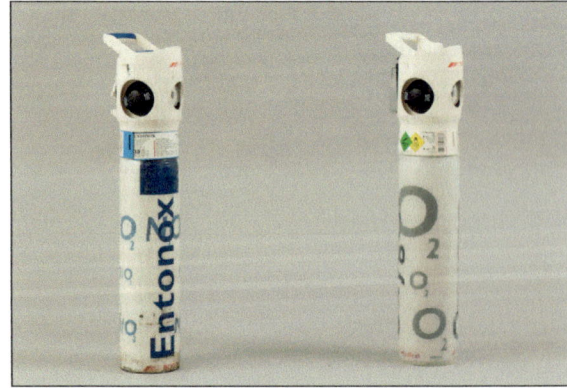

Figure 11.6 Medical gases. Entonox on the left, oxygen on the right

Note: Entonox is usually only provided as the smaller, portable cylinder.

Oxygen behaves differently from air, compressed air, nitrogen and other inert gases. It is very reactive. Pure oxygen, at high pressure, such as from a cylinder, can react violently with common materials such as oil and grease. Other materials may catch fire spontaneously. Nearly all materials including textiles, rubber and even metals will burn vigorously in oxygen [HSE, 2013b].

Even a small increase in the oxygen level in the air to 24% can create a dangerous situation. It becomes easier to start a fire, which will then burn hotter and more fiercely than in normal air. It may be almost impossible to put the fire out. A leaking valve or hose in a poorly ventilated room or confined space can quickly increase the oxygen concentration to a dangerous level.

The main causes of fires and explosions when using oxygen are [HSE, 2013b]:
- oxygen enrichment from leaking equipment
- use of materials not compatible with oxygen
- use of oxygen in equipment not designed for oxygen service
- incorrect or careless operation of oxygen equipment.

2.3 *Medical gas cylinder storage*

Most ambulance stations have a medical gas cylinder store (Figure 11.7). It should meet all of the following requirements [DoH, 2006]:

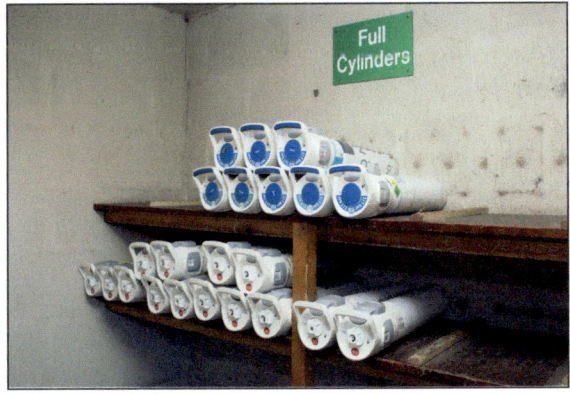

Figure 11.7 An ambulance station medical gas cylinder store

- on ground level, as close as possible to delivery point
- clearly identifiable, so it can easily be located in an emergency
- not close to any installation that may cause a fire risk (such as the fuel pump)
- have a level floor, made of concrete or other non-combustible material
- well-ventilated
- contain only medical gases
- adequate means of securing large cylinders to prevent falling
- clear and separate areas for full and empty cylinders
- kept free from naked flames and marked with signage such as 'No Smoking'
- not prone to excessively hot or cold temperatures
- contain shelving to store smaller cylinders horizontally
- be secure enough to prevent theft and misuse.

Depending on local arrangements, you may be able to replace your empty oxygen cylinder from this store. However, it is probably more practicable to exchange empty cylinders with the ambulance on scene.

2.4 *Anatomy of a medical gas cylinder*

Integrated valve cylinders (Figure 11.8) are the most common type found in UK ambulance services and are covered in this section. You may find, however, that your service still uses the older-style cylinders, which require a regulator head to be fitted before they can be used, and you should seek guidance on their use.

There is a British Standard (BS EN 1089-3:2011) relating to the labelling of medical gases to ensure that they are easy to identify and so inappropriate administration is avoided [BSI, 2011]. Medical gases always have a white body, but sometimes have different-coloured collars to indicate the type of gas. The most commonly encountered gases that you will find while responding are oxygen (white collar) and Entonox (blue and white collar).

Chapter 11 – *Breathing*

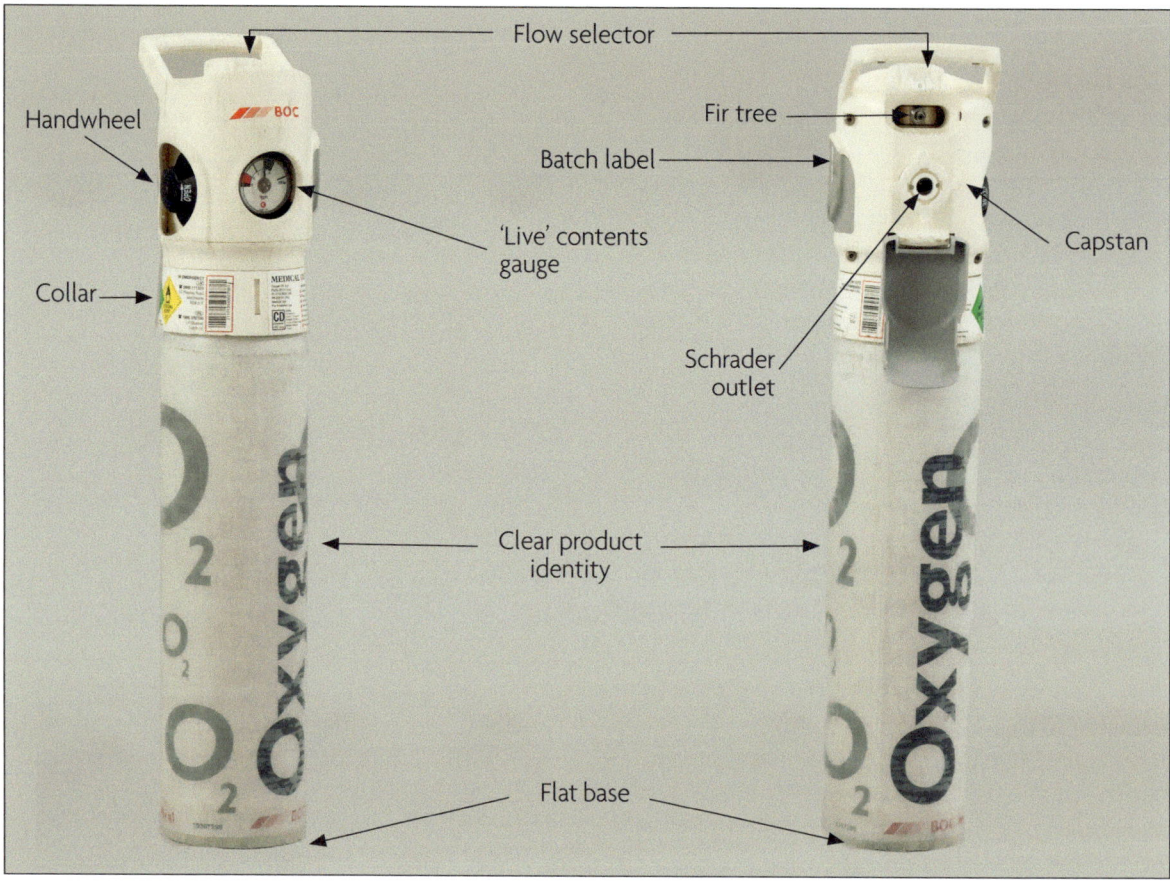

Figure 11.8 Example of portable integrated valve oxygen cylinder

Important components of the cylinder are [BOC, 2022]:
- collar
  - Identifies the gas type and/or gas mixture if there is more than one gas present
- flow selector
  - desired flow rate can be selected by rotating the dial
  - positive 'click' between flow rates to ensure correct setting is chosen
- 'live' contents gauge
  - shows contents of cylinder, even when turned off
  - green = full
  - red = low/empty
- handwheel
  - simple on/off dial – no spanner required
  - turn anti-clockwise to open
  - turn clockwise to close
- clear product identity
  - name of gas is written on cylinder collar and body
- flat base
  - easier to handle
  - improves stability
- firtree
  - attachment point for oxygen tubing
- batch label
  - located on guard or collar
  - shows expiry date
  - required when reporting cylinder defect
- Schrader outlet
  - push-fit connector for other methods of administration/connection to artificial ventilators
  - gas-specific to avoid inadvertent inappropriate administration
  - out sleeve (capstan) can be twisted to release.

Using medical gases safely

2.5 Safety first

Prior to using a medical gas, there are a number of safety checks required [BOC, 2022]:
- Make sure your hands are clean. If you have used an alcohol-based hand rub, ensure that it has evaporated completely.
- Check the cylinder to ensure it is clean and free from damage.
- Ensure the cylinder is free from oil and grease, especially around the Schrader and firtree outlets.
- Both oxygen and Entonox are non-flammable, but strongly support combustion. Keep away from naked flames, sources of ignition and combustible materials.

If the medical gas is Entonox, check that it has not been allowed to get too cold. Below -6°C the nitrous oxide will separate from the gas mixture. To prevent this, it should be stored above 10°C for at least 24 hours prior to use. If this is not possible and the bottle is of a portable size, warm the bottle to 10°C and then invert three times prior to use to mix the gases.

2.6 Preparing a new cylinder for use

Procedure

The following steps apply to both oxygen and Entonox cylinders [BOC, 2022; BOC, 2013]:

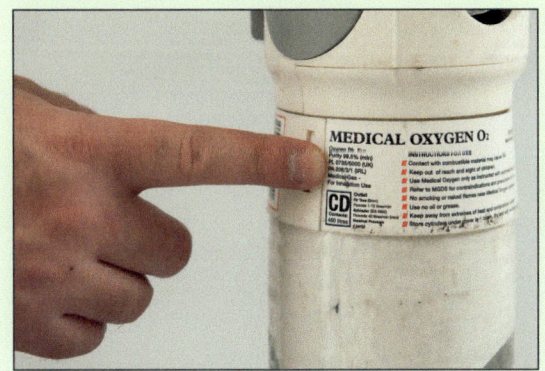

1. Ensure you have the correct medical gas by checking the cylinder label.

Procedure – *cont*

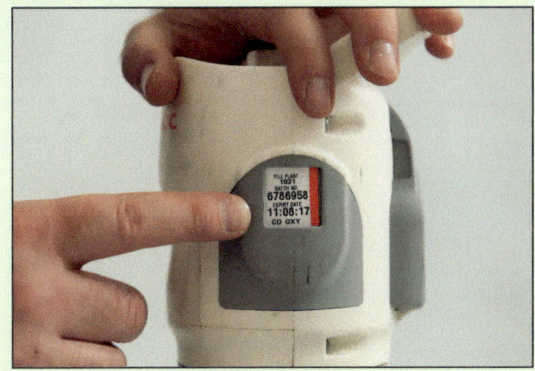

2. Check the expiry date on the batch label fitted to the cylinder.

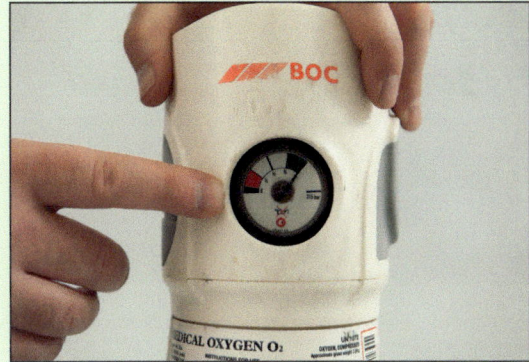

3. Make sure the contents gauge is in the green zone. This indicates that the cylinder is full.

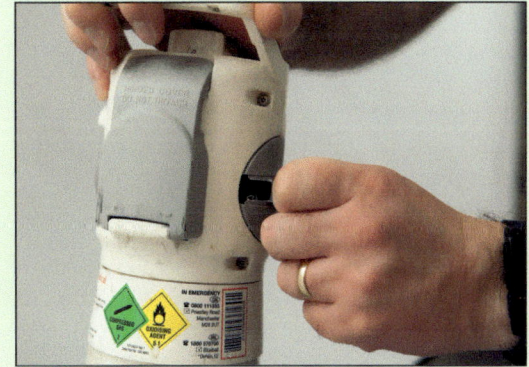

4. Remove the tamper-evident handwheel cover by pulling the tear ring.

Chapter 11 – Breathing

Procedure – *cont*

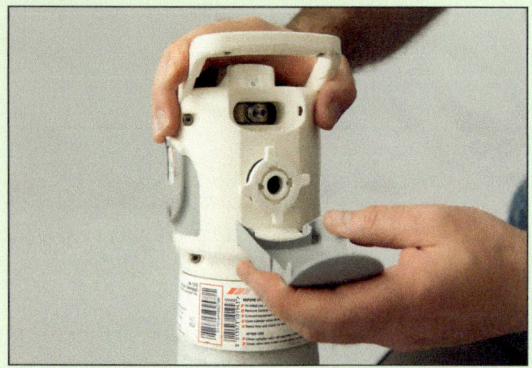

5. Remove the valve outlet cover. Pull the grey cover downwards. It stays attached to the cylinder.

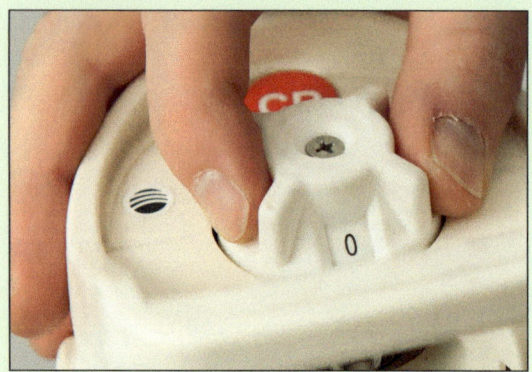

6. Ensure the flow selector on top of the cylinder is set to zero and the handwheel is turned off before connecting equipment.

2.7 Oxygen delivery devices

The firtree connector (Figure 11.9) is used to connect oxygen tubing to the cylinder, which in turn can provide oxygen to a BVM, oxygen-driven nebuliser, oxygen masks and nasal cannulae (Figure 11.10).

Note: The masks and nasal cannulae all require the patient to be spontaneously breathing in order to work. If the patient is not breathing effectively, they require assisted and artificial ventilation, most commonly with a BVM.

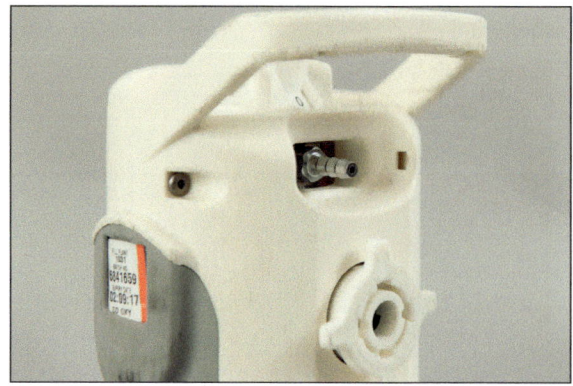

Figure 11.9 Oxygen firtree connector

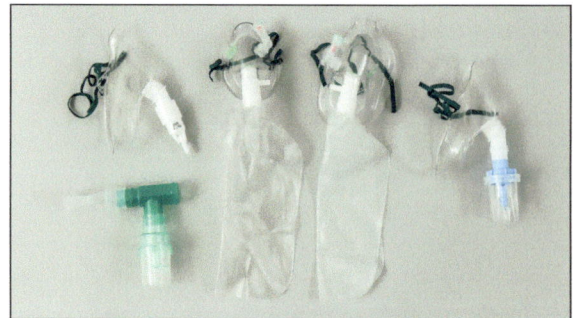

Figure 11.10 A variety of devices to administer oxygen

2.7.1 Preparing an oxygen cylinder for administration

Procedure

Follow the steps below to provide oxygen from the appropriate oxygen delivery device [BOC, 2022]:

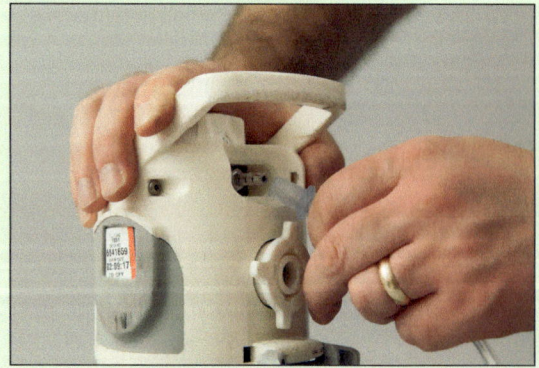

1. Attach tubing from mask or nasal cannulae to the firtree outlet. Ensure the tubing is pushed on securely.

Using medical gases safely

2.7.2 Supplemental oxygen delivery devices

Non-rebreathe mask

This mask is used when the patient requires a high concentration of oxygen. At 15 l/min, the mask can deliver up to 85% inspired oxygen. It consists of a mask and reservoir bag that is fitted with a one-way valve, ensuring that the patient can only inhale oxygen from it and not exhale into the bag. The bag must be inflated in order to ensure maximum inspired oxygen.

Medium concentration face mask (simple face mask)

This face mask has ports on either side to allow room air to be drawn inside. At 10 l/min, it will deliver around 40% oxygen, but this is variable depending on how well fitting the mask is.

Venturi mask

This mask also draws in (or entrains) room air, but allows for more accurate oxygen delivery than the medium concentration face mask. It comes with a variety of spigots, which are capable of delivering a variety of oxygen concentrations. The percentage of oxygen and flow rate required are usually clearly marked on the spigot. They are particularly useful when providing oxygen to patients with COPD.

Nasal cannulae

These deliver oxygen via two nasal prongs, which sit just inside the patient's nostrils. Oxygen flow rates are typically limited to 1–4 l/min as higher rates lead to irritation of the nasal lining. They are often used by patients on long-term oxygen therapy and may be preferred by patients who do not tolerate a face mask.

Nebuliser

This is used to deliver aerosolised drugs. The pressurised chamber when powered by oxygen turns the liquid drug inside (usually salbutamol or ipratropium) into a mist (i.e. aerosolises the drug), which is then inhaled by the patient. Some nebulisers (particularly if the patient has one at home) are powered using compressed room air.

Procedure – *cont*

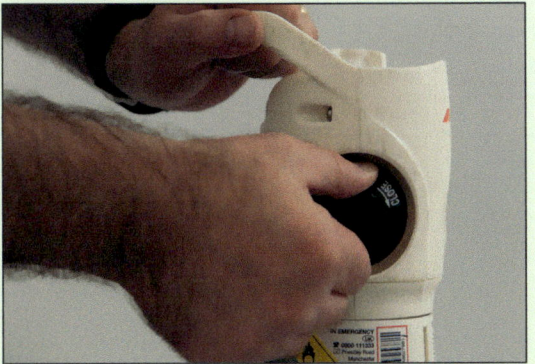

2. Slowly turn on the cylinder by rotating the handwheel anti-clockwise until it comes to a complete stop. Do not use excessive force.

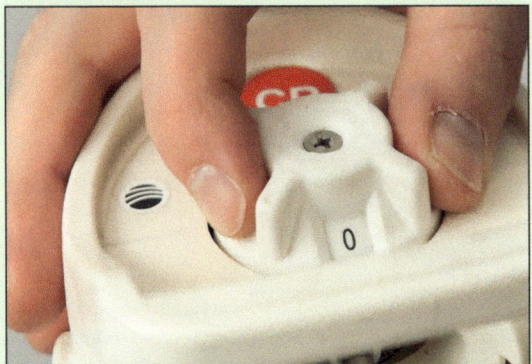

3. Set the prescribed flow by rotating the flow selector dial. Ensure that the correct flow rate number is clearly visible in the flow selector window. Check the gas is flowing.

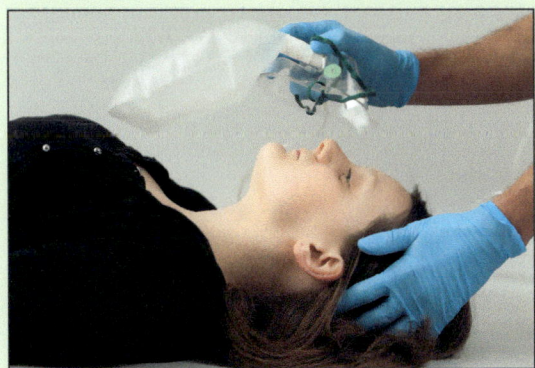

4. Place oxygen mask or nasal cannulae on the patient.

Chapter 11 – Breathing

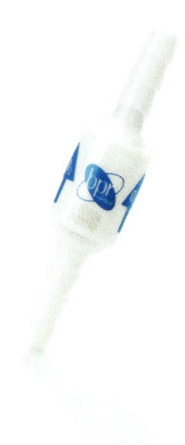

Figure 11.11   A Firesafe

Firesafe
You may notice a small device inserted into a patient's tubing if they are on home oxygen (Figure 11.11). This is a Firesafe, a cannula valve that is designed to cut the oxygen supply to the patient in the event of a fire. It will not affect the oxygen flow to the patient as long as it is inserted the correct way around (the arrow shows the direction of gas flow).

2.8   Assisted ventilation

Patients who are breathing inadequately (for example, because they have a slow respiratory rate or an irregular pattern of respiration) and patients whose breathing is too shallow or who are not breathing at all require assisted ventilation. Assisted ventilation can be provided with a pocket mask, BVM or oxygen-powered ventilation device. In most circumstances, you will be using a BVM.

2.8.1   Gastric distension

In contrast to the normal way we breathe (i.e. the negative pressure inside the chest cavity draws air into the chest), assisted and artificial ventilation require the use of PPV, i.e. actively blowing air into the lungs. This has some disadvantages as high inflation pressures can result in air going into the stomach instead of the lungs, leading to gastric distension. This is more likely if:
- high inflation pressures are used
- ventilations are performed too fast
- the airway is partially obstructed.

A distended stomach is bad for the patient as vomit can rise up into the airway and be inhaled (aspirated). It also pushes up the diaphragm, reducing the amount of space for lung expansion.

2.8.2   Mouth-to-mouth ventilation

The most basic ventilation device is your mouth and lungs, using mouth-to-mouth ventilation. However, healthcare professionals and members of the public are sometimes reluctant to perform mouth-to-mouth on people they do not know. In addition, there are risks relating to exposure to blood and other body fluids through direct contact with the patient's mouth and nose. In certain cases, direct mouth-to-mouth contact is not appropriate, such as in cases of poisoning [RCUK, 2021a].

Procedure

Take the following steps to perform mouth-to-mouth ventilation [SJA, 2021]:
1. Place the patient on their back (supine).
2. Open the airway using a head tilt–chin lift, or jaw thrust if cervical spine injury is suspected.
3. Pinch the patient's nose to close the nostrils.
4. Take a breath and seal your lips over the patient's mouth.
5. Blow steadily for about one second, just enough to make the chest rise.
6. While maintaining the head tilt–chin lift, take your mouth away from the patient and watch the chest fall.
7. Repeat, aiming to provide a breath to an adult every six seconds.

Note: If the patient is not breathing and has no signs of life, commence chest compressions, not ventilations (this is covered in Chapter 20, 'Cardiac Arrest').

2.8.3 Facial shields

To provide some protection for yourself, it may be possible to use a face shield, which provides a plastic barrier between you and the patient. Face shields are also fitted with a filter that fits over the patient's mouth. As with mouth-to-mouth ventilation, this method does not allow for the administration of supplemental oxygen. The technique is the same for mouth-to-mouth ventilation.

2.8.4 Mouth-to-mask ventilation

Using a pocket mask to provide mouth-to-mask ventilation uses your lungs as before, but does not require direct contact with the patient's mouth. The one-way valve also prevents you coming into contact with blood and secretions from the patient's mouth. You use both hands to hold the mask to the patient's face, which makes it easier to get a good seal and deliver effective ventilations (Figure 11.12).

Some pocket masks also have an oxygen port, allowing administration of supplemental oxygen. Even with pocket masks without an oxygen port, oxygen tubing can be placed under one side of the mask.

Procedure

Take the following steps to perform mouth-to-mask ventilation [RCUK, 2021a]:
1. Place the patient supine with their head in the sniffing position (neck slightly flexed and head extended).
2. Apply the mask to the patient's face using the thumbs of both hands.
3. Grip the jaw and perform a jaw thrust, while pressing down with the thumbs to make a tight seal.
4. Blow gently for one second through the valve and watch the chest rise.
5. Stop inflation and watch the chest fall.
6. Repeat every six seconds or as instructed by the senior clinician.

Leaks between the face and pocket mask can be reduced by increasing the jaw thrust, or changing finger position and pressure being applied. Oxygen, if available, should run at 10 l/min.

2.8.5 BVM ventilation

The BVM consists of a self-inflating bag, one-way valve and mask. When used without oxygen, it delivers room air (21% oxygen). This can be increased to 45% when high-flow oxygen is attached, but it should generally be used with a reservoir bag attached, as this can result in oxygen concentrations of around 85% (Figure 11.13) with oxygen supplied at 10 l/min [RCUK, 2021a].

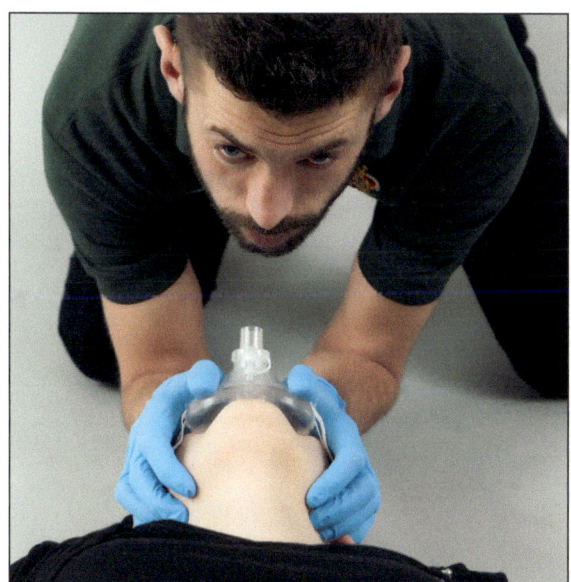

Figure 11.12 Mouth-to-mask ventilation

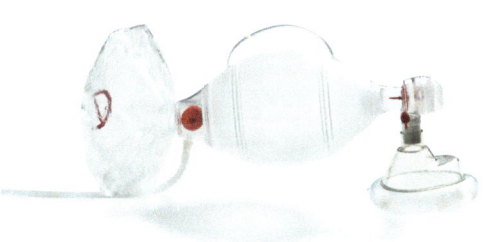

Figure 11.13 BVM with oxygen reservoir bag attached and inflated

Chapter 11 – Breathing

The BVM can be used by one person, but this requires considerable skill. Where possible, a two-person technique is generally recommended [Monsieurs, 2015]. In addition, an oropharyngeal airway should be inserted prior to using a BVM.

Indications
- Patient requiring ventilation.

Contra-indications
- None in the emergency situation.

Advantages
- Can be performed by one clinician (although two-person technique preferred).
- No need for complex equipment.
- Supplemental oxygen is easy to administer.

Disadvantages
- Difficult technique to master and maintain.
- Challenging to perform in some patient groups, for example obese or bearded patients, or those with a maxillofacial injury.

Procedure - single-handed BVM ventilation

Take the following steps to perform single-handed BVM ventilation:
1. Don appropriate PPE, and undertake appropriate hand hygiene.
2. Open the airway and position the patient's head into the 'sniffing the morning air' position (head extended and neck flexed) unless they have a suspected cervical spine injury. In this case a jaw thrust can be used to minimise movement.

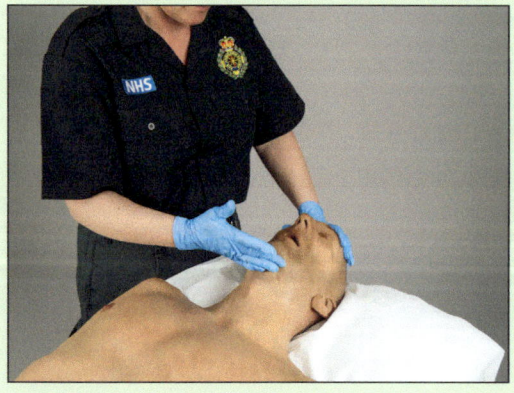

Procedure – cont
3. Perform a quick visual check of the oropharynx to see if you can detect a foreign body, unless there is an indication in the history that a foreign body might be present, in which case laryngoscopy should be performed by the senior clinician.

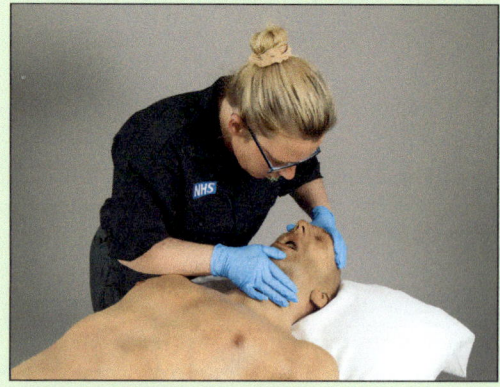

4. The ventilating clinician should locate themselves at the head of the patient, facing the feet.

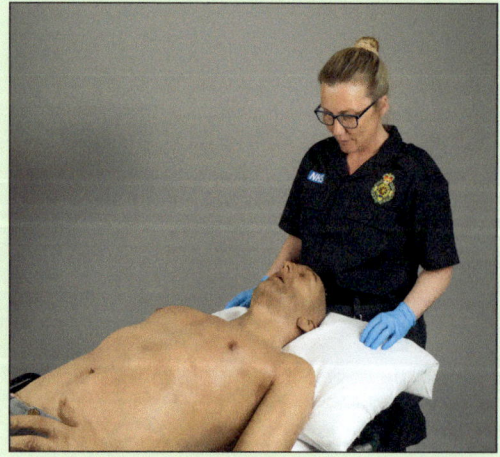

5. Use the mnemonic ROMAN to assess the patient for signs that they may be difficult to ventilate with a BVM:
    - Radiation/restriction
    - Obesity/obstruction/obstructive sleep apnoea
    - Mask seal/Mallampati/male sex
    - Age more than 55 years
    - No teeth.

Using medical gases safely

Procedure – *cont*

6. Insert an appropriately sized OPA, or NPA(s) if an OPA cannot be used for any reason.

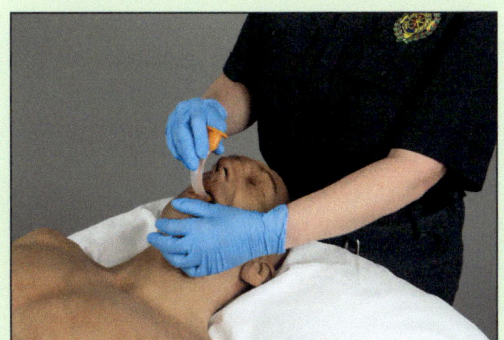

7. Select the most appropriately sized mask. The lower edge of the mask should rest in the groove between the patient's chin and lower lip, and the upper edge should rest across the bridge of the nose.

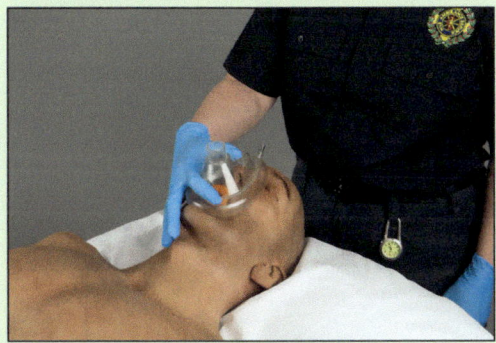

8. Connect mask to bag, capnography (where available) and oxygen supply.
9. Position the mask on the patient's face and ensure an adequate seal. Apply the mask to the groove formed by the chin and lower lip first, and then the bridge of the nose.
10. Form a 'C' shape with the thumb and index finger and rest this on top of the mask; place the middle and ring fingers on the ridge of the jaw and the little finger behind the angle of the jaw.

Procedure – *cont*

11. Gently squeeze the bag just enough to see the chest rise. Each ventilation should consist of an inspiratory component lasting 1 second. If capnography is available, aim for a ventilatory rate that results in normal end-tidal carbon dioxide (normocapnia). Otherwise, ventilate at a rate of 10–12 ventilations per minute.

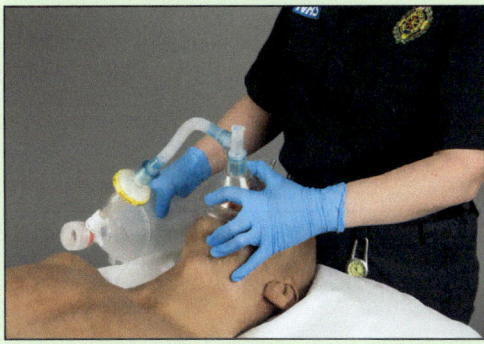

12. If ventilation is difficult, try gently flexing and extending the airway until you can successfully ventilate. If this fails, the senior clinician may consider upgrading the airway to a supraglottic airway device.
13. Frequently reassess the adequacy of the ventilation and escalate airway management if required.
14. Document the procedure.

Chapter 11 – Breathing

Procedure - two-handed BVM ventilation

Take the following steps to perform two-handed BVM ventilation:
1. Don appropriate PPE, and undertake appropriate hand hygiene.
2. Open the airway and position the patient's head in the 'sniffing the morning air' position (head extended and neck flexed) unless they have a suspected cervical spine injury. In this case a jaw thrust can be used to minimise movement.

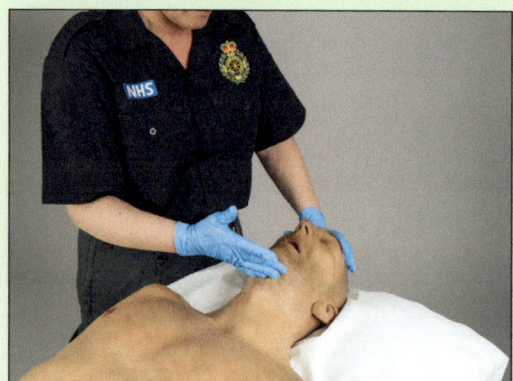

3. Perform a quick visual check of the oropharynx to see if you can detect a foreign body, unless there is an indication in the history that a foreign body might be present, in which case laryngoscopy should be performed by the senior clinician.

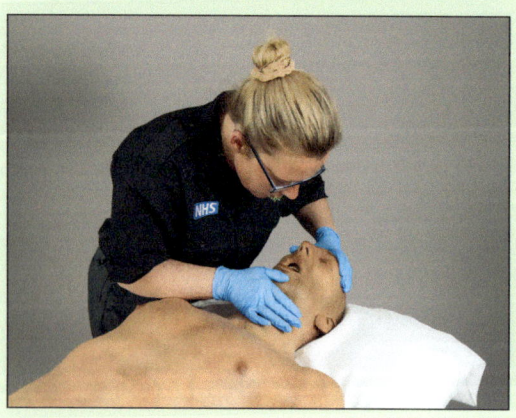

Procedure – *cont*

4. The clinician responsible for holding the mask in position should be located at the head of the patient, facing the feet.

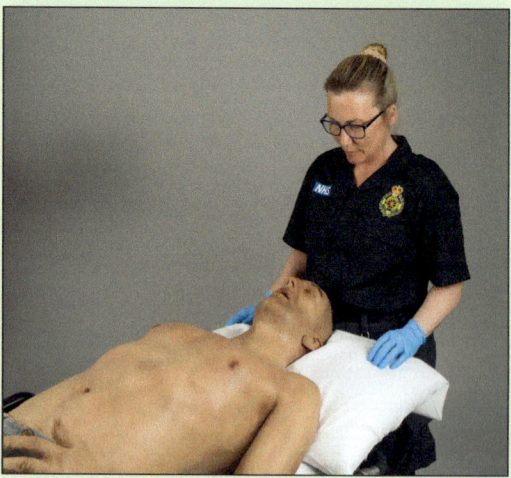

5. Use the mnemonic ROMAN to assess the patient for signs that they may be difficult to ventilate with a BVM:
   - Radiation/restriction
   - Obesity/obstruction/obstructive sleep apnoea
   - Mask seal/Mallampati/male sex
   - Age more than 55 years
   - No teeth.
6. Insert an appropriately sized OPA or NPA(s) if an OPA cannot be used for any reason.

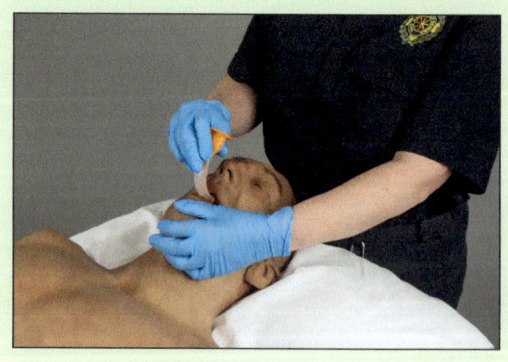

Using medical gases safely

Procedure – *cont*

7. Select the most appropriately sized mask. The lower edge of the mask should rest in the groove between the patient's chin and lower lip, and the upper edge should rest across the bridge of the nose.

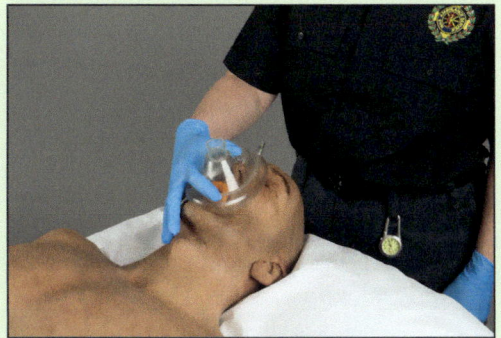

8. Connect mask to bag, capnography (where available) and oxygen supply.
9. Position the mask on the patient's face and ensure an adequate seal. Apply the mask to the groove formed by the chin and lower lip first, and then the bridge of the nose.
10. The mask-holding clinician should place both thenar eminences on top of the mask with their thumbs facing the patient's feet (caudally). The fingers should then grasp the mandible and pull it forward to meet the mask.

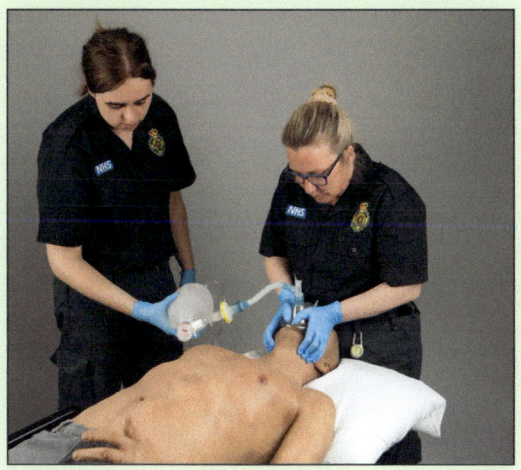

Procedure – *cont*

11. The clinician who is not holding the mask should gently squeeze the bag just enough to see the chest rise. Each ventilation should consist of an inspiratory component lasting 1 second. If capnography is available, aim for a ventilatory rate that results in normal end-tidal carbondioxide (normocapnia). Otherwise, ventilate at a rate of 10–12 ventilations per minute.

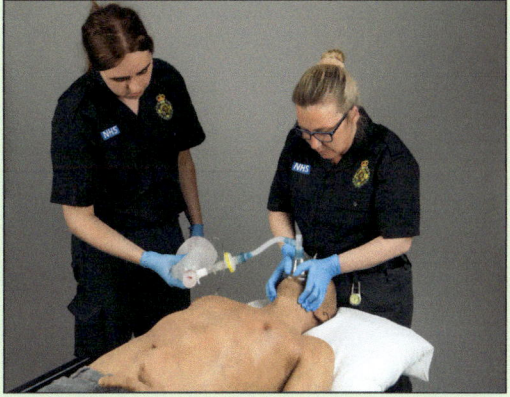

12. If ventilation is difficult, try gently flexing and extending the airway until you can successfully ventilate. If this fails, the senior clinician may consider upgrading the airway to a supraglottic airway device.
13. Frequently reassess the adequacy of the ventilation and escalate airway management if required.
14. Document the procedure.

2.9 *Oxygen administration*

The UK Ambulance Services Clinical Practice Guidelines [JRCALC, 2023] have divided oxygen administration for adults into four categories, which are provided here. However, you MUST follow local instruction about oxygen administration.

Note: Children are not included here. They should always receive high-concentration oxygen if they have a significant illness or injury. Follow local guidance.

Chapter 11 – Breathing

Indications
- Critical illnesses requiring high levels of supplemental oxygen.
- Serious illnesses requiring moderate levels of supplemental oxygen if the patient is hypoxaemic.
- COPD and other conditions requiring controlled or low-dose oxygen therapy.
- Conditions for which patients should be monitored closely but oxygen therapy is not required unless the patient is hypoxaemic.

Contra-indications
- Explosive environments.

Cautions
- Oxygen increases the fire hazard at the scene of an incident.
- Defibrillation – ensure pads are firmly applied to reduce spark hazard.

Side effects
- Non-humidified oxygen is drying and irritating to mucous membranes over a period of time.
- In patients with COPD there is a risk that even moderately high doses of inspired oxygen can produce increased carbon dioxide levels, which may cause respiratory depression and in turn may lead to respiratory arrest.

Dosage and administration
- Measure oxygen saturation (SpO_2) in all patients using pulse oximetry.
- For the administration of moderate levels of supplemental oxygen, nasal cannulae are recommended in preference to simple face masks as they offer a more flexible dose range.
- Administer the initial oxygen dose until a reliable oxygen saturation reading is obtained.
- If the desired oxygen saturation cannot be maintained with a simple face mask, change to a reservoir (non-rebreathe) mask.
- For dosage and administration of supplemental oxygen, refer to Table 11.1 for patients with critical illnesses, Table 11.2 for serious illnesses and Table 11.3 for patients who need controlled or low-dose oxygen therapy.
- For conditions where NO supplemental oxygen is required unless the patient is hypoxaemic, refer to Table 11.4.

Table 11.1 High levels of supplemental oxygen for adults with critical illnesses

Administer the initial oxygen dose until the vital signs are normal, then reduce oxygen dose and aim for target saturation within the range of 94–98%.		
Condition	**Initial dose**	**Method of administration**

- Cardiac arrest or resuscitation:
  – basic life support
  – advanced life support
  – foreign body airway obstruction
  – traumatic cardiac arrest
  – maternal resuscitation
- Carbon monoxide poisoning
	Maximum dose until vital signs are normal	Bag-valve-mask (BVM)

- Major trauma:
  – abdominal trauma
  – burns and scalds
  – electrocution
  – head trauma
  – limb trauma
  – spinal injury and spinal cord
	15 l/min	Non-rebreathe mask

Using medical gases safely

Condition	Initial dose	Method of administration
– pelvic trauma – immersion – thoracic trauma – trauma in pregnancy • Anaphylaxis • Major pulmonary haemorrhage • Sepsis, e.g. meningococcal septicaemia • Shock • Drowning		
• Active convulsion • Hypothermia	Administer 15 l/minute until a reliable SpO_2 measurement can be obtained and then adjust oxygen flow to aim for target saturation within the range of 94–98%	Non-rebreathe mask

Table 11.2 Moderate levels of supplemental oxygen for adults with serious illnesses if the patient is hypoxaemic

Administer the initial oxygen dose until a reliable SpO_2 measurement is available, then adjust oxygen flow to aim for target saturation within the range of 94–98%.

Condition	Initial dose	Method of administration
• Acute hypoxaemia (cause not yet diagnosed) • Deterioration of lung fibrosis or other interstitial lung disease • Acute asthma • Acute heart failure • Pneumonia • Lung cancer • Post-operative breathlessness • Pulmonary embolism • Pleural effusions • Pneumothorax • Severe anaemia • Sickle cell crisis	**SpO_2 < 85%** 10–15 l/minute **SpO_2 85–93%** 2–6 l/minute **SpO_2 85–93%** 5–10 l/minute	Non-rebreathe mask Nasal cannulae Simple face mask

Chapter 11 – Breathing

Table 11.3 Controlled or low-dose supplemental oxygen for adults with COPD and other conditions

Administer the initial oxygen dose until a reliable SpO$_2$ measurement is available, then adjust oxygen flow to aim for target saturation within the range of 88–92% or pre-specified range as detailed on the patient's alert card.

Condition	Initial dose	Method of administration
• Chronic obstructive pulmonary disease (COPD) • Exacerbation of cystic fibrosis	4 l/minute Increase flow rate to 6 l/minute if respiratory rate is > 30 breaths/minute (i.e. 50% above minimum specified for the mask)	28% Venturi mask (or patient's own)
• Chronic neuromuscular disorders • Chest wall disorders • Morbid obesity	4 l/minute	28% Venturi mask (or patient's own)
Note: If the oxygen saturation remains below 88%, change to simple face mask	5–10 l/minute	Simple face mask
Note: Critical illness AND COPD or other risk factors for hypercapnia	As for Table 11.1	As for Table 11.1

Table 11.4 No supplemental oxygen required for adults with these conditions unless the patient is hypoxaemic, but patients should be monitored closely

If hypoxaemic (SpO$_2$ < 94%), administer the initial oxygen dose, then adjust oxygen flow to aim for target saturation within the range of 94–98% as per the table below.

Condition	Initial dose	Method of administration

• Myocardial infarction and acute coronary syndromes
• Stroke
• Cardiac rhythm disturbance
• Non-traumatic chest pain/discomfort
• Implantable cardioverter defibrillator firing
• Pregnancy and obstetric emergencies:
  – birth imminent
  – haemorrhage during pregnancy
  – pregnancy-induced hypertension
  – vaginal bleeding
• Abdominal pain
• Headache
• Hyperventilation syndrome or dysfunctional breathing
	SpO$_2$ < 85%
	10–15 l/minute
	
	SpO$_2$ 85–93%
	2–6 l/minute
	
	SpO$_2$ 85–93%
	5–10 l/minute
		Non-rebreathe mask
		
		Nasal cannulae
		
		Simple face mask

Using medical gases safely

Condition	Initial dose	Method of administration
• Most poisonings and drug overdoses (see Table 11.1 for carbon monoxide poisoning and special cases below for paraquat poisoning) • Metabolic and renal disorders • Acute and sub-acute neurological and muscular conditions producing muscle weakness (assess the need for assisted ventilation if SpO$_2$ ‹ 94%) • Post-convulsion • Gastrointestinal bleeds • Glycaemic emergencies • Heat exhaustion/heat stroke **SPECIAL CASES** • Poisoning with paraquat • Poisoning with bleomycin Patients with paraquat or bleomycin poisoning may be harmed by supplemental oxygen so avoid oxygen unless the patient is hypoxaemic Target saturation 85–88%		

2.9.1 Actions after oxygen administration

Procedure

Once you have finished administering oxygen to a patient, take the following steps [BOC, 2022]:

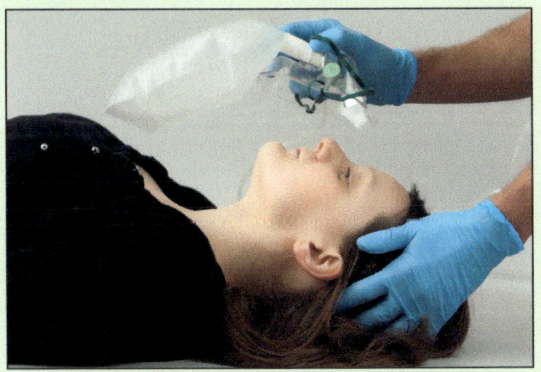

1. Remove the mask or nasal cannulae from the patient.

Procedure – *cont*

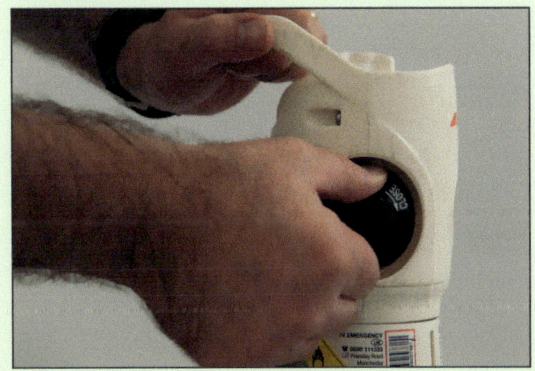

2. Turn off the cylinder by rotating the handwheel clockwise until it comes to a stop. Do not use excessive force.

Chapter 11 – Breathing

Procedure – *cont*

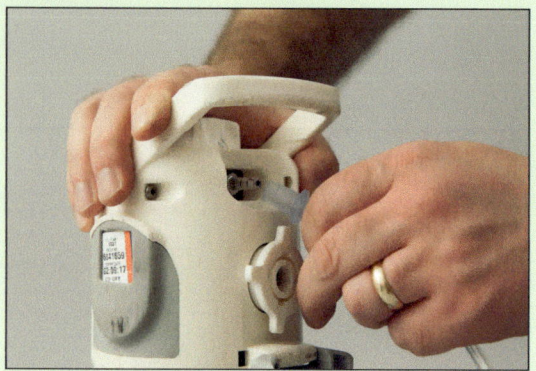

3a. Disconnect equipment. Remove the tubing by firmly pulling the tube while holding the cylinder handle.

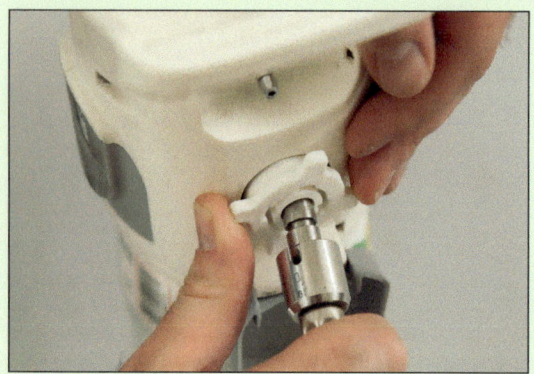

3b. If you have used the Schrader valve, release by twisting the capstan clockwise.

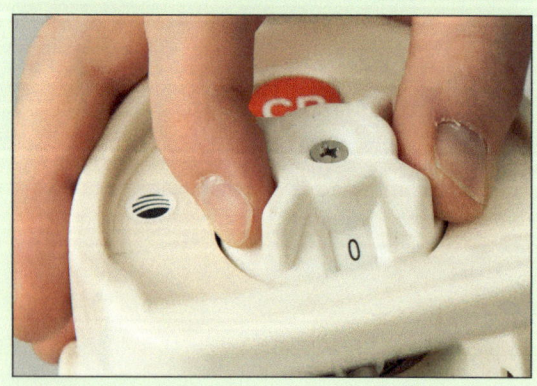

4. Turn the flow selector to zero.

Procedure – *cont*

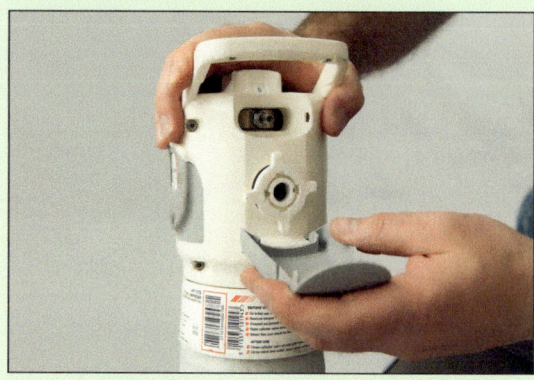

5. Replace the outlet cover by pulling up the hinged grey cover.

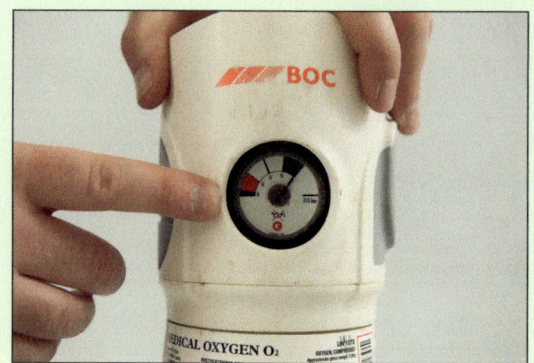

6. Check the cylinder gauge and replace if necessary.

2.10 Entonox administration

Entonox is a combination of 50% nitrous oxide and 50% oxygen. The cylinders that contain Entonox have a blue and white collar (Figure 11.14).

The UK Ambulance Services Clinical Practice Guidelines [JRCALC, 2023] for Entonox administration are as follows:

Indications
- Moderate to severe pain.
- Labour pains.

Contra-indications
- Chest injury with a clinically suspected pneumothorax.

Using medical gases safely

- Severe head injuries with impaired consciousness due to possible presence of intracranial air.
- Decompression sickness (the bends) where nitrous oxide can cause nitrogen bubbles within the blood stream to expand, aggravating the problem further. Consider anyone who has been diving within the previous 24 hours to be at risk.
- Violently disturbed psychiatric patients.
- An intraocular injection of gas within the last 8 weeks. Check to see if these patients have an information leaflet, card or wristband. The information leaflet may advise that nitrous oxide can be administered less than 8 weeks after this treatment.
- Abdominal pain where intestinal obstruction is suspected.

Action
- Inhaled analgesic agent.

Caution
- Any patient at risk of having a pneumothorax, pneumomediastinum and/or a pneumoperitoneum, e.g. polytrauma, penetrating torso injury.

Side effects
- Minimal side effects.

Dosage and administration
- **Adults:** Entonox should be self-administered via a face mask or mouthpiece, after suitable instruction. It takes about 3–5 minutes to be effective, but it may be 5–10 minutes before maximum effect is achieved.
- **Children:** Entonox is effective in children provided they are capable of following the administration instructions and can activate the demand valve.

Additional information
- Administration of Entonox should be in conjunction with pain score monitoring.
- Entonox's advantages include:
  - rapid analgesic effect with minimal side effects
  - no cardio-respiratory depression
  - self-administered
  - analgesic effect rapidly wears off
  - the 50% oxygen concentration is valuable in many medical and trauma conditions
- Entonox can be administered while preparing to deliver other analgesics.

2.10.1 Preparing Entonox for administration

Procedure

Take the following steps to prepare Entonox for administration [BOC, 2013]:

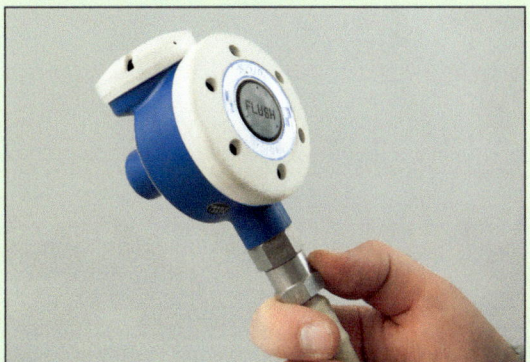

1. Ensure the demand valve is clean and ready for use.

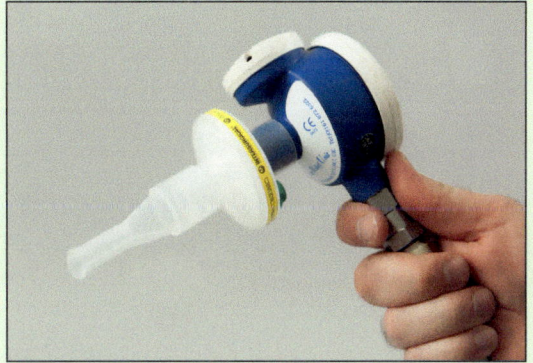

2. Fit a new microbial and mouthpiece to the demand valve. They are single use.

Chapter 11 – *Breathing*

Procedure – *cont*

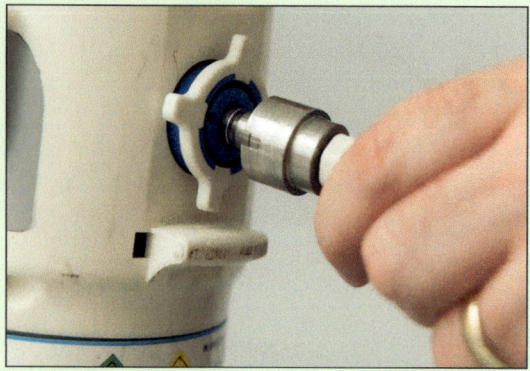

3. Insert the probe on the hose connected to the demand valve into the Schrader outlet on the Entonox cylinder. Push firmly to ensure the probe clicks into place.

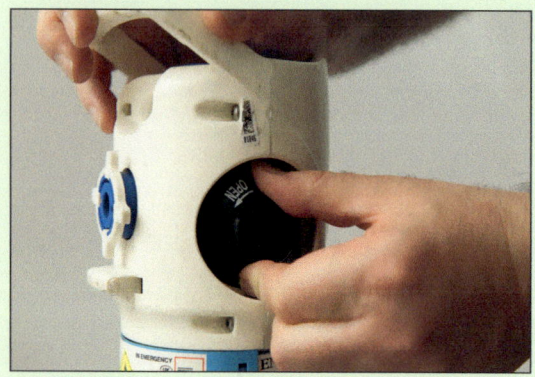

4. Slowly turn the cylinder on by rotating the handwheel anti-clockwise until fully open. Do not use excessive force.

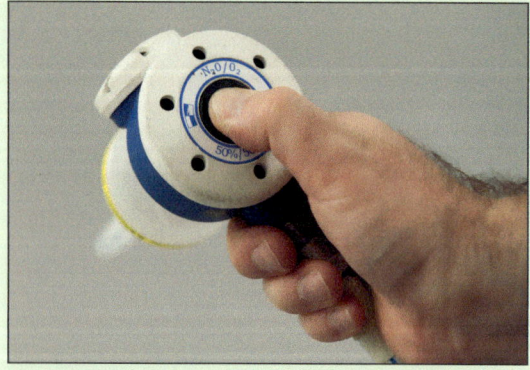

5. Check the demand valve is operative by pushing the 'test button'. You should hear the gas flowing.

Procedure – *cont*

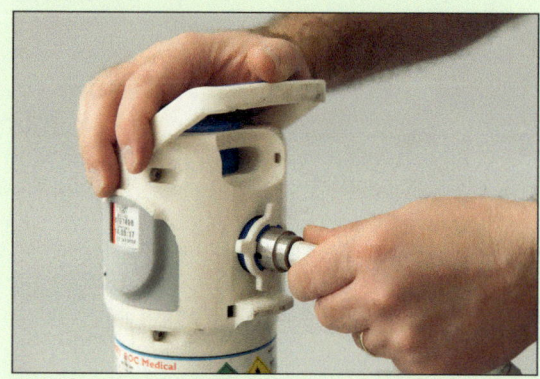

6. Check for leaks which may be indicated by a hissing sound. If you suspect that there is a leak, turn off the cylinder and check the equipment is properly connected. Turn on the cylinder and re-check for leaks. If the leak continues, turn off and remove the cylinder from service. Report it using your ambulance service equipment defect procedure.

2.10.2 Actions after Entonox administration

Procedure

Take the following steps once the patient has finished using the Entonox [BOC, 2013]:

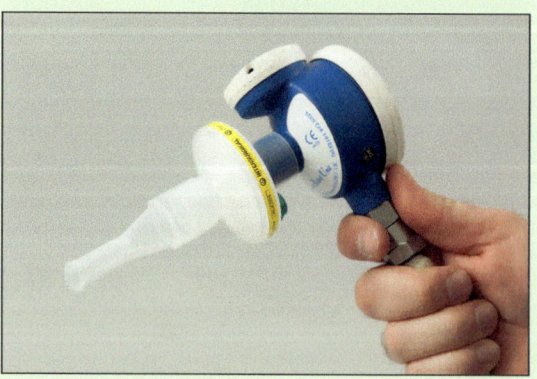

1. Remove the demand valve from the patient. Dispose of the filter and mouthpiece.

Procedure – *cont*

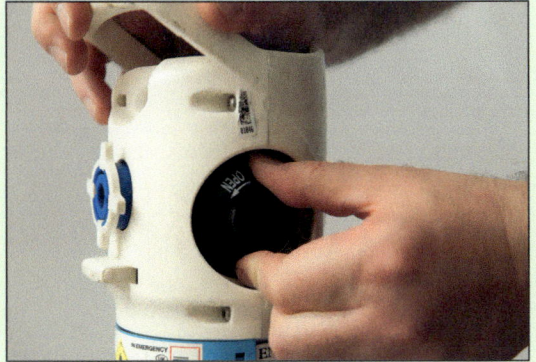

2. Turn off the cylinder by rotating the handwheel clockwise until it comes to a stop. Do not use excessive force.

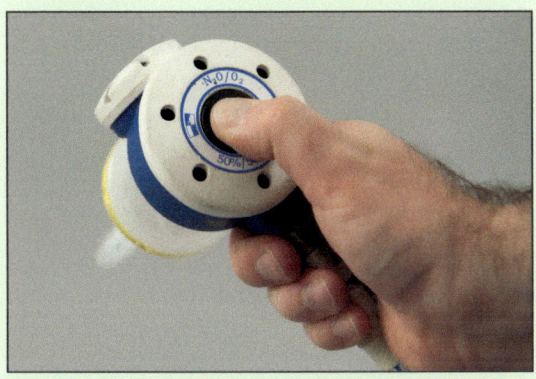

3. Vent any residual gas in the hose by pressing the test button on the demand valve. Keep pressing until the gas has stopped venting.

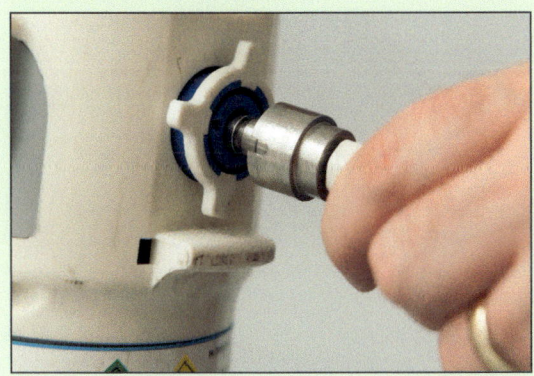

4. Disconnect the probe from the cylinder outlet. Holding the probe, twist the capstan and withdraw the probe from the Schrader outlet.

Procedure – *cont*

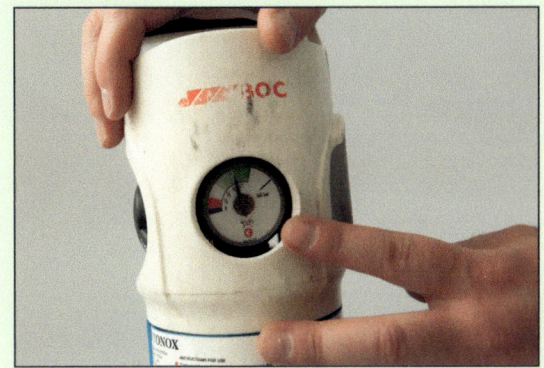

5. Replace the outlet cover by pulling up the hinged grey cover. Check the cylinder gauge and replace if empty.

3 Assessment of breathing

3.1 *Learning objectives*

By the end of this section you will be able to:
- record the following observations:
  - respiratory rate
  - oxygen saturations.

3.2 *Respiratory rate*

A normal adult respiratory rate is 12–20 breaths per minute (breaths/min) [RCUK, 2021a]. Patients with a respiratory rate of less than 10 breaths/minute or more than 30 breaths/minute may need assisted ventilation, so inform a senior clinician immediately or update the EOC [JRCALC, 2023].

3.2.1 Measuring respiratory rate

How fast are you breathing now? Before considering this question, it is likely that you weren't even thinking about your respiratory rate. So it is with patients. Don't tell them that you are going to record their respiratory rate!

Indications
- Any patient requiring a physiological assessment.
- Before and after the administration of medication that might alter respiratory function, for example beta-2 agonist drugs, opiates and benzodiazepines.

Chapter 11 – Breathing

Contra-indications
- Prior to correction of a life-threatening airway/breathing/circulation (ABC) problem, for example occluded airway, tension pneumothorax or catastrophic haemorrhage.
- Suspected cardiac arrest.

Advantages
- Respiratory rate can provide an early warning of severe illness.
- A routine observation to assess patient physiology.

Disadvantages
- Does not provide indication of efficacy of either oxygenation or ventilation.

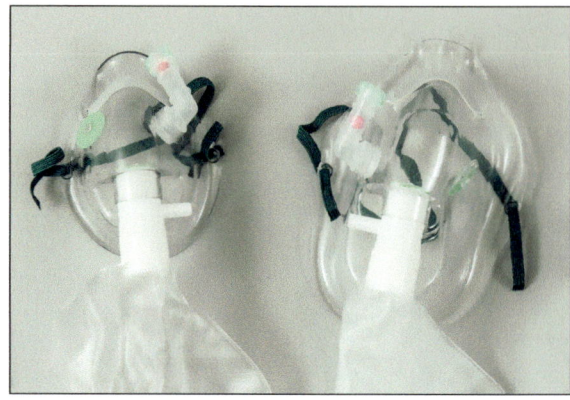

Figure 11.14 Non-rebreathe masks with integral respiratory rate indicator

> **Procedure**
>
> Take the following steps to record a respiratory rate [Pilbery & Lethbridge, 2022]:
> 1. Do not inform the patient you are intending to record their respiratory rate.
> 2. Don appropriate PPE, if required.
> 3. If possible, position the patient so their chest is clearly visible and not obscured by baggy clothing.
> 4. Using a watch or clock with a second hand, or a timer, count the respiratory rate for a full minute. This can be achieved by watching the rise and fall of the chest, or by using an alternative method such as an oxygen mask with an integrated respiratory rate indicator Figure 11.14.
> 5. Document the respiratory rate.

3.3 Oxygen saturations

Most oxygen is transported around the body bound to haemoglobin in the blood (oxyhaemoglobin), as it travels from the lungs to the body's tissues. Oxygen saturation is the ratio of oxyhaemoglobin to the total amount of haemoglobin and is usually shown as a percentage [Tortora, 2017].

Oxygen saturations are measured in two ways: invasively and non-invasively. In hospital, it is common for critically ill patients to have an arterial blood gas sample taken, whereby a small amount of blood from an artery (often the radial) is taken and the arterial oxygen saturation measured (SaO_2). However, this is not a practical method of measurement to undertake in the out-of-hospital setting, so oxygen saturations are measured non-invasively using a technique known as pulse oximetry (SpO_2) [O'Driscoll, 2017].

3.3.1 Pulse oximetry

Pulse oximetry works by shining red and infrared light through a part of the body that is relatively translucent and has an arterial pulse, such as a finger, toe or earlobe. The amount of light transmitted through the tissue depends on the amount of oxyhaemoglobin present; this enables the pulse oximeter to calculate the oxygen saturation and will also provide the pulse rate. The target saturation for most patients is 94–98%.

Indications
- As part of a cardiovascular or respiratory assessment of a patient.
- Titration of oxygen delivery.

Contra-indications
- None.

Cautions
- Pulse oximeters do not instantaneously reflect changes in blood oxygenation.
- Can give false values in the presence of carboxyhaemoglobin and methaemoglobinaemia.
- Using probes in different anatomical areas or age groups than specified can result in significant measurement errors.

Assessment of breathing

Advantages
- Non-invasive and easy to measure.
- Can assist in accurate titration of oxygen.
- Provides an estimate of arterial oxygenation.

Disadvantages
1. Not as accurate as invasive methods of measuring oxygenation.
2. Does not provide sufficient information about adequacy of ventilation.
3. Can give erroneous readings in cases of carbon monoxide poisoning and methaemoglobinaemia, in the presence of poor peripheral perfusion, nail varnish, and during excessive motion.

Procedure

Take the following steps to record a patient's oxygen saturations with pulse oximetry [Pilbery & Lethbridge, 2022]:

1. Explain the procedure and obtain consent if appropriate to do so.
2. Don appropriate PPE, and undertake appropriate hand hygiene.
3. Turn the pulse oximeter on.

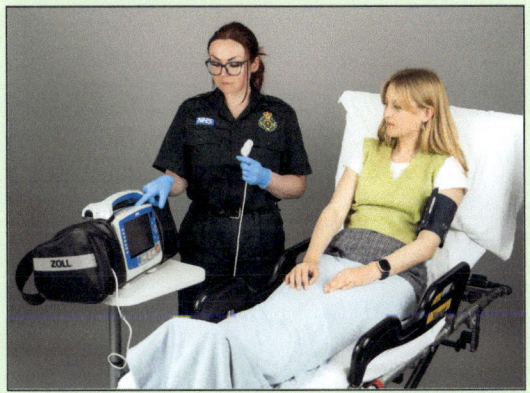

4. Select the appropriate probe with particular attention to correct sizing and where it will go (usually the finger, toe or ear). If used on a finger or toe, make sure the area is clean. Do not place probes designed for adults on babies or finger probes on ears, and vice versa. If present, consider removing nail varnish or rotating the probe by 90°.

Procedure – *cont*

5. Connect the probe to the pulse oximeter.
6. Position the probe securely and, if possible, avoid the arm being used for blood pressure monitoring.

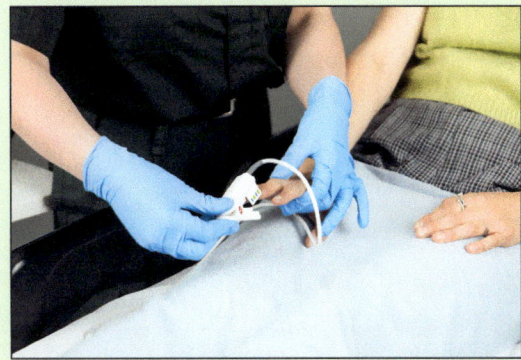

7. Allow several seconds for the pulse oximeter to detect the pulse and calculate the oxygen saturation. Look for the displayed pulse indicator or waveform to indicate that the device has detected the pulse reliably. In addition, if your device can measure the perfusion index (PI), this should be above the manufacturer's minimum (1.0 for the X-Series). If it is not, try another finger or limb.

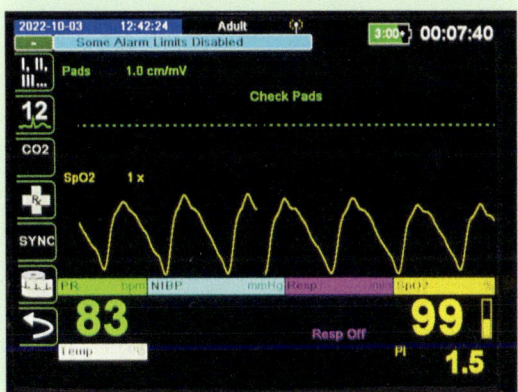

8. Once the unit has detected a good pulse, the oxygen saturation and pulse rate will be displayed. Like all machines, oximeters may occasionally give a false reading – if in doubt, rely on clinical judgement rather than the machine. You can check the pulse oximeter is working properly by placing it on your own finger.
9. Document your findings.

4 Common respiratory conditions

4.1 Learning objectives

By the end of this section you will be able to:
- describe the following conditions of the respiratory system:
  - asthma
  - COPD
  - pneumonia
  - pulmonary embolism.

4.2 Asthma

4.2.1 Definition

Asthma is a condition characterised by intermittent, reversible, airway obstruction [Simon, 2010].

4.2.2 Pathophysiology

Asthma is caused by a chronic inflammation of the bronchi, making them narrower. The muscles around the bronchi become irritated and contract, causing sudden worsening of the symptoms. The inflammation can also cause the mucus glands to produce excessive sputum, which further blocks the air passages.

The obstruction and subsequent wheezing are caused by three factors within the bronchial tree:
- increased production of bronchial mucus
- swelling of the mucosal cells that line the bronchi and bronchioles
- spasm and constriction of bronchial muscles.

These three factors combine to cause blockage and narrowing of the small airways in the lung. Because inspiration is an active process involving the muscles of respiration, the obstruction of the airways is overcome on breathing in. Expiration occurs with muscle relaxation and is severely delayed by the narrowing of the airways in asthma. This generates the wheezing on expiration that is characteristic of this condition.

4.2.3 Medication

Asthma is managed with a variety of inhaled and tablet medications. Inhalers are divided into two broad categories: preventer and reliever.

Preventer

The preventer inhalers are normally anti-inflammatory drugs. These include steroids and other milder anti-inflammatories such as nedocramil sodium (Tilade). The common steroid inhalers are beclomethasone (Becotide), budesonide (Pulmicort) and fluticasone propionate (Flixotide). These drugs act on the smooth muscles of the bronchi and bronchioles over a period of time to reduce the inflammatory reaction that causes asthma. Regular use of these inhalers often eradicates all symptoms of asthma and allows for a normal lifestyle.

Reliever

The reliever inhalers include salbutamol (Ventolin), terbutaline (Bricanyl), tiotropium bromide (Spiriva) and ipratropium bromide (Atrovent). These inhalers work rapidly on the bronchi and bronchioles to relax the smooth muscle spasm when the patient feels wheezy or tight-chested. They are used in conjunction with preventer inhalers. Inhalers are often used through large plastic spacer devices (Figure 11.15). This allows the drug to spread into a larger volume and enables the patient to inhale it more effectively. In mild and moderate asthma attacks some patients may be treated with high doses of 'relievers' through a spacer device [SIGN/BTS, 2019].

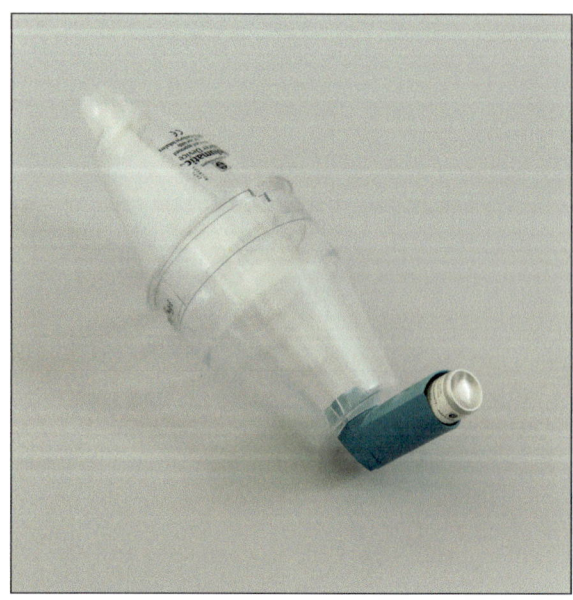

Figure 11.15 An inhaler with a spacer device

Common respiratory conditions

4.2.4 Signs and symptoms

History
Patients will typically tell you about increasing shortness of breath with wheezing over the past 6–48 hours, with increasing inhaler use. The reliever inhalers may also be proving less effective than normal.

Ask specifically about:
- repeated attendances at ED for asthma care in the past year
- previous admissions for asthma
- previous near-fatal asthma, e.g. previously required ventilation/intensive care
- heavy use of reliever inhalers
- brittle asthma.

Assessment of severity
The signs and symptoms of asthma are organised according to their severity [SIGN/BTS 2019]. Table 11.5 shows the broad categories of asthma severity, which in turn will determine the most appropriate interventions for your patient [JRCALC, 2023].

Table 11.5 Assessing asthma severity

Moderate	**Severe**	**Life-threatening**
$SpO_2 \geq 92\%$	$SpO_2 \geq 92\%$	$SpO_2 < 92\%$
Adults: Respiratory rate < 25 breaths/min Heart rate < 110 beats/min	**Adults:** Respiratory rate ≥ 25 breaths/min Heart rate ≥ 110 beats/min	**Adults:** Silent chest Poor respiratory effort Exhaustion Altered consciousness Cyanosis Arrhythmia Hypotension
Children > 5 years Able to talk Respiratory rate ≤ 30 breaths/min Heart rate ≤ 125 beats/min	**Children > 5 years** Too breathless to talk Using accessory neck muscles Respiratory rate > 30 breaths/min Heart rate > 125 beats/min	**Children > 5 years** Silent chest Poor respiratory effort Agitation Altered consciousness Cyanosis
Children 2–5 years Able to talk Respiratory rate ≤ 40 breaths/min Heart rate ≤ 140 beats/min	**Children 2–5 years** Too breathless to talk Using accessory neck muscles Respiratory rate > 40 breaths/min Heart rate > 140 beats/min	**Children 2–5 years** Silent chest Poor respiratory effort Agitation Altered consciousness Cyanosis
Children < 2 years Audible wheezing Using accessory muscles Still feeding	**Children < 2 years** Cyanosis Marked respiratory distress Too breathless to feed	**Children < 2 years** Apnoea or poor respiratory effort Bradycardia

Note: Only one sign or symptom is required to qualify a patient for a higher severity. For example, an SpO_2 of 91% would place a patient in the life-threatening column, irrespective of other observations.

4.2.5 Management

The management of asthma depends on the assessment of severity and the patient's response to treatment [SIGN/BTS, 2019; JRCALC, 2023]. Encourage patients to use their own reliever inhalers, such as salbutamol, and administer high-flow oxygen. Patients with life-threatening asthma may require assisted ventilation if they lose consciousness.

4.3 COPD

4.3.1 Definition

COPD is an umbrella term for a range of respiratory diseases that result in airflow obstruction. This obstruction is usually progressive and, unlike asthma, is not fully reversible and does not change markedly over several months [NICE, 2019].

The two most important respiratory diseases related to COPD are chronic bronchitis and emphysema. Chronic bronchitis is defined clinically as a persistent cough with sputum production for at least 3 months of the year for 2 consecutive years [Hickin, 2015]. Emphysema, on the other hand, is a permanent enlargement of the air spaces below the terminal bronchioles as a result of the destruction of the alveolar walls.

4.3.2 Pathophysiology

COPD

The most important causative factor in chronic bronchitis and emphysema is smoking, although only 15% of smokers develop COPD [Hickin, 2015]. The general effects of smoking in COPD are:

- Inflammation resulting from activation of inflammatory cells which release substances that trigger an immune system response. This activates enzymes that can damage lung tissue, although normally these are kept in check. However, in COPD so many enzymes are produced that they overwhelm the neutralising mechanism, and lung tissue is digested and destroyed. This is thought to be particularly important in the development of emphysema.
- Inflammation as a direct result of inhaling oxidants in cigarette smoke (free radicals) which damage the cells directly.

Both of these mechanisms lead to alveolar destruction and the production of excess mucus, which is made worse by the impairment of the respiratory cilia, hair-like projections that line the airways and move debris and mucus upwards and out of the respiratory tract [Tortora, 2017].

Chronic bronchitis

Cigarette smoking, occupational exposure and/or recurrent bronchial infections lead to inflammation that narrows the airways, and an increase in mucus secretions coupled with inhibition of the cilia. This in turn leads to the accumulation of secretions and bronchoconstriction due to irritant receptor activation, which also causes the chronic productive cough [Hickin, 2015].

Emphysema

In emphysema, the walls of the alveoli are destroyed by enzymes called proteases. These are usually kept under control by another group of enzymes called anti-proteases. Once the balance is upset (due to smoking, for example) destruction of the alveoli occurs, leading to a collapse of the airways, resulting in obstruction. In addition, as the walls of the alveoli are destroyed, bullae (small, blister-like air pockets) form on the lung. If these bullae form, air can directly enter the pleural cavity, causing a pneumothorax and collapse of the lung on the affected side [Hickin, 2015].

4.3.3 Oxygen and COPD

Research studies and audits suggest that over-oxygenation increases mortality and morbidity, but careful pre-hospital titration of oxygen administration to patients with COPD can significantly reduce mortality [Austin, 2010]. This is why the oxygen guidelines recommend titrating oxygen administration to patients with COPD between 88–92% [O'Driscoll, 2017].

4.3.4 Signs and symptoms

Patients will usually call for an ambulance during an acute infective exacerbation (sudden worsening) of their COPD.

Features of an acute infective exacerbation of COPD include [JRCALC, 2023]:
- increased dyspnoea (difficulty breathing)
- increased sputum production/purulence (containing pus)
- increased cough
- upper airway symptoms, such as cold and sore throat
- increased wheeze
- reduced exercise tolerance
- fluid retention
- increased fatigue
- acute confusion
- worsening of a previously stable condition.

Features that warn of a severe episode of COPD include [JRCALC, 2023]:
- marked dyspnoea
- tachypnoea (increased respiratory rate)
- pursed-lip breathing
- use of accessory muscles
- acute confusion
- new-onset cyanosis
- new-onset peripheral oedema
- marked reduction in activities of daily living.

Despite the lists above, it is not always clear that the patient with difficulty breathing has COPD. Therefore, you should consider this as a possibility for any patient who meets the following criteria [NICE, 2019]:
- over 35 years of age
- smoker (or ex-smoker)
- has any of the following symptoms:
  - exertional breathlessness
  - chronic cough
  - regular sputum production
  - frequent winter 'bronchitis'
  - wheeze.

4.3.5 Management

The management of the patient with COPD depends on the presence of any time-critical features:
- major ABCD problems
- extreme breathing difficulty (compared to normal)
- cyanosis (although peripheral cyanosis can be normal)
- exhaustion
- hypoxia unresponsive to oxygen (in COPD patients hypoxia is considered to be an SpO_2 below 88%).

These patients require an urgent transfer to the nearest ED and may also require suction, airway management and assisted ventilation, so be sure to update the EOC [JRCALC, 2023].

For patients with no time-critical features, you should ask if they have a treatment plan and follow this, if available. Treatments typically include [JRCALC, 2023]:
- **Oxygen:** Target range of 88–92%. Venturi masks are a good choice for delivering accurate percentages of oxygen, although nasal cannulae may be better tolerated by patients. If you are using a Venturi mask and the patient's respiratory rate is greater than 30 breaths/minute, remember to increase the recommended flow rate by 50%. So if the flow rate should be set at 4 l/min, then increase this to 6 l/min.
- **Bronchodilators:** Salbutamol and ipratropium (once only). If the nebuliser is powered by oxygen, nebulisation should be limited to 6 minutes. Note: This will normally be administered by a clinician, carer or the patient.
- Patients may need taking to hospital, but depending on how well they respond to treatment, they may be suitable for referral to their GP, respiratory team or advanced paramedic. The ambulance staff will decide the most appropriate management.

4.4 Pneumonia

4.4.1 Definition

Pneumonia is an infection of the terminal bronchioles and alveoli [Hickin, 2015]. It is more common in the elderly and during the winter months [Simon, 2010]. It is often classified in three main ways, although the first is the most commonly used [Dunn, 2005; Osler, 2012]:
- **Setting:** i.e. hospital- or community-acquired pneumonia.

Chapter 11 – *Breathing*

- **Anatomy:** Lobar, if the infection is localised to a lobe of the lung, or bronchopneumonia, if the infection is more widespread.
- **Organism:** Bacterial, viral, fungal.

4.4.2 Risk factors for community-acquired pneumonia (CAP)

These are factors that undermine the lung's natural defences and so increase the risk of pneumonia [Hickin, 2015]:
- excessive alcohol
- cigarette smoking
- chronic heart and lung diseases
- bronchial obstruction
- immunosuppression (e.g. due to chemotherapy for cancer)
- drug abuse.

4.4.3 Pathophysiology

This inflammatory process is typically due to a bacterial or viral infection, which has usually entered the lungs having been inhaled from the environment or nasopharynx. Normally, these organisms should be destroyed by the body's lung defences, but infection results if they survive and multiply. This leads to a build-up of fluid and blood cells (red and white) in the alveoli, known as consolidation [Porth, 2014].

4.4.4 Signs and symptoms

When taking a history, the following symptoms are suggestive of pneumonia [Johnson, 2012]:
- fever with or without rigors (exaggerated shivering or shaking)
- cough (often productive with green, bloodstained or rusty-coloured sputum)
- pleuritic chest pain
- muscle or joint pain
- when examining a patient, you may notice the following signs:
  - high temperature (pyrexia)
  - increased respiratory rate (tachypnoea)
  - increased heart rate (tachycardia).

4.4.5 Management

Not all patients with pneumonia need to go to hospital. However, while waiting for an ambulance, patients who have difficulty breathing should receive oxygen.

4.5 *Pulmonary embolism*

4.5.1 Definition

An embolus is a foreign body in the blood (including air) that is transported from one part of the circulation to another, lodging in a vessel that is too small to allow the embolus to pass. When the embolus lodges in the pulmonary vessels, it is termed a pulmonary embolism (PE) [Hickin, 2015]. Deep vein thrombosis (DVT) and pulmonary embolism represent the spectrum of one disease known as venous thromboembolism (VTE) [Tapson, 2008]. Although an embolus can consist of air, fat or amniotic fluid, for example, the most common is a clot from a DVT [Porth, 2014; Konstantinides, 2020].

4.5.2 Risk factors

The risk factors for developing a VTE are well known and can help to identify patients who may have a PE [Konstantinides, 2020]:
- high risk:
  - fracture (hip or leg)
  - major general surgery
  - major trauma
  - spinal cord injury
- moderate risk:
  - chronic heart or respiratory failure
  - chemotherapy
  - hormone replacement therapy
  - cancer
  - oral contraceptive therapy
  - paralytic stroke
  - post-partum
  - previous VTE
  - thrombophilia
- low risk:
  - bed rest for more than 3 days
  - immobility due to sitting (e.g. prolonged car or air travel)

- increasing age
- obesity
- pregnancy
- varicose veins.

4.5.3 Pathophysiology

Thrombi (blood clots) most often form in the deep veins of the calf (hence the name, deep vein thrombosis) and can grow to lengths of 30–50 cm [Tapson, 2008]. The proximal end of the thrombus can extend into the popliteal vein, where the risk of embolisation is greater. Once the thrombus (or a portion) breaks off, it becomes an embolus, travelling up the femoral vein and into the iliac veins. From there it is free to ascend via the inferior vena cava to the heart. It continues into the right atrium, the ventricle and finally into the lungs via the pulmonary trunk and left and right pulmonary arteries (the only arteries to carry deoxygenated blood), which divide and sub-divide until they form capillaries around the alveoli. In healthy patients, an obstruction of up to 25% of the pulmonary arterial bed will only cause mild respiratory symptoms, such as shortness of breath. Once this increases to 30–50% there will also be cardiovascular compromise, including potentially cardiac arrest. Patients with pre-existing respiratory and/or cardiovascular disease will be symptomatic at much lower percentages [Konstantinides, 2020].

4.5.4 Signs and symptoms

Common signs and symptoms of PE include dyspnoea (difficulty breathing) and tachypnoea (rapid breathing). Pleuritic chest pain is the most common symptom [JRCALC, 2023].

Other signs and symptoms include:
- signs:
    - respiratory rate greater than 20 breaths/min
    - pulse rate greater than 100 beats/min
    - SpO_2 less than 92% on air
    - signs of a DVT, which include pain, swelling and/or tenderness on only one leg, often in the calf [Simon, 2010].
- symptoms:
    - dyspnoea
    - pleuritic chest pain
    - substernal chest pain
    - cough
    - haemoptysis (blood from the respiratory tract, usually coughed up)
    - syncope (faint).

4.5.5 Management

Patients with suspected PE need swift transport to hospital. Treatment is mainly supportive of the ABCs (airway, breathing and circulation). Place the patient in a position of comfort (often sitting up, unless they have low blood pressure), provide oxygen if required (to maintain the SpO_2 in the range 94–98%) and be prepared for cardiac arrest [JRCALC, 2023].

Chapter 12 Circulation

1 Cardiovascular system anatomy and physiology

1.1 Learning objectives
By the end of this section, you will be able to:
- state the functions of the cardiovascular system
- describe the anatomy and function of the heart
- state the components of the electrical pathway of the heart
- explain the difference between arteries and veins
- describe the stages of the cardiac cycle.

1.2 Introduction
At the most basic level, the cardiovascular system is composed of blood vessels that transport blood around the body thanks to the work of a pump, the heart. The heart is actually two pumps (the ventricles), each with its own reservoir (the atria), which normally serve two different circulations. The right side of the heart pumps blood to the pulmonary circulation, which travels around the lungs, enabling the blood to take up oxygen and give up carbon dioxide. This blood then returns to the left side of the heart, where it is pumped into the systemic circulation to be transported all around the body via the largest artery in the body, the aorta. Both these pumps operate simultaneously and, thanks to valves in the heart, in one direction.

The main functions of the cardiovascular system are [Evans, 2012]:
- transport of oxygen and nutrients, such as glucose (sugar), fatty acids and water
- removal of waste products from metabolic processes, such as carbon dioxide, urea and creatine
- hormonal control, by delivering hormones to their target organs (and secreting some of its own)
- regulation of temperature by controlling heat distribution between the core and skin of the body
- reproduction, by producing penile erection and providing nutrition for the unborn fetus
- host defence, by transporting immune cells and other mediators.

1.3 Heart
The heart is relatively small, considering the work it has to do; it is only about the size of your fist. It sits within the mediastinum, a region in the thoracic cavity that extends from the sternum to the vertebral column, and is positioned between the lungs. About two-thirds of the heart sits to the left of the body's midline. It is cone-shaped, with the pointed apex orientated anteriorly (to the front), inferiorly (downwards) and to the left, and the flat base directed posteriorly (to the back), superiorly (upwards) and to the right [Tortora, 2017].

1.3.1 Pericardium and heart wall
The pericardium is a fibrous sac that surrounds and protects the heart, keeping it fixed within the mediastinum, but allowing for the vigorous contractions required to move blood around the pulmonary and systemic circulations [Tortora, 2017]. The outer, parietal, layer is fixed to the fibrous pericardium, whereas the inner, visceral, layer (also called the epicardium) forms the outer layer of the heart wall.

The wall of the heart is made up of three layers:
- **Epicardium:** Also known as the visceral layer of the pericardium.
- **Myocardium:** The heart muscle, which makes up most of the bulk of the heart and is responsible for the pumping action that moves blood around the body.
- **Endocardium:** The smooth inner layer which also covers the valves of the heart and is continuous with the innermost lining

Chapter 12 – Circulation

(endothelium) of the blood vessels attached to the heart.

1.3.2 Chambers of the heart

The heart has four chambers. The two superior chambers are called atria and the two inferior chambers are called ventricles (Figure 12.1) [Tortora, 2017; Evans, 2012].

Right atrium

The right atrium receives deoxygenated blood from the body, via large veins called the superior and inferior vena cavae, and from the coronary (heart) circulation via the coronary sinus. It is separated from the left atrium by a thin partition known as the interatrial septum, and from the right ventricle by the tricuspid valve, so called because it is made up of three cusps. This valve is also sometimes referred to as the right atrioventricular (AV) valve.

Right ventricle

The right ventricle makes up most of the anterior surface of the heart and receives blood from the right atrium via the tricuspid valve. To prevent this valve from everting (turning inside out like an umbrella in strong winds) during contraction of the ventricles, the valve is anchored by tendon-like cords known as the chordae tendineae, which connect to papillary muscles. Like the atria, the ventricles are separated by a partition, known as the interventricular septum.

Blood leaves the ventricle via the pulmonary valve, where it enters the pulmonary trunk, which splits into the left and right pulmonary arteries. These arteries are unusual because they transport deoxygenated blood.

Left atrium

The left atrium makes up the majority of the base of the heart. Blood enters the atrium from the lungs via four pulmonary veins and exits through the bicuspid (two cusps) valve. This is also known as the mitral valve (because of the valve's resemblance to a bishop's mitre or hat) and the left AV valve.

Left ventricle

This forms the apex of the heart and also contains the chordae tendineae and papillary muscle assembly to secure the mitral valve. Blood exits via the aortic valve, where it travels up the ascending aorta. Some blood leaves here and enters the coronary arteries to provide oxygen and nutrients to the heart itself. The remaining blood is transported throughout the body.

1.3.3 Electrical conduction pathway

In order to ensure an effective pumping action of the heart, there is a network of specialised auto-rhythmic (self-excitable) muscle cell fibres that trigger co-ordinated muscle contraction (Figure 12.2), forcing blood around the heart chambers in the direction dictated by the heart valves.

Sinoatrial (SA) node

The SA node is the main pacemaker of the heart and in textbooks is typically shown as a small area of tissue at the junction of the superior vena cava (SVC) with the right atrium. However, electrophysiology studies have shown that the pacemaker site can spontaneously move down

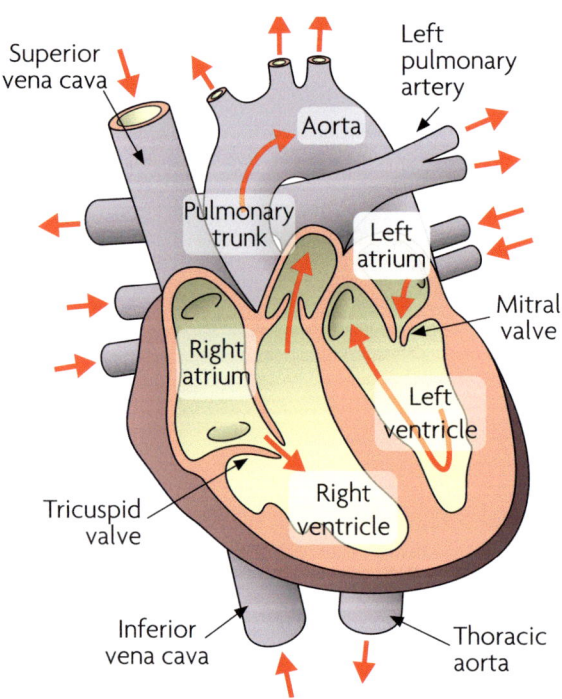

Figure 12.1 Chambers of the heart and related anatomy

Cardiovascular system anatomy and physiology

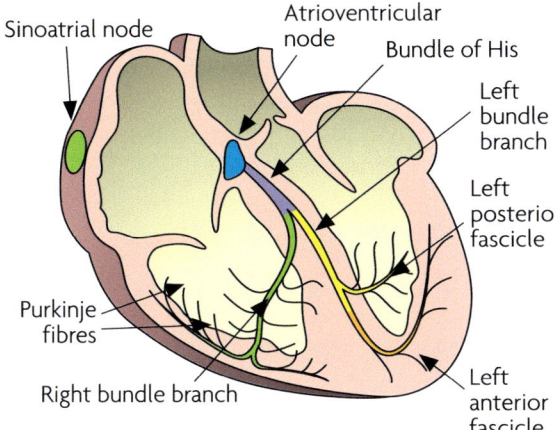

Figure 12.2 The electrical conduction pathway of the heart

the terminal crest of the right atrium, giving rise to the phenomenon of the wandering pacemaker and suggesting that there is a much larger area of pacemaker cells [Boyett, 2009]. Electrical impulses travel from the SA node to the AV node and also cross the interatrial septum via a set of specialised cells known as Bachmann's bundle.

AV node and bundle of His

The AV node is found in the right atrial wall, close to the opening of the coronary sinus and septal leaflet of the tricuspid valve. Its primary function is to delay the electrical impulse from the SA node long enough for atrial muscle contraction to squeeze additional blood into the ventricles (known as the atrial kick). Between the AV node and bundle branches is the bundle of His, which originates in the wall of the right atrium and straddles the interventricular septum. In normal physiology, this is the only way electrical impulses can pass between the atria and ventricles [Garcia, 2015].

Left bundle branch

The left bundle branch starts at the end of the bundle of His, travelling through the interventricular septum, providing fibres which innervate the left ventricle and left side of the interventricular septum. It splits into two fascicles: anterior and posterior. The left posterior fascicle is a fan-like structure that provides innervation to the posterior and inferior left ventricle via the Purkinje system. Being so widely distributed, it is hard to completely block. The left anterior fascicle, on the other hand, is a single strand, innervating the anterior and superior portions of the left ventricle [Garcia, 2015].

Right bundle branch

The right bundle branch also originates from the bundle of His and sprouts fibres that innervate the right ventricle and right face of the interventricular septum, stimulating the Purkinje fibres. These fibres (named after a Czech physiologist, Jan Purkinje) consist of individual cells located just under the endocardium, and directly innervate the myocardial cells [Boyett, 2009].

1.3.4 Coronary arteries

The heart requires its own blood supply in order to function properly. There are two main arteries that serve the heart, the right and left coronary arteries, which originate at the base of the ascending aorta (Figure 12.3).

Right coronary artery (RCA)

The RCA runs down the right side of the heart in the coronary sulcus (depression) between the right atrium and ventricle. Most people (around 80%) are right dominant; the RCA gives rise to the posterior descending artery (PDA). In around 8% however, the PDA arises from the left circumflex

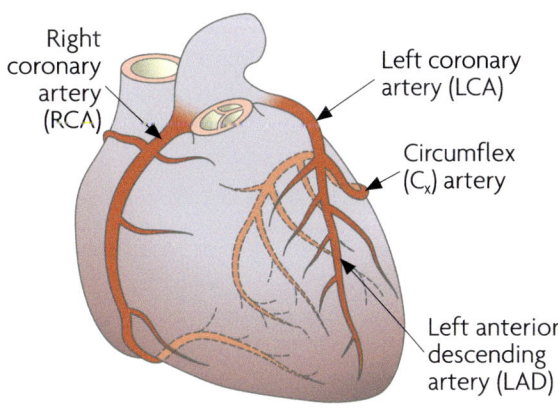

Figure 12.3 Coronary artery anatomy

(Cx) artery instead (termed left dominance), with the remainder (12%) being served by both arteries [Goldberg, 2007]. The PDA serves the inferior wall of the left ventricle and the inferior part of the septum.

Left coronary artery (LCA)
The LCA passes behind the pulmonary trunk and splits almost immediately into two branches, the anterior interventricular branch (often referred to as the left anterior descending artery, LAD) and the Cx. The LAD descends obliquely towards the apex of the heart in the anterior interventricular sulcus, supplying the anterior part of the septum and anterior wall of the left ventricle via one or two diagonal branches [Drake, 2019].

1.4 Blood

Blood is a connective tissue consisting of a liquid (plasma) and cells performing a range of essential functions for the body [Tortora, 2017]:
- Plasma makes up around 55% of blood and carries antibodies (an important part of the immune system) and nutrients to the body's tissues, and removes waste products.
- The formed elements make up the remaining 45% and consist of red and white blood cells, and platelets.
- Red blood cells (erythrocytes) carry oxygen to the tissues and remove carbon dioxide.
- White blood cells (leukocytes) are an important part of the immune and inflammatory processes.
- Platelets (thrombocytes) along with clotting factors are an essential component of normal blood clotting, particularly in cases of bleeding.

1.5 Blood vessels

There are five main types of blood vessels in the body. The largest are the elastic **arteries** that leave the heart before subdividing into medium-sized muscular arteries. These further subdivide into even smaller arteries known as **arterioles**. These are important vessels as they control blood flow into the **capillaries**, thin-walled vessels that allow for the exchange of substances between the blood and tissues. The capillaries unite to form small veins, known as **venules**, which subsequently merge to form larger and larger **veins** that return blood to the heart [Tortora, 2017].

1.5.1 Vessel structure

Most blood vessels (except capillaries) are made up of three layers or tunics (Figure 12.4). The internal layer (tunica intima or interna) consists of a smooth inner layer (the endothelium), a basement membrane and, in medium-sized arteries, a layer of elastic tissue that helps to maintain blood pressure. Ordinarily, the endothelial layer is the only one that comes into contact with blood in the lumen of the artery.

The medium-sized veins have one-way valves formed from the endothelial layer. These are designed to prevent blood flow from travelling in the wrong direction (i.e. away from the heart). They resist gravity-induced pooling, particularly in the lower limbs (i.e. the legs).

The next layer is the tunica media. This is made up of smooth muscle and elastic fibres, and is most developed in the medium-sized arteries and least developed in the veins. In the aorta and other large arteries there is a higher proportion of elastic

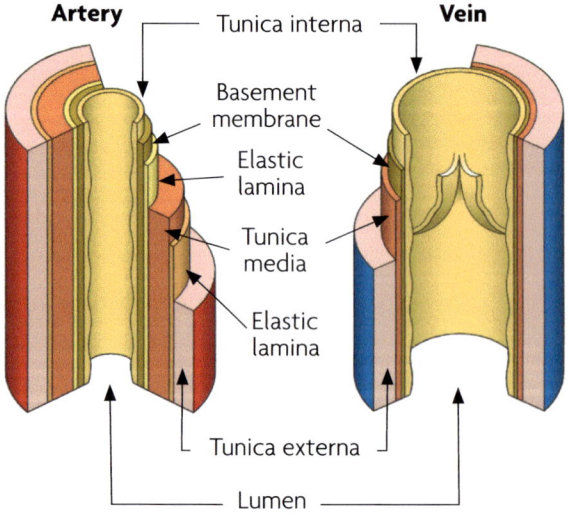

Figure 12.4 The structure of blood vessels

Cardiovascular system anatomy and physiology

fibres, making the walls highly compliant and able to stretch easily without tearing when subjected to pressure changes. This is advantageous because, as blood is ejected from the heart, the walls of the aorta stretch, acting as a pressure reservoir which can ensure blood flow continues, even when the ventricles are relaxed [Tortora, 2017].

The final layer is the tunica externa, which is constructed mostly from elastic and collagen fibres, but is also home to the vasa vasorum (the blood supply to the arteries) and nervi vasorum (motor nerves).

1.5.2 Arteries

Figure 12.5 shows the main arteries that branch from the aorta. It is not necessary to remember them all.

1.5.3 Veins

Figure 12.6 shows the main veins that are drained by the superior and inferior vena cavae.

1.6 *Cardiac cycle*

During a single cardiac cycle, both the atria and ventricles take it in turns to contract and relax, forcing blood from an area of high pressure (due to the contracted muscle) to low pressure. The cycle is short, just 0.8 seconds in a person with an average heart rate of 75 beats/minute [Garcia, 2015; Tortora, 2017].

1.6.1 Atrial systole

This takes about 0.1 second. It starts with the SA node generating an action potential (electrical

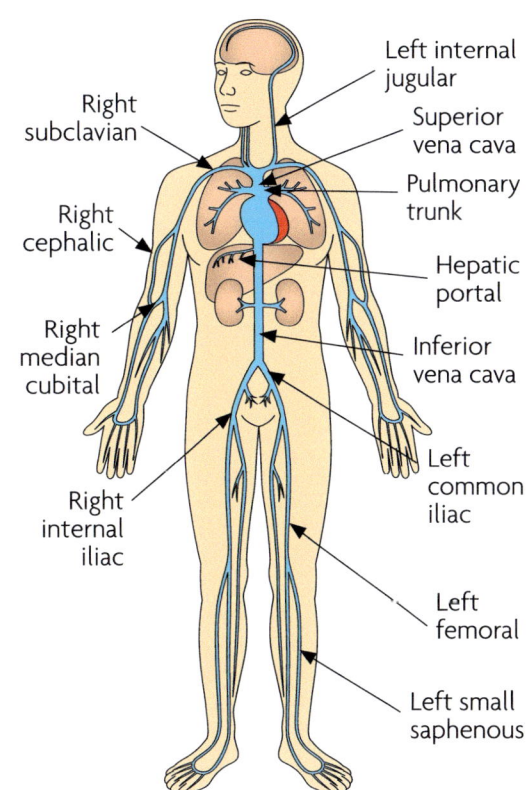

Figure 12.5 The aorta and its branches

Figure 12.6 Veins of the body

signal) when it depolarises (its voltage changes from negative to positive). This in turn causes the depolarisation of the atrial cardiac muscle cells, which contract (atrial systole). Blood is forced out of the atria, through the AV valves and into the ventricles, topping them up.

During this period, the electrical impulses from the SA node reach the AV node, pause to allow for atrial muscle contraction and then continue down the bundle of His, the bundle branches and into the Purkinje fibres, leading to ventricular depolarisation.

1.6.2 Ventricular systole

This lasts about 0.3 seconds, and during this time the atrial muscle relaxes (atrial diastole). Ventricular depolarisation causes the ventricular muscles to contract, and as the pressure inside the ventricles increases, the AV valves close and there is a brief period where all four valves of the heart are shut. This is known as isovolumetric contraction and lasts 0.05 seconds.

Contraction of the ventricles continues and eventually overcomes the pressure in the pulmonary and systemic circulations, causing the pulmonary and aortic valves (collectively known as the semilunar valves) to open. Blood is ejected into the pulmonary trunk and ascending aorta.

Meanwhile, the cardiac cells reset their voltage from positive (depolarised) to negative, a process known as repolarisation.

1.6.3 Relaxation period

This is the longest period in a cardiac cycle (around 0.4 seconds) and now both the atria and the ventricles are relaxed. This period is the most shortened when heart rate increases.

Ventricular repolarisation leads to relaxation of the ventricles (ventricular diastole), and as the pressure inside the ventricles falls, the semilunar valves close. As with systole, there is a brief period where all four valves are closed (isovolumetric relaxation). The pressure continues to fall, leading to the AV valves reopening, and passive filling of the ventricles begins. By the end of diastole, the ventricles will be 75% full, just in time for another action potential from the SA node to start the process all over again.

1.7 Electrocardiograms

The electrical signals that are responsible for the muscle contraction and relaxation during the cardiac cycle can be recorded on an electrocardiogram (ECG) (Figure 12.7). They are useful for determining cardiac rhythm disturbances (arrhythmias) and detecting myocardial injury, such as occurs during a heart attack (myocardial infarction).

As the heart's muscle cells depolarise and repolarise during the cardiac cycle, a potential difference (voltage) is generated, which can be detected on the surface of the body. Each cell generates its own electrical impulse, which has a strength and direction. The sum of all of these vectors is known as the heart's electrical axis and this is recorded on the ECG.

Recording the ECG is achieved with the use of electrodes that are placed in specific locations on the body, to capture the electrical activity of the heart. They are often compared to cameras placed around the heart to build up a three-dimensional picture. In reality, we do not refer to these electrical views as cameras but as leads, which are not to be confused with the physical leads that the electrodes are attached to. To record a 12-lead ECG, for example, you will only actually place 9 or 10 physical leads on the patient.

1.7.1 The ECG complex

An ECG complex is made up of a series of waves (a deflection from the baseline), segments and intervals which represent electrical events in the heart (Figure 12.8) [Garcia, 2015]:
- **P wave:** Atrial depolarisation.
- **PR segment:** This is the part of the complex between the end of the P wave and the start of the QRS wave. It should be along the baseline (the line from one TP segment to the next).
- **QRS wave:** It should be 0.12–0.20 seconds (three to five small squares).

Assessment of circulation

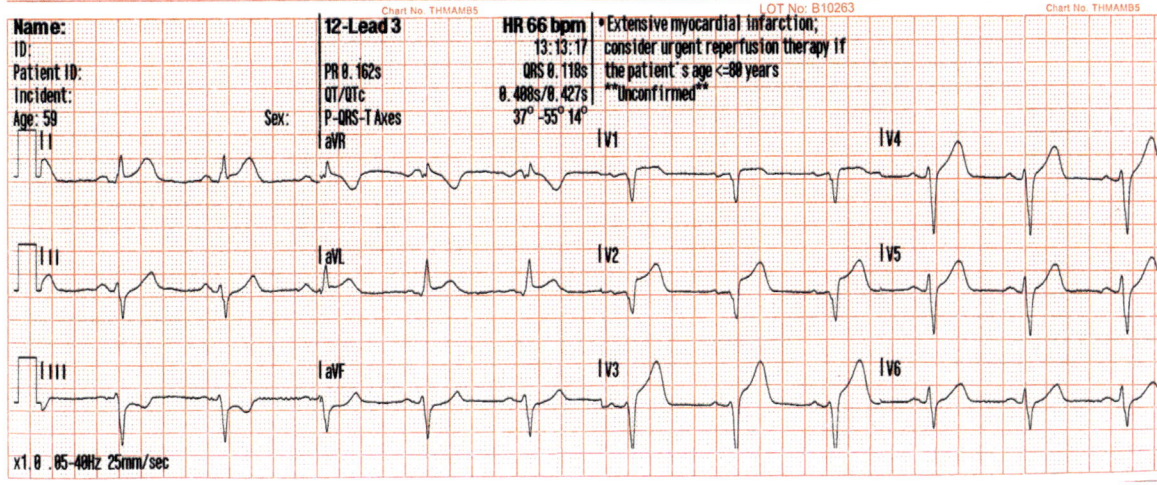

Figure 12.7 An example of a 12-lead ECG

- **QRS complex:** This represents ventricular depolarisation and is typically made up of a Q, R and S wave. It should be less than 0.12 seconds or three small squares in duration.
- **ST segment:** This is the part of the complex between the end of the QRS wave and the start of the T wave. The point at which the QRS wave ends and the ST segment begins is known as the J point. The ST segment should be on the baseline.
- **T wave:** This wave represents ventricular repolarisation and is the first deflection (positive or negative) that occurs after the ST segment. It should begin in the same direction as the QRS complex.

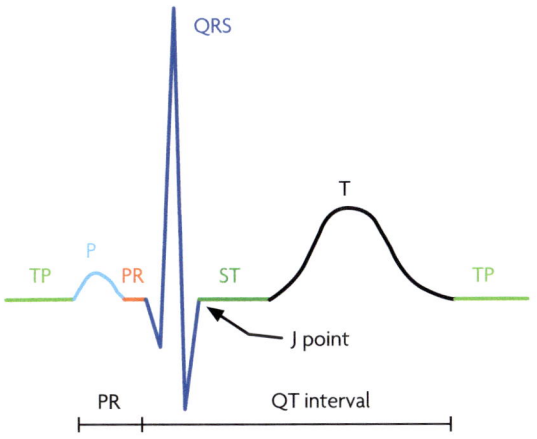

Figure 12.8 Basic components of an ECG complex

2 Assessment of circulation

2.1 Learning objectives

By the end of this section you will be able to:
- describe how to accurately measure the following:
  - pulse
  - capillary refill time
  - blood pressure (BP).

2.2 Introduction

If you are asked to assess a patient's pulse, or obtain a manual BP, you have been given a big responsibility, since only you will know how fast, regular and strong the pulse feels, or when you can hear the Korotkoff sounds in your stethoscope as the BP cuff is deflating.

Treatment decisions are made on the basis of clinical observations, so make sure you record observations accurately.

2.3 Pulse

The alternating expansion and recoil of the elastic arteries after ventricular systole creates a pressure wave, called a pulse, that can be felt in any artery that lies near the surface of the body and which can be compressed against a bone or other firm structure [Tortora, 2017].

Chapter 12 – Circulation

2.3.1 Pulse locations

Pulses are palpable all over the body, but you should be able to confidently locate the radial, brachial and carotid pulses (Figure 12.9). The other sites are useful for specific conditions, for example checking that a patient with a leg fracture has a dorsalis pedis pulse.

Radial pulse
The radial artery can be palpated at the wrist, on the radial side (thumb side) of the palmar (inner) aspect of the forearm. It is lateral to the long flexor tendons of the forearm (Figure 12.10) [Allan, 2004].

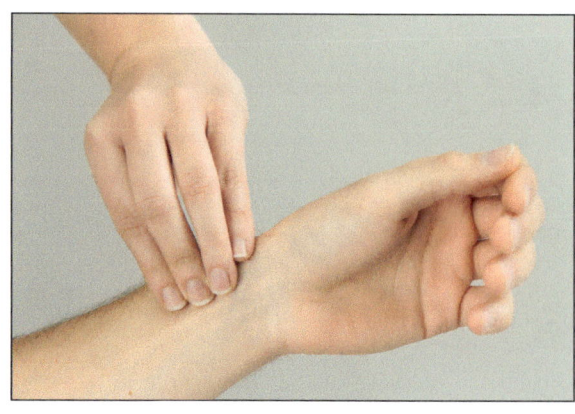

Figure 12.10 Palpating a radial pulse

Brachial pulse
There are two locations for measuring this pulse. The first is in the mid-arm and can be found

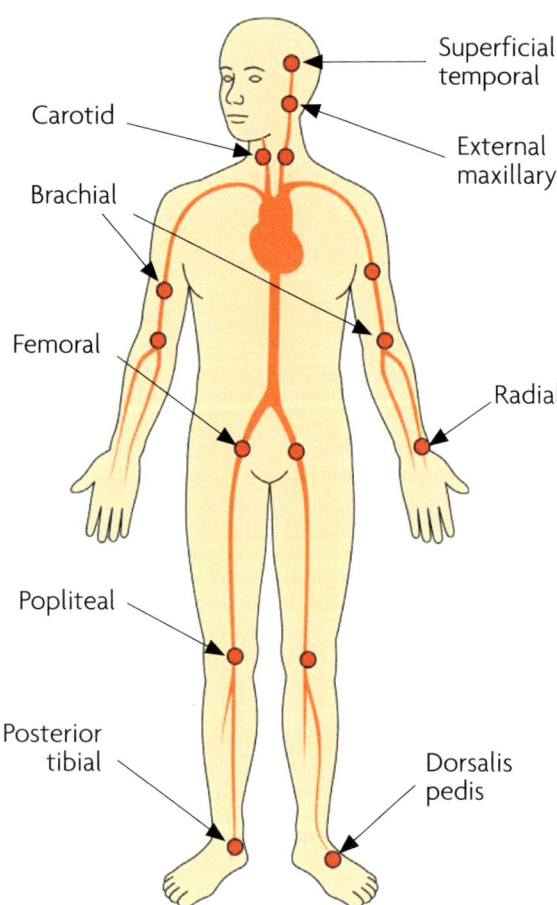

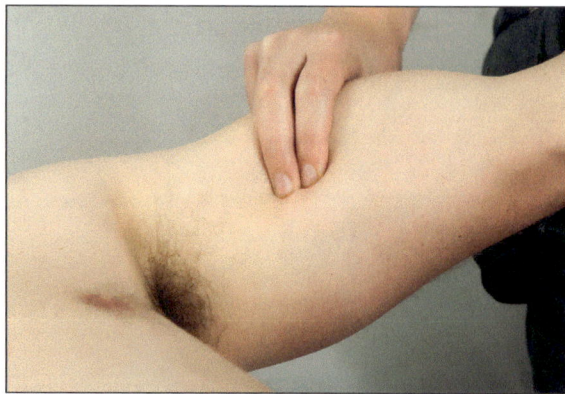

Figure 12.11 Palpating a brachial pulse between the biceps and triceps muscles

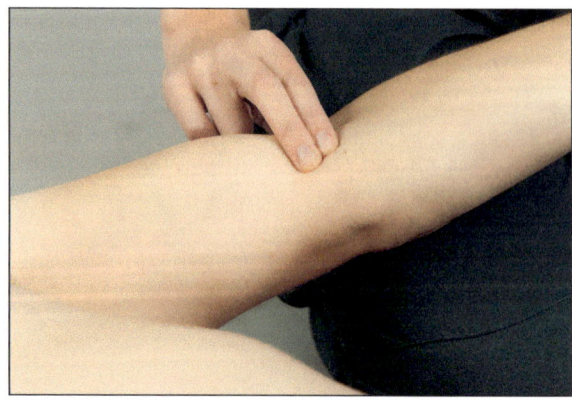

Figure 12.9 The location of commonly palpable pulses

Figure 12.12 Palpating a brachial pulse in the crease of the elbow

Assessment of circulation

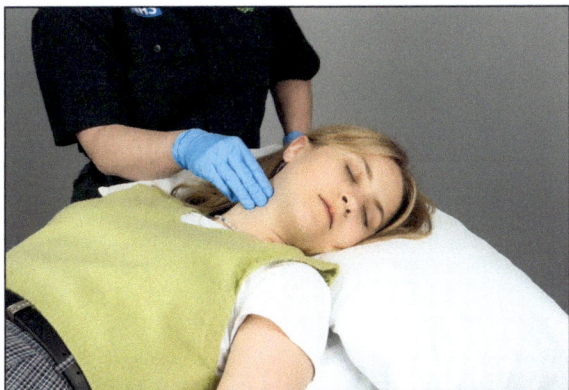

Figure 12.13 Palpating a carotid pulse

medially (towards the midline of the body) in the cleft between the biceps and triceps muscles (Figure 12.11). However, this is where a BP cuff is usually placed, so in that instance you can also palpate the pulse in the crease of the elbow (antecubital fossa, Figure 12.12). The pulse can be palpated just medial to the biceps tendon [Drake, 2019].

Carotid pulse
The carotid artery can be palpated between the larynx and the sternocleidomastoid muscle. Gently press to feel the pulse (Figure 12.13).

2.3.2 Assessment
When you assess a patient's pulse, you are looking for four things:
- rate
- rhythm
- volume
- character.

Rate
The normal pulse rate for an adult is 60–100 beats/min [Allan, 2004]. If the pulse rate is less than 60 beats/min, this is termed bradycardia, and if greater than 100 beats/min, tachycardia [Talley, 2006].

Causes of bradycardia include:
- sleep
- athletic training
- hypothyroidism (under-active thyroid gland)
- medications such as beta-blockers
- hypothermia
- some types of arrhythmia (abnormal electrical activity within the heart).

Causes of tachycardia include:
- exercise
- pain
- excitement/anxiety
- hyperthyroidism (over-active thyroid gland)
- fever
- some types of stimulant drugs, such as caffeine and cocaine
- some arrhythmias.

Rhythm
In healthy patients, the rhythm should be regular. However, in certain arrhythmias this regularity can be interrupted. Try to identify whether the irregularity is regular, i.e. seems to occur in a pattern, or the beats are apparently completely random, i.e. irregularly irregular [RCUK, 2021a].

Volume and character
The volume reflects the strength of the pulse. A high volume is typically noted during times when the cardiac output is high, such as during exercise, stress, heat and pregnancy. On the other hand, a low-volume pulse can be due to heart failure or peripheral vascular disease. A weak (also described as 'thready') pulse is most often seen in patients with a decreased blood volume (hypovolaemia, or shock) [Douglas, 2005].

The character of the pulse is slightly different, as you need to picture how the pulse changes during the cardiac cycle. This is tricky to master and will require practice.

2.3.3 Pulse measurement
Indications
- As part of initial assessment to determine whether the patient is in cardiac arrest.
- Routine cardiovascular physiological assessment.

Contra-indications
- None.

Advantages
- Gives early indication of the adequacy of cardiac output.
- Greater accuracy when estimating the rate of irregular heart rhythms than electronic devices (if count conducted over 60 seconds).

Chapter 12 – Circulation

Disadvantages
- Requires physical contact with the patient and the use of one hand, making other simultaneous activities difficult.
- Can take up to 60 seconds to perform accurately.

Procedure

Take the following steps to record a pulse [Pilbery & Lethbridge, 2022]:
1. Explain the procedure and obtain consent if appropriate to do so.
2. Don appropriate PPE, and undertake appropriate hand hygiene.
3. Place your index and middle fingers (and your ring finger, optionally) along the artery and press gently.

   As a general rule for adults, palpate the radial pulse first in conscious patients and the carotid pulse first in unconscious patients.

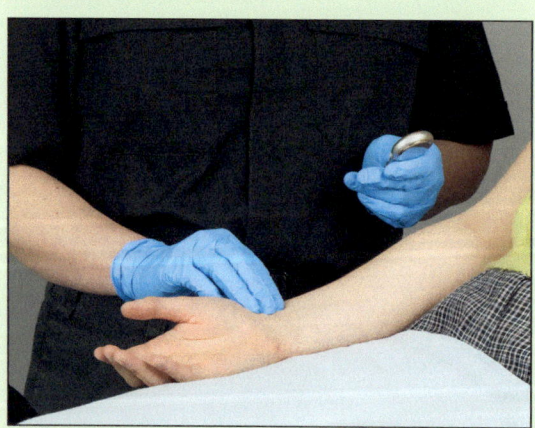

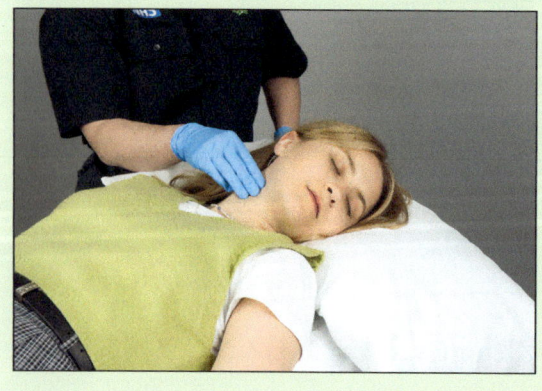

Procedure – *cont*
4. If the pulse has a regular rhythm, count for 15 seconds and then multiply by four. If the pulse is very fast or slow, or irregular, then count for a full 60 seconds.
5. Document the procedure.

2.4 Capillary refill time (CRT)

CRT is defined as the time taken for a distal capillary bed to regain its colour after pressure has been applied to cause blanching (turning pale) [Pickard, 2011]. It was introduced during World War II to estimate the degree of shock in battlefield survivors. In 1981, an upper limit of 2 seconds was arbitrarily chosen as the acceptable upper limit; this has become the acceptable normal value and is published widely [King, 2014].

This presents a problem because subsequent research has generally determined that it is not a good indicator of the degree of hypovolaemia in seriously ill and injured adult patients, and should not be used [Lewin, 2008].

It does have a place in the assessment of children, although it should not be taken in isolation, i.e. take into account the other aspects of patient assessment that you will undertake, such as pulse rate, respiratory rate, work of breathing, level of consciousness, etc. [King, 2014].

Because the usefulness of CRT is uncertain, you will need to follow local guidance about when to use CRT and in which age group.

2.4.1 Assessment

Be aware of the following external factors that can affect the accuracy of CRT measurement in children and neonates [King, 2014]:
- **Temperature:** Children in cool environments will have a prolonged CRT, even when they are completely healthy. There is no evidence that CRT is affected by a child's body temperature, such as when they are feverish due to an illness.
- **Ambient light:** Assessing CRT in poor light leads to errors. Ensure you are somewhere well lit.

Assessment of circulation

- **Site:** CRT is longer in neonates if the heel is used. One study demonstrated that fingertip and sternum CRTs are different in children [Crook, 2013]. Current paediatric guidelines advocate using only the sternum to assess CRT in children [RCUK, 2021b].
- **Pressure application:** It is not known how long pressure should be applied prior to assessing CRT, but current paediatric guidelines suggest pressing on the sternum for 5 seconds [RCUK, 2021b].
- **Observer:** When different people (observers) measure CRT at the same time, on the same child, they end up with different results. As a rule of thumb, try to ensure that the same clinician assesses CRT each time.

2.4.2 CRT measurement

Indications
- Part of the circulatory assessment of a patient.
- Suspicion of dehydration.
- Assessment of response to treatment.

Contra-indications
- Very sick children where distress may lead to decline of current condition, for example life-threatening asthma.
- Low-ambient light makes accurate assessment difficult.

Advantages
- Does not require equipment to perform.
- Provides some measure of circulatory adequacy when BP measurement is not possible.

Disadvantages
- Sick infants or children can have a normal CRT.
- Does not predict mild-to-moderate hypotension in adults and its usefulness in adults has been questioned.
- Accuracy can be affected by ambient temperature and light, the site and poor inter-observer agreement.

Procedure

Take the following steps to measure the CRT [Pilbery & Lethbridge, 2022]:

1. Explain the procedure to the patient and the patient's caregiver (depending on age) and obtain consent if appropriate to do so.
2. Don appropriate PPE, and undertake appropriate hand hygiene.
3. Ensure the environment is warm and well lit. Choose one person to record all CRT measurements.
4. Select either the upper part of the sternum (manubrium) or the fingertip pulp as the site for measurement.

    Site specific advice:
    - **Sternum:** Place your index finger on the patient's manubrium.
    - **Fingertip:** Place the fingertip pulp between your thumb and index finger and hold the hand at the level of the patient's heart.

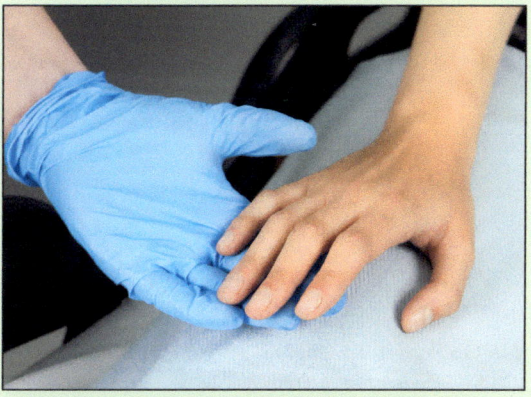

5. Provide sufficient pressure to make the tip of your nail blanch. Press for 5 seconds.

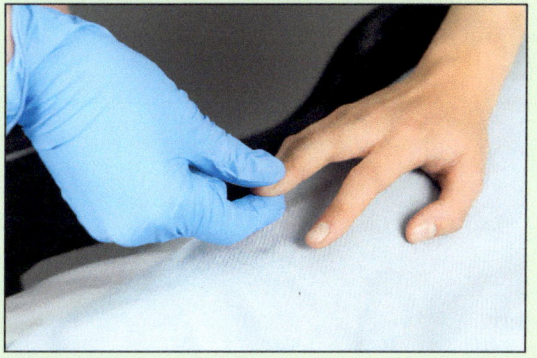

Chapter 12 – Circulation

Procedure – *cont*

6. Remove the pressure and immediately count aloud how long it takes for the skin to return to the pre-test colour.

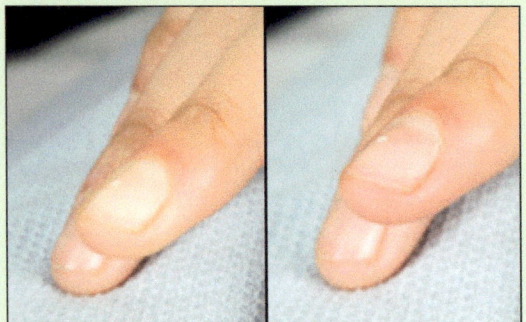

7. Consider repeating steps 4–5 and then average the results.
8. Document the procedure. A normal CRT is 2–3 seconds. A CRT of more than 3 seconds in a child is clinically important.

2.5 Blood pressure (BP)

BP is the measurement of the pressure exerted by the blood on the walls of a blood vessel. It is highest in the aorta and large systemic arteries and lowest in the large veins [Tortora, 2017].

A BP that you record consists of two measurements:
- **Systolic BP:** The BP during the systole phase of the cardiac cycle, when the ventricles contract and blood is forced out of the heart. This is the higher reading of BP.
- **Diastolic BP:** The BP during the diastole phase of the cardiac cycle, when the ventricles are relaxed. This is the lower reading of BP.
- It is usually measured in millimetres of mercury (mmHg) and recorded as the systolic value over the diastolic, for example 120/80 mmHg.

2.5.1 Assessment

BP values

The normal range for adult BP is a systolic value of 120–129 mmHg and/or diastolic of 80–84 mmHg. Hypertension (high BP) is defined as a systolic value of 140 mmHg or higher and/or a diastolic of 90 mmHg or higher [Williams, 2018]. Hypotension is usually defined as a systolic BP of less than 90 mmHg in adults [JRCALC, 2023].

Measurement of BP

Blood pressure can be measured directly, by inserting a sensor into a patient's artery, or indirectly, using a cuff, which is applied to a patient's arm. The advantage of direct measurement is that it is accurate and continuous; it is typically used in hospital intensive care units. This method is not practicable outside of hospital and so non-invasive methods are used.

Non-invasive BP (NIBP) measurement

There are two methods of NIBP measurement used by the ambulance service:
- **Auscultatory:** This method uses a stethoscope and an aneroid sphygmomanometer, a device consisting of an inflatable cuff and an aneroid manometer to measure the pressure on a dial (Figure 12.14).
- **Automated:** This consists of an inflatable cuff with a sensor that detects the oscillations generated by turbulent blood flow and calculates systolic and diastolic values using an algorithm.

Korotkoff sounds

When using the auscultatory method of measuring BP, you will place a stethoscope over the patient's brachial artery and listen for turbulent blood flow, known as the Korotkoff sounds, after a Russian surgeon, Nikolai Korotkoff, who first described them in 1905 [Talley, 2006].

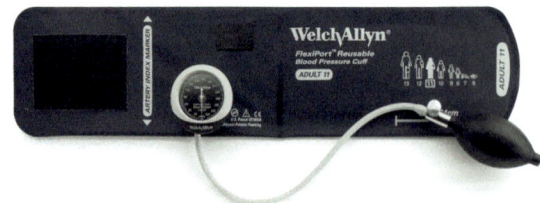

Figure 12.14 An aneroid sphygmomanometer
Image reproduced courtesy of Welch Allyn.

Assessment of circulation

The sounds are split into five phases [O'Brien, 2003]:
1. The first appearance of faint, repetitive, clear tapping sounds that gradually increase in intensity for at least two consecutive beats is the systolic blood pressure. This corresponds to the restoration of blood flow, and is confirmed by the presence of a palpable pulse.
2. A brief period may follow during which the sounds soften and acquire a swishing quality. In some patients, sounds may disappear altogether for a short time.
3. The return of sharper sounds, which become crisper, to regain or even exceed the intensity of phase 1 sounds.
4. The distinct, abrupt muffling of sounds, which become soft and blowing in quality.
5. The point at which all sounds finally disappear completely is the diastolic pressure.

Note that in some groups of patients, the phase 4 sounds may be heard until the BP measurement reaches 0 mmHg. In these cases, the onset of phase 4 is taken to be the diastolic BP measurement [O'Brien, 2003].

2.5.2 BP measurement

Manual BP measurement

Indications
- Need to undertake a cardiovascular assessment of a patient.
- Patient showing signs of shock.
- Assessment of a patient's response to treatment.

Contra-indications
- Patients who have an arteriovenous shunt should not have a BP recorded in the ipsilateral (same side of the body) arm.

Caution
- Korotkoff sounds are not reliably audible in infants under 6 months and in some older infants and children. Automated BP measurement is preferable in these age groups.

Advantages
- Provides reliable assessment of BP in the presence of slow or irregular heart rhythms, such as atrial fibrillation.
- Mechanical process (no need for electrical power).

Disadvantages
- Not as accurate as invasive BP monitoring.
- Takes time to perform with no opportunity for conducting other clinical care at the same time.

Procedure

Take the following steps to manually record a BP [Pilbery & Lethbridge, 2022]:
1. Explain the procedure and obtain consent if appropriate to do so.
2. Don appropriate PPE, and undertake appropriate hand hygiene.
3. If possible, allow the patient to sit for 3–5 minutes before measuring their BP, with feet flat on the floor and legs uncrossed. Ideally, the patient should have an empty bladder and have not experienced acute exposure to cold temperatures.

    The patient should have their back and arm supported, with the arm at the level of their heart (level with the mid-sternum).

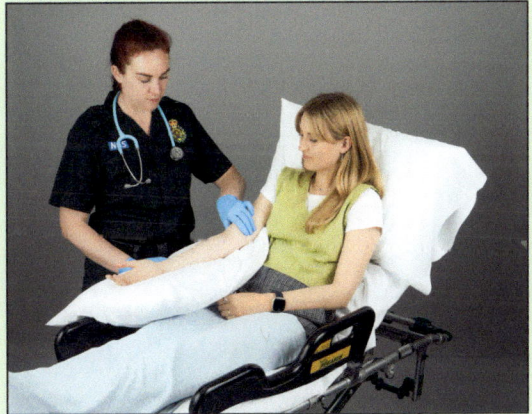

4. Ask about any medical conditions that might prevent a BP being recorded on a particular arm, such as paretic (partially paralysed) limbs, for example due to stroke, or arteriovenous shunts in dialysis patients.

Chapter 12 – Circulation

Procedure – *cont*

5. Ensure the arm is free of restrictive clothing.

   Do not apply a cuff over clothes, if possible.

6. Palpate the brachial artery. This can be found by placing the pads of the index and middle fingers of one hand on the biceps tendon and then moving medially and pressing deeply.

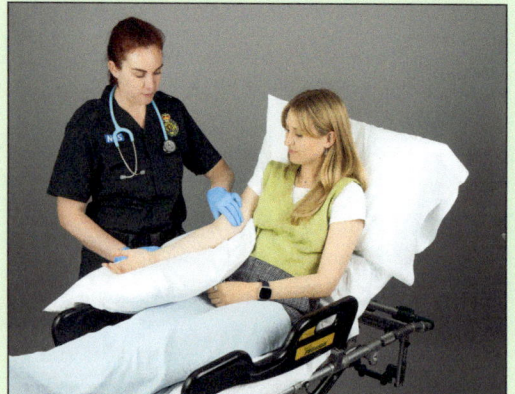

7. Select the appropriate cuff size. A standard bladder is 12–13 cm wide and 35 cm long, but ensure you have smaller and larger sizes available.

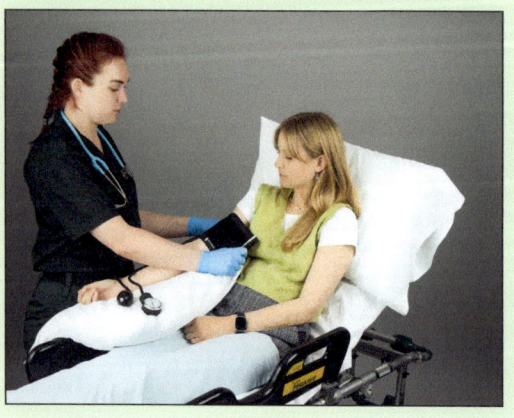

Procedure – *cont*

8. Place the artery marker on the cuff over the patient's brachial artery. The artery marker should be located within the sizing markers on the cuff.

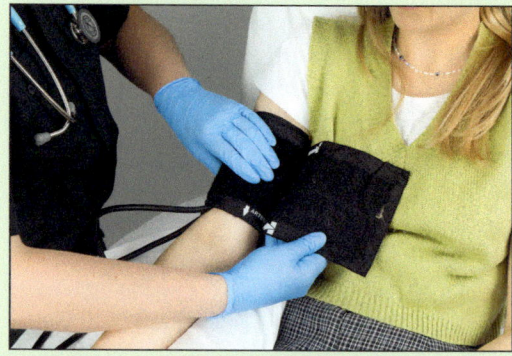

9. Wrap the cuff snugly around the patient's upper arm, with the lower edge of the cuff 2–3 cm above the palpated brachial artery. Ensure it is clear of the antecubital fossa and does not touch the stethoscope.

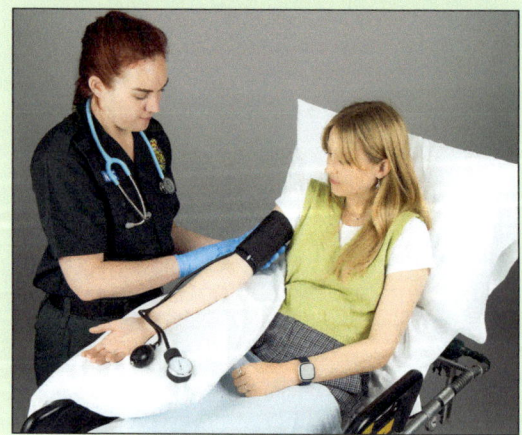

10. Ask the patient to remain still and not talk during the BP measurement.

Assessment of circulation

Procedure – *cont*

11. Palpate the brachial artery and inflate the cuff until the pulse disappears. Continue to inflate to 20–30 mmHg above this point.

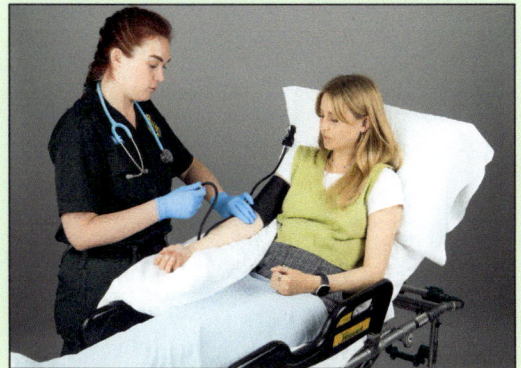

12. Slowly deflate the cuff and note when the pulse returns. This gives an estimation of the systolic BP.
13. Wait for 30 seconds. Then put the diaphragm of the stethoscope in position. Place it firmly, but not with too much pressure, over the brachial artery.

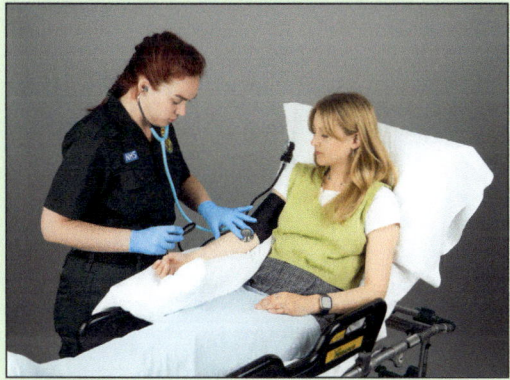

14. Rapidly inflate the cuff to 20–30 mmHg above your estimation of the systolic BP.
15. Deflate at a rate of 2–3 mmHg per pulse beat.

Procedure – *cont*

16. Note the pressure at which you first hear the Korotkoff sounds (phase 1, the systolic BP), the point at which they become muffled (phase 4) and then disappear (phase 5). The disappearance of sounds is usually taken to be the diastolic BP. If phase 5 does not occur until 0 mmHg, then the onset of phase 4 measurement should be taken as the diastolic value.

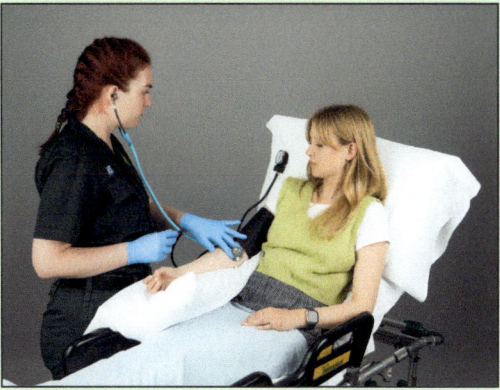

17. Document the BP as soon as possible, including the position of the patient and which arm the measurement was taken from, since these can affect the BP result.

Automated BP measurement

Indications
- Need for general physiological assessment of a patient.
- Patient showing signs of shock.
- To assess response to treatment.

Contra-indications
- Patients who have an arteriovenous shunt should not have BP recorded in the ipsilateral (same side of the body) arm.

Caution
- Some automated BP devices (for example, LifePak15 and Corpuls3) will not give an accurate reading when the patient has an irregular pulse (arrythmia).

Chapter 12 – Circulation

Advantages
- Provides reliable assessment of BP in infants under 6 months and in some older infants and children.
- Allows the clinician to undertake other tasks simultaneously.
- Unaffected by environments where there is excessive noise or lack of light.

Disadvantages
- Not as accurate as invasive BP monitoring.
- Requires batteries or external power source to function.

Procedure

Generic steps to obtain an accurate automated BP are presented here. However, you should follow the manufacturer's instructions for device-specific guidance [Pilbery & Lethbridge, 2022]:

1. Explain the procedure and obtain consent if appropriate to do so.
2. Don appropriate PPE, and undertake appropriate hand hygiene.
3. If possible, allow the patient to sit for 3–5 minutes before measuring their BP, with feet flat on the floor and legs uncrossed. Ideally, the patient should have an empty bladder and have not experienced acute exposure to cold temperatures.
   The patient should have their back and arm supported, with the arm at the level of their heart (level with the mid-sternum).
4. Ask about any medical conditions that might prevent a BP being recorded on a particular arm, for example paretic (partially paralysed) limbs or arteriovenous shunts in dialysis patients.
5. Ensure the arm is free of restrictive clothing. Do not apply a cuff over clothes, if possible.

Procedure – *cont*

6. Select the appropriate cuff size. If the cuff has sizing range markers or lines, ensure that the cuff ends between the range markings. If it doesn't, select a larger or smaller cuff. If the cuff is not fully deflated, squeeze any remaining air out of the cuff.

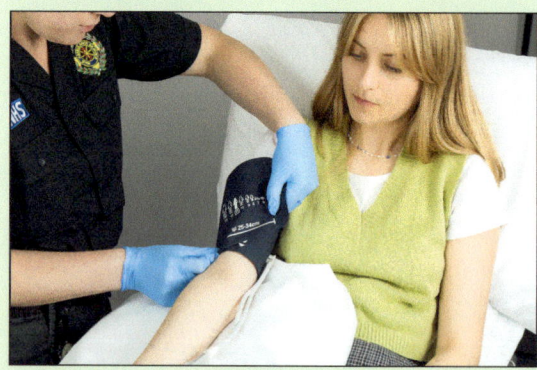

7. Connect the inflation tubing hose to the cuff and the monitor.

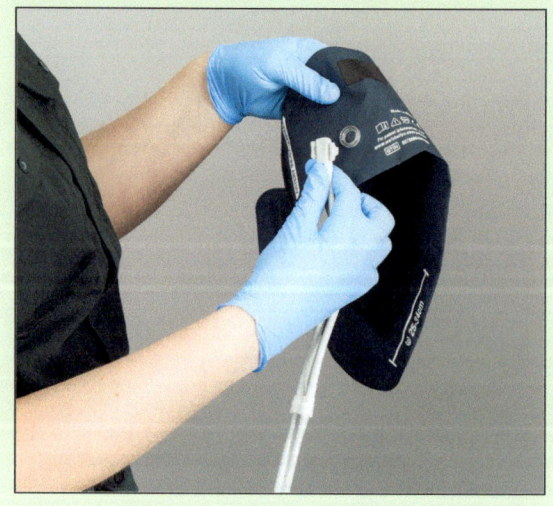

Assessment of circulation

Procedure – *cont*

8. Wrap the cuff snugly around the patient's upper arm, with the lower edge of the cuff 2–3 cm above the elbow crease. If the cuff has an artery marker, this should be placed over the brachial artery with the arrow pointing towards the hand.

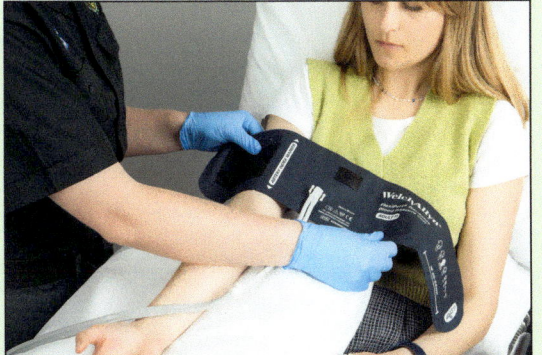

9. Check that the correct inflation setting has been selected.

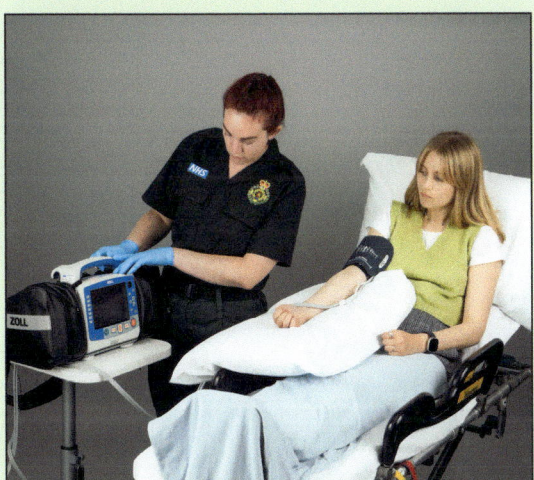

10. Ask the patient to remain still and not talk during the BP measurement.

Procedure – *cont*

11. Press the appropriate button on the monitor to measure the BP.

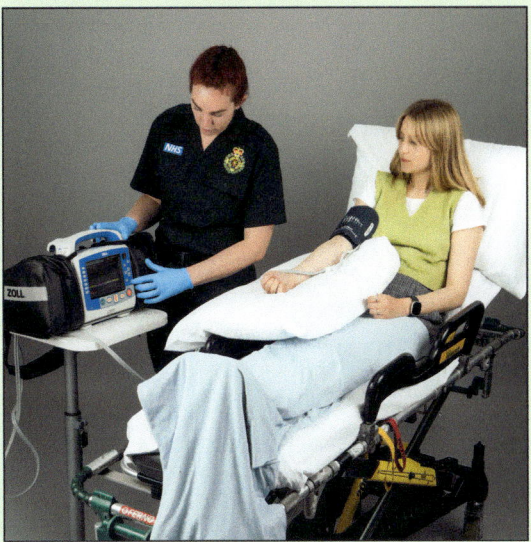

12. Document the BP as soon as possible, including the position of the patient and which arm the measurement was taken from, since these can affect the BP result.

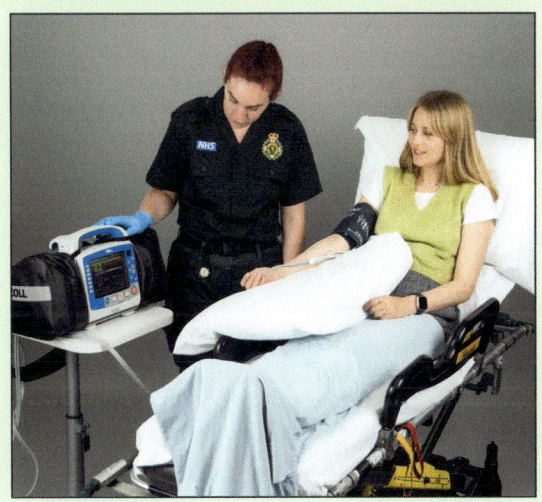

3 Cardiovascular system disorders

3.1 Learning objectives

By the end of this section you will be able to:
- describe the following conditions of the cardiovascular system and their management:
  - coronary artery disease (CAD)
  - stable angina
  - acute coronary syndromes (ACS)
  - heart failure
- explain the types and causes of shock and their management.

3.2 Introduction

Many of the cardiovascular conditions you are going to learn about in this section are most commonly caused by the consequences of ischaemic heart disease (IHD), which is the most common cause of death worldwide, with around 1.8 million people dying of it each year in Europe [Byrne, 2023]. However, this section will also cover some other conditions that affect the cardiovascular system.

3.3 Coronary artery disease (CAD)

CAD, sometimes referred to as IHD, is almost always caused by atherosclerosis of the coronary arteries. This is a systemic, lipid-(fat-)driven immune/inflammatory-disease of the medium and large arteries. Over time (usually decades), atherosclerosis causes the formation of plaques: collections of lipids and cholesterol that accumulate in the intimal layer of arteries, some of which attract macrophages (a type of white blood cell). The macrophages secrete protein-dissolving enzymes and engulf the lipids, leaving behind a lipid-rich 'necrotic core' [Falk, 2003].

The interface between the plaque and the lumen of the artery is known as the fibrous cap. If it becomes thickened, it can cause narrowing of the artery lumen (stenosis). If significant, this leads to cardiac ischaemia, particularly when myocardial oxygen demand rises, such as when the patient exercises. This can lead to stable or exertional angina. If the plaque ruptures, the artery can become occluded (blocked), leading to an acute coronary syndrome [Aaronson, 2012].

3.4 Angina

Angina is a pain or discomfort usually felt across or in the centre of the chest as a tightness or indigestion-like ache. This can radiate to one or both arms, the neck, back or epigastrium (the portion of the abdomen between the diaphragm and umbilicus, or belly button). It can be accompanied by belching, which may be wrongly assumed to be due to indigestion [RCUK, 2021a]. It is caused by significant stenosis (>70%) of at least one coronary artery due to CAD. This causes narrowing of the artery, which at rest still allows sufficient oxygenated blood to the myocardium. However, during exercise or stress, coronary oxygen demand increases. This demand can be met by increasing blood flow through increasing the diameter of the arteries. But this is not possible in stenosed vessels and the resulting imbalance of oxygen supply and demand leads to myocardial ischaemia [Aaronson, 2012].

Angina can be classified as stable or unstable. Unstable angina is defined as myocardial ischaemia at rest or on minimal exertion. It is characterised by specific clinical findings of prolonged (>20 minutes) angina at rest; new onset of severe angina; angina that is increasing in frequency, longer in duration, or lower in threshold; or angina that occurs after a recent heart attack. Stable angina is, in turn, split into three clinical classifications [Knuuti, 2020]:
- Typical angina: This has all of the following presenting characteristics:
  - constricting discomfort in the front of the chest or in the neck, jaw, shoulder or arm
  - caused by physical exertion
  - relived by rest or the administration of nitrate drugs within 5 minutes.
- Atypical angina: Patients report two of the characteristics of typical angina.
- Non-anginal chest pain: Has one (or sometimes none) of the characteristics of typical angina.

Note that research conducted since 2015 suggests that the most common presentations of stable angina are now atypical and non-anginal chest pain [Knuuti, 2020].

Cardiovascular system disorders

3.5 *Acute coronary syndrome (ACS)*

ACS represents a spectrum of three dangerous conditions, all of which constitute medical emergencies and result from a sudden decrease in coronary artery blood flow [Aaronson, 2012]. These three conditions, in order of increasing severity, are:
- unstable angina (UA)
- non-ST-elevation myocardial infarction (NSTEMI)
- ST-elevation myocardial infarction (STEMI).

Since the treatment of UA and NSTEMI is similar, they are usually considered together. The ST-segment in NSTEMI and STEMI refers to the portion of an ECG complex which may rise or elevate (STEMI) or not (NSTEMI) during a myocardial infarction (MI, heart attack).

3.5.1 Pathophysiology

The steps that lead to an ACS consist of [Aaronson, 2012]:
1. Rupture of the fibrous cap leads to platelet aggregation (clumping together).
2. Intraplaque thrombus (blood clot) expands the plaque and can occlude the artery if large enough.
3. Intraluminal thrombus resulting in partial or complete occlusion of the artery.
4. Release of vasoconstricting substances associated with platelet aggregation, which makes the vessel constrict.
5. Endothelial damage promotes further vasoconstriction.

3.5.2 Assessment

The most common presentation of ACS is chest pain felt just under the sternum (sub-sternal) that may be described as heavy, squeezing, crushing or tight, that has lasted for more than 20 minutes and has not been relieved by glyceryl trinitrate (GTN). Excessive sweating, epigastric pain/indigestion, and shoulder or arm pain are commonly associated symptoms in both men and women. Some symptoms are more common in women with ACS and include [Byrne, 2023]:
- dizziness/syncope
- nausea and vomiting
- jaw/neck pain
- shortness of breath
- pain between the shoulder blades
- palpitations
- fatigue.

Note that a small proportion of patients will not present with chest pain [Valensi, 2011]. These are more likely to be women, and have diabetes or a history of heart failure [Canto, 2012].

3.5.3 Aspirin

The indications and contra-indications listed below are taken from the UK Ambulance Services Clinical Practice Guidelines [JRCALC, 2023]. However, you should be familiar with your own service guidelines as restrictions on administration may exist.

Presentation
- 300 milligrams aspirin (acetylsalicylic acid) in tablet form. Dispersible or chewable.

Actions
- Has an antiplatelet action which reduces clot formation.

Indications
- Adults with clinical or ECG evidence suggestive of MI or ischaemia.

Contra-indications
- Known aspirin allergy or sensitivity.
- Children under 16 years.
- Active gastrointestinal bleeding.
- Haemophilia or other known clotting disorders.
- Severe hepatic (liver) failure with jaundice.

Cautions
- As the likely benefits of a single 300 milligram aspirin tablet outweigh the potential risks, aspirin may be given to patients with:
  - asthma
  - pregnancy
  - renal (kidney) failure
  - moderate hepatic disease without jaundice
  - gastric or duodenal ulcer
  - current treatment with anticoagulants.

Side effects
- Increased risk of gastric bleeding.
- Wheezing in some asthmatics.

Chapter 12 – Circulation

Dosage and administration
- Route: oral – chewed or dissolved in water.
- 300 milligram tablet, no repeat dose.
- 300 milligrams must be given unless the patient has already had 300 milligrams for this episode. If the patient has had a smaller dose that day (less than 300 milligrams), a dose of 300 milligrams should be given.

⚠ 3.5.4 Glyceryl trinitrate (GTN)

The indications and contra-indications listed below are taken from the UK Ambulance Services Clinical Practice Guidelines [JRCALC, 2023]. However, you should be familiar with your own service guidelines as restrictions on administration may exist.

Presentation
- Sublingual spray containing 400 micrograms GTN per metered dose.
- Sublingual tablets containing GTN 300, 500 or 600 micrograms per tablet.

Actions
- A potent vasodilator drug resulting in:
  - dilatation of coronary arteries/relief of coronary spasm.
  - dilatation of systemic veins resulting in lower pre-load.
  - reduced BP.

Indications
- Cardiac chest pain due to angina or MI, when systolic blood pressure is greater than 90 mmHg.

Contra-indications
- Hypotension (systolic blood pressure <90 mmHg).
- Hypovolaemia.
- Head trauma.
- Cerebral haemorrhage.
- Sildenafil (Viagra) and other related drugs – GTN must not be given to patients who have taken sildenafil or related drugs within the previous 24 hours. Profound hypotension may occur.
- Unconscious patients.
- Known severe aortic or mitral stenosis.

Side effects
- Headache.
- Hypotension.

Dosage and administration
- Route: sublingual tablet/spray (administer under the patient's tongue and close mouth).
- Sublingual spray: 1–2 sprays providing 400–800 micrograms of GTN.
- Sublingual tablet: 2, 3 or 5 milligram tablet.
- Repeat every 5–10 minutes.
- The effect of the first dose should be assessed over 5 minutes; further doses can be administered provided the systolic blood pressure is >90 mmHg. Remove the tablet if side effects occur, for example hypotension.
- Note: The oral mucosa must be moist for GTN absorption; moisten if necessary.

3.5.5 Management

The management of ACS includes [JRCALC, 2023]:
- correction of major <C>ABCD problems
- oxygen, if the patient has oxygen saturations of less than 94% on air
- administration of aspirin
- assisting the patient to take their own GTN
- being prepared to resuscitate the patient if they have a cardiac arrest.

3.6 Heart failure

Heart failure is a clinical syndrome consisting of cardinal signs (e.g. elevated jugular venous pressure, pulmonary crackles, and peripheral oedema) and symptoms (e.g. breathlessness, ankle swelling, and fatigue). It is due to a structural and/or functional abnormality of the heart that results in elevated intracardiac pressures and/or inadequate cardiac output at rest and/or during exercise [McDonagh, 2021].

Patients who have been living with heart failure for some time are classed as having chronic heart failure. If their signs and symptoms have not changed in the past month, then it is considered to be stable. On the other hand, if there is an acute deterioration in these patients, they are considered to be in acute decompensated heart failure (often just called acute heart failure, AHF) [Allen, 2007].

Although the most common cause of AHF is sudden worsening of chronic heart failure (sometimes referred to as 'acute on chronic heart failure'), about

20–30% of cases are new-onset heart failure, with a small percentage due to malignant hypertensive crisis (BP that is high enough to damage the body's organs) or cardiogenic shock. Up to 25% of cases are caused by an ACS, although these are normally considered separately from 'typical' AHF because of the differing presentation, pathophysiology and treatment [Howlett, 2011].

3.6.1 Assessment

Heart failure can be difficult to diagnose in the pre-hospital environment, since many of the symptoms are non-specific (Table 12.1), making it difficult to differentiate AHF from other conditions such as pneumonia, COPD and pulmonary oedema [Williams, 2013]. The more specific symptoms (such as orthopnoea [shortness of breath when lying flat], paroxysmal nocturnal dyspnoea [PND, shortness of breath that awakens a patient from sleep] and haemoptysis [coughing up blood from the lungs]) are less common [Dobson, 2009].

3.6.2 Management

The management of AHF includes [JRCALC, 2023]:
- correction of major <C>ABCD problems
- patient positioning: sit the patient fully upright as soon as possible
- oxygen, if the patient has oxygen saturations of less than 94% on air.

Table 12.1 History, signs and symptoms of heart failure

History	Signs	Symptoms
Patient age	Tachypnoea	Shortness of breath
Coronary artery disease	Crackles	Dyspnoea
Hypertension	Dullness to percussion	Orthopnoea
High cholesterol	Reduced SpO_2	Fatigue
Valvular disease (e.g. mitral regurgitation or aortic stenosis)	Haemoptysis	PND
Known heart failure or myocardial injury	Tachycardia	Reduced exercise tolerance
Loop diuretic use (e.g. furosemide)	Peripheral oedema	Ankle swelling
Arrhythmias	Enlarged liver	
	Reduced urine output	

3.7 Shock

Shock is a clinical state in which the delivery of oxygenated blood (and other nutrients, such as glucose) to the body's tissues is not adequate to meet metabolic demand [RCUK, 2021b]. While the cause of shock may not originate in the cardiovascular system, it will cause an impact, sometimes life-threatening, on the system.

The types of shock vary between textbooks, but five types are included here:
- hypovolaemic shock
- distributive shock
- cardiogenic shock
- obstructive shock
- dissociative shock.

3.7.1 Hypovolaemic shock

This is an acute loss of circulating blood volume either from dehydration (loss of fluids and electrolytes) or from bleeding (haemorrhage) externally or internally. Shock due to blood loss (haemorrhagic shock) has been classified into four classes (stages) [NAEMT, 2020]:
- Class 1: The body is able to cope with losses and there are no obvious clinical signs.
- Class 2: This is the compensated stage. Blood loss is more significant, but the body has mechanisms to maintain blood pressure despite the reduction in blood volume.
- Class 3: This is the decompensated stage. Despite the compensatory mechanisms, blood loss is now too severe to maintain blood pressure. These patients require blood and urgent surgical intervention to stop the bleeding.
- Class 4: The irreversible stage. Even if the circulation is restored, the patient is still likely to die.

Signs of hypovolaemic shock

The classic signs of hypovolaemic shock include [JRCALC, 2023]:
- pallor
- cool peripheries
- anxiety and abnormal behaviour
- increased heart and respiratory rates.

Note that these signs may not appear until 1,000–1,500 ml of blood has been lost, and even later in some patient groups, such as pregnant women, patients on medication such as beta-blockers, and fit individuals.

3.7.2 Distributive shock

This type of shock is caused by widespread dilation of the peripheral vascular system because of dilation of the arterioles and/or venules. This in effect creates a larger container for the same blood volume, leading to decreased tissue perfusion. In addition, in causes such as anaphylaxis and sepsis, the vessels become 'leaky', allowing fluid to escape into the tissues and so being removed from the general circulation.

Common causes of distributive shock include:
- anaphylaxis
- sepsis
- nervous system-related causes such as spinal cord injury.

3.7.3 Cardiogenic shock

This is due to a primary cardiac problem when the heart is unable to circulate sufficient blood to meet the body's metabolic needs. This is most common following a MI, but can also be caused by acute heart failure or arrhythmia.

3.7.4 Obstructive shock

This is an uncommon cause of shock and is due to an obstruction of blood flow to/from the heart. It can be caused by a tension pneumothorax, cardiac tamponade or a massive pulmonary embolism [Evans, 2012].

3.7.5 Dissociative shock

This occurs when the oxygen-carrying capacity of the blood is affected because of inadequate numbers of red blood cells available to carry sufficient oxygen (anaemia) or when competing molecules take up space on the red blood cells that would normally be used to carry oxygen, such as in cases of carbon monoxide poisoning [RCUK, 2021b].

3.7.6 Management

Your management of shock will include the following steps [JRCALC, 2023; Zideman, 2021]:
1. Identify and control sources of external bleeding (note that the management of life-threatening external bleeding is covered in Chapter 16, 'Trauma').
2. Administer high levels of supplemental oxygen via a non-rebreathe mask to target oxygen saturations of 94–98% or 88–92% if the patient is known to have COPD.
3. Place patients supine and, if there is no history of trauma, raise their legs. Note that this is only likely to provide transient improvement in vital signs (typically less than 7 minutes).

13 Disability

1 Nervous system anatomy and physiology

1.1 Learning objectives

By the end of this section you will be able to:
- state the functions of the nervous system
- describe the anatomy and physiology of the nervous system.

1.2 Introduction

The nervous system performs three main functions in order to carry out a complex range of tasks including controlling body movements, regulating heart rate, creating memories and producing speech [Tortora, 2017; Briar, 2003]:

- **Sensory function (perception):** Receptors located around the body detect internal stimuli, such as a change in blood pressure, and external stimuli, such as a bad odour, and transmit them via afferent nerves through the cranial and spinal nerves and into the brain and spinal cord.
- **Information transfer and processing:** Nerve cells (neurons) have special projections (axons) that allow the conduction of electrical impulses. These can be delivered to other neurons, and/or modified by or integrated with other impulses to create a complex web that can process sensory information received from afferent neurons.
- **Motor function:** This is the nervous system's response to the processing stage and is communicated via efferent nerves, which carry electrical impulses from the brain via cranial or spinal nerves. This enables the brain to control the body's movements as well as control ventilation and circulation.

1.3 Anatomy and physiology

The nervous system (Figure 13.1) consists of the brain and spinal cord (generally referred to as the central nervous system, CNS) and a network of peripheral nerves either originating from the brain (as 12 pairs of cranial nerves) or the spinal cord (as 31 pairs of spinal nerves). Together with small collections

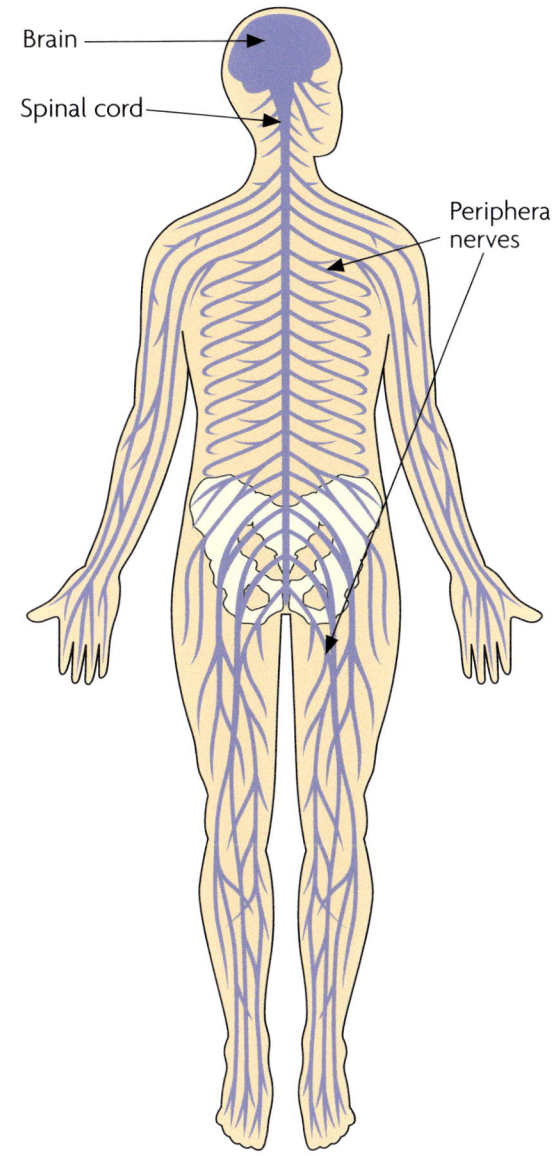

Figure 13.1 The nervous system

of neurons known as ganglia, these form the peripheral nervous system (PNS).

The PNS consists of two divisions. The first is the sensory, or afferent, division, which is composed of large numbers of sensory receptors in the skin. Their nerve impulses are conveyed by somatic sensory fibres, as well as internally around the body (impulses from which are transmitted by visceral sensory fibres), and an extensive network of neurons around the gastrointestinal (GI) tract, collectively known as the enteric plexus, which helps regulate digestion. The other division of the PNS is the motor, or efferent, division. This is split into the somatic nervous system and the autonomic nervous system (ANS) [Marieb, 2019; Tortora, 2017].

1.4 Brain

The portion of the CNS that is contained within the skull is known as the brain. The brain occupies 80% of the cranial vault, with the remaining 20% made up of cerebral blood (12%) and cerebral spinal fluid (CSF, 8%). It has a wide range of functions in addition to serving as the centre for intellect, emotions, behaviour and memory. The brain is generally divided into four major sections (Figure 13.2) [Tortora, 2017]:
- brain stem
- cerebellum
- diencephalon
- cerebrum.

1.4.1 Brain stem

The brain stem consists of the medulla oblongata, pons and midbrain. Their functions include:
- medulla oblongata:
  - relays sensory and motor input between other parts of the brain and spinal cord
  - together with pons and midbrain, controls level of consciousness
  - contains centres to manage heart rate, BP and breathing
  - contains the origins of a number of cranial nerves
- pons:
  - relays nervous impulses from one side of the cerebellum to the other and between the medulla and midbrain
  - contains the origins of a number of cranial nerves
  - contains centres to regulate breathing
- midbrain:
  - relays motor output from the cerebral cortex and sensory input from the spinal cord to the thalamus
  - controls and co-ordinates movement
  - contains the origins of two cranial nerves.

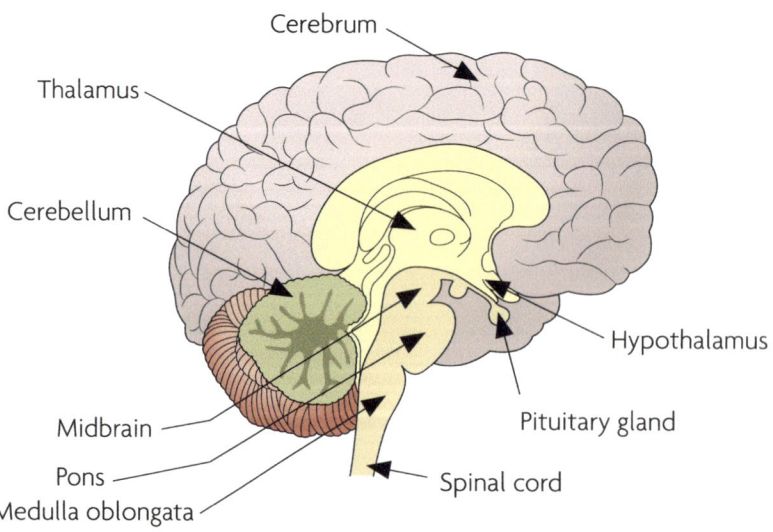

Figure 13.2 The brain

1.4.2 Cerebellum

This part of the brain is responsible for co-ordinating complex and skilled movements, and regulates posture and balance.

1.4.3 Diencephalon

Located deep within the brain, underneath the cerebrum, the diencephalon is the link between the nervous system and the endocrine system. The diencephalon comprises:
- thalamus:
  - relays sensory input to the cerebral cortex
  - provides perception of touch, pressure, pain and temperature
- hypothalamus:
  - controls and integrates ANS activity
  - regulates behavioural patterns and circadian rhythms
  - controls body temperature
  - regulates eating and drinking behaviour.

1.4.4 Cerebrum

The cerebrum allows you to read, write and speak. Various regions are responsible for a range of other functions:
- Sensory areas are involved in perception of sensory information.
- Motor areas control muscular movements.
- Association areas are responsible for complex functions such as memory, personality and intelligence.

The cerebrum is split into two hemispheres and consists of an outer rim of grey matter and an internal region of white matter. The outer rim of grey matter contains the cerebral cortex which, although thin, contains billions of neurons. Each hemisphere can also be further divided into four lobes: frontal, parietal, occipital and temporal.

1.4.5 Meninges

In addition to the skull, the brain is protected by the meninges. There are three of them [Tortora, 2017]:

- **Dura mater:** Tough outer layer consisting of connective tissue.
- **Arachnoid mater:** Middle layer. The subarachnoid space (between arachnoid and pia layers) is filled with CSF.
- **Pia mater:** Delicate inner layer containing small blood vessels that supply oxygen and nutrients to the brain.

1.4.6 Cerebral spinal fluid (CSF)

CSF is a clear, colourless liquid, which protects the brain and spinal cord from physical and chemical injury. It also carries oxygen, glucose and other nutrients that are essential for normal brain function, as well as removing waste products [Tortora, 2017].

1.5 Spinal cord

The vertebral column consists of 33 vertebrae: 7 cervical, 12 thoracic, 5 lumbar, 5 sacral and 4 coccygeal. Part of their function is to provide physical protection for the spinal cord, which the vertebrae encapsulate. Additional protection is provided by vertebral ligaments, meninges and the CSF [Tortora, 2017]. Rather confusingly, there are 31 pairs of spinal nerves: 8 cervical, 12 thoracic, 5 lumbar, 5 sacral and 1 coccygeal (Figure 13.3).

The spinal cord is almost cylindrical in shape, although slightly squashed in the anterior-posterior dimension. Its average diameter is just 12 mm, and in adults it extends from the medulla oblongata to the superior border of the second lumbar vertebra (L2), i.e. it does not extend the full length of the vertebral column. Instead, it tapers to form a cone-like structure called the conus medullaris [Tortora, 2017]. Nerves that originate distal to the conus medullaris form the cauda equina (meaning horse's tail). These nerves have a dorsal root containing afferent fibres, which transmit sensation, and a ventral root containing efferent motor fibres [Gitelman, 2008].

1.6 Somatic nervous system

The somatic nervous system is also sometimes known as the voluntary nervous system, since it

Chapter 13 – Disability

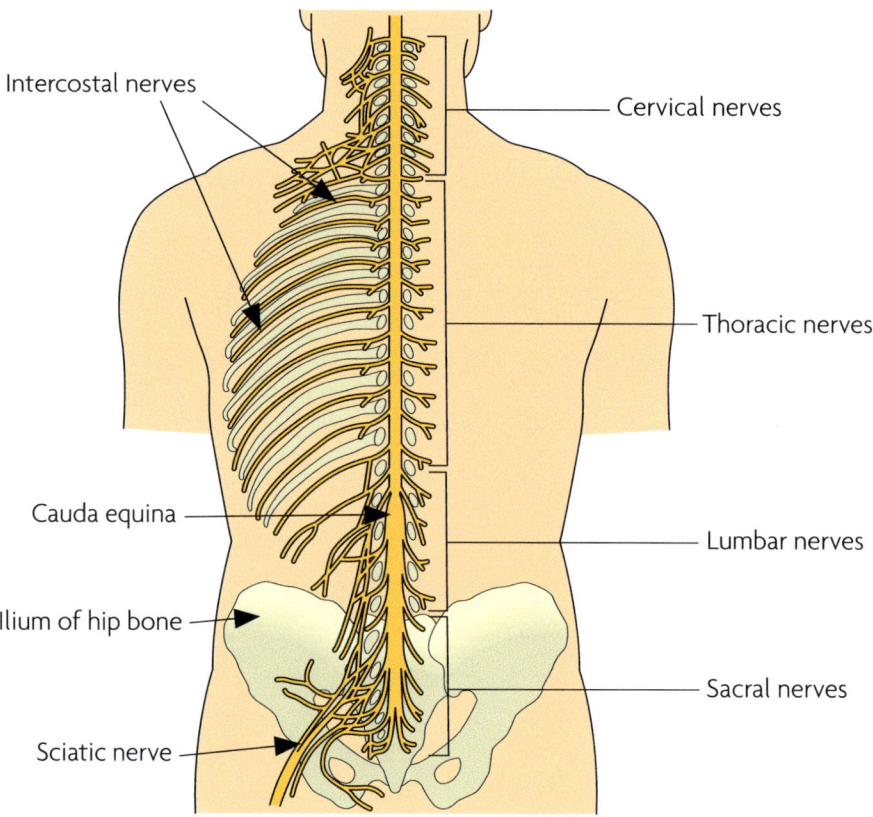

Figure 13.3 Spinal nerves

allows the person to consciously control their skeletal muscles thanks to somatic nerve fibres that conduct impulses from the CNS to skeletal muscles [Marieb, 2019]. However, the somatic nervous system also includes an involuntary component: reflexes. These are primarily a protective mechanism, for instance removing your hand when you touch something hot [Tortora, 2017].

1.7 *Autonomic nervous system (ANS)*

The ANS is divided into three parts. These are the sympathetic, parasympathetic and enteric nervous systems. They are called autonomic because it was originally believed that they functioned completely independently from the CNS. However, it is now known that the hypothalamus and brain stem regulate ANS activity [Tortora, 2017]. The enteric division is an extensive network of neurons which reside within the walls of the GI tract, pancreas and gall bladder. It has a sensory nervous function enabling the monitoring of the mechanical state of the alimentary canal and the chemical status of the stomach and intestines. In addition, it can output motor signals to modify the motility and secretions of the gut, as well as controlling the diameter of local blood vessels [Briar, 2003].

The sympathetic and parasympathetic divisions of the ANS are often thought of as being at either end of a see-saw. This is true in some organs, such as the heart, but in reality this is rather a simplistic view. Some parts of the body receive inputs from only one division, whereas in others the effects of the sympathetic and parasympathetic divisions are similar. However, their actions are carefully controlled and co-ordinated by the hypothalamus.

1.7.1 Sympathetic and parasympathetic divisions

The sympathetic division is often referred to as the fight-or-flight division, as its actions prepare the body to respond to stress, facilitating sudden strenuous exercise and increased vigilance. In addition, it helps control blood pressure, thermoregulation, and gut and urogenital function.

The parasympathetic division is often referred to as the rest-and-digest division. Actions of the parasympathetic division include antagonising some effects of the sympathetic division, for example heart rate, gut motility and bronchiole diameter, and controlling many body functions in non-stress states, such as GI secretion to aid digestion, micturition (emptying the bladder of urine) and defecation.

Another important difference between the sympathetic and parasympathetic divisions is their structure. Parasympathetic neurons are clustered at either end of the spinal cord, whereas the sympathetic neurons originate from the thoracolumbar section.

2 Assessment of disability

2.1 Learning objectives

By the end of this section you will be able to:
- describe how to undertake and record a face, arm, speech, time (FAST) test.

2.2 Introduction

A complete assessment of the nervous system is involved and requires a number of tests, which is beyond the scope of the responder. However, there are a couple of useful and simple tests that you can perform, which will uncover the presence of serious neurological problems in your patient and help determine the most appropriate management for them. You have already met one of them, AVPU, in Chapter 9, 'Patient Assessment'. The other, is the FAST test.

2.3 FAST test

With the advent of clot-busting drugs (thrombolytics) and mechanical removal of clots (thrombectomy) for the management of acute stroke, the need for prompt recognition of stroke has never been greater. A simple tool that can be used to identify a patient having a stroke is the FAST test [JRCALC, 2023].

2.3.1 Procedure

Indications
- Patient with suspected stroke or transient ischaemic attack.

Contra-indications
- None.

Advantages
- Quick and straightforward to undertake.
- Can facilitate direct referral to hyper-acute stroke pathways in eligible patients.

Disadvantages
- Does not detect symptoms such as unilateral leg weakness or vision loss.
- Requires the patient to be able to understand and follow commands.

Procedure

Take the following steps to undertake a FAST test [Pilbery & Lethbrige, 2022]:

Action
1. Explain the procedure to the patient and obtain consent.

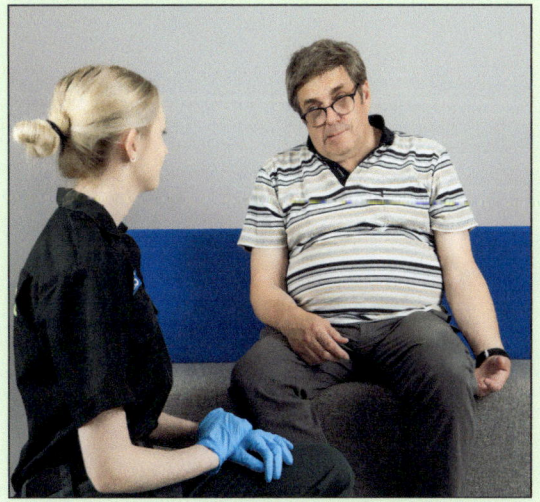

2. Don appropriate PPE, and undertake appropriate hand hygiene.

Chapter 13 – Disability

Procedure – *cont*

3. Ask the patient to smile or show their teeth. Look for a new lack of symmetry. This is positive if there is an unequal smile, grimace or obvious facial asymmetry.

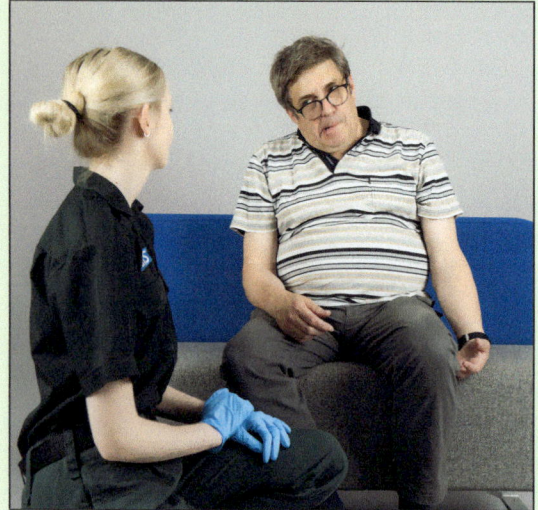

4. Lift the patient's arms together to 90° (45° if they are lying on their back) with palms uppermost. Ask them to hold that position for 5 seconds. Look for one arm drifting or falling rapidly.

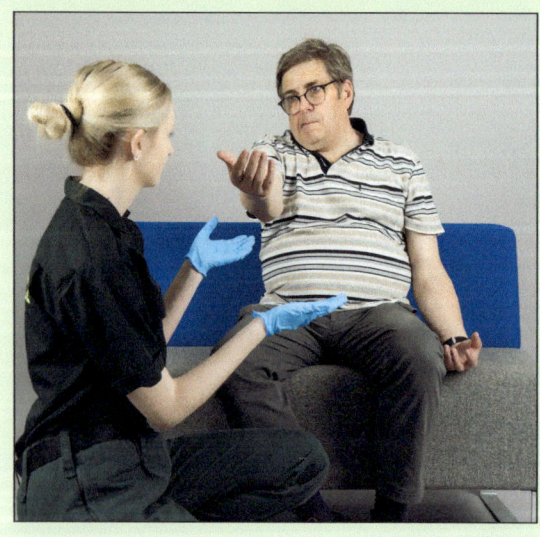

Procedure – *cont*

5. During conversation (if the patient can speak), look for new speech disturbance. This may require asking someone who knows the patient. Specifically, look for slurred speech and word-finding difficulties. Ask the patient to identify common objects (such as keys, a cup, a chair or a pen). If the patient has a severe visual disturbance, place the object in the patient's hand and ask them to name it.

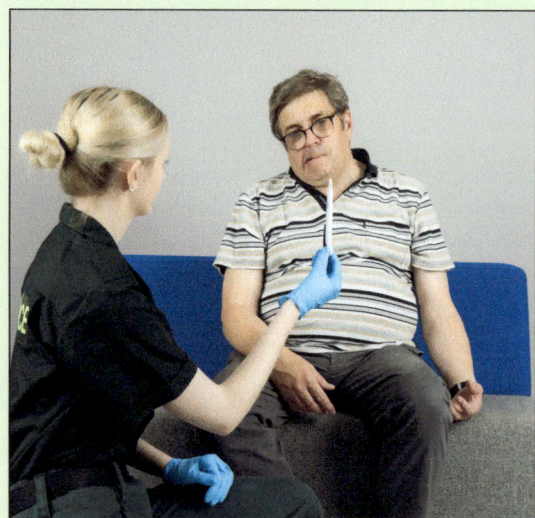

6. Document the procedure including the time of onset, if known; the presence of one or more of the signs above constitutes a positive test.

3   Disorders of the nervous system

3.1   *Learning objectives*

By the end of this section you will be able to:
- explain the pathophysiology relating to a range of neurological disorders
- describe the management of a range of neurological disorders
- list several causes of coma.

3.2 Introduction

In this section, you will learn about a range of nervous system disorders. The nervous system is extremely complex and you will learn about only a few of the many disease processes. However, it is important to be able to recognise patients with epilepsy, stroke and meningococcal disease and patients who are unconscious. Timely and appropriate management can result in a better outcome: in some cases, literally the difference between life and death, and/or life-altering disability.

3.3 Convulsions

Epilepsy is not a single condition, but a term used to describe a tendency to have recurrent, unprovoked convulsions (also called seizures and fits). It is the commonest of the serious neurological conditions [Smithson, 2012].

Convulsions result from the synchronised and excessive activation of neurons in the cerebral cortex. How this presents clinically depends on where this activity starts and how far and fast it spreads through the brain [Briar, 2003]. Convulsions are divided into two broad categories:

- **Partial (focal) convulsions:** As the name suggests, these originate from a specific area of the cortex, typically the temporal or frontal lobes. They are split into two sub-types [Smithson, 2012; Briar, 2003]:
    - **Simple partial:** Patients remain conscious but may complain of 'butterflies' in their stomach, fear, illusions and hallucinations. These are usually brief.
    - **Complex partial:** Complex refers to an altered level of consciousness and is characterised by the patient chewing, lip-smacking and fiddling with their hands. These usually resolve within a few minutes.
- **Generalised convulsions:** These convulsions are also divided into two sub-types:
    - **Tonic–clonic:** These convulsions consist of two phases. In the tonic phase, the patient goes stiff (and may cry out), falls (if standing) and bites their tongue as the jaw clenches. This is followed by the clonic phase, characterised by regular jerking movements, which start in the upper limbs. These eventually slow and stop, which may herald the onset of incontinence. Patients typically experience a post-ictal (post-convulsion) period following a tonic–clonic convulsion, where they may be sleepy and confused. This usually resolves within 20 minutes.
    - **Absence convulsions:** These typically begin in childhood and adolescence and consist of 'day-dreaming', with a few seconds of staring into space, eyelid fluttering, swallowing and head flopping.

3.3.1 Febrile convulsions

Patients with febrile convulsions are not considered to have epilepsy, since the convulsion is provoked by a sudden increase in temperature. The most commonly affected age group is from 6 months to 6 years. They are not associated with an increased risk of developing epilepsy in later life [Lissauer, 2007].

3.3.2 Convulsive status epilepticus

Convulsive status epilepticus is defined as a generalised convulsion that has not stopped after 5 minutes, or a series of such convulsions without recovery in between which lasts for 5 minutes or more [JRCALC, 2023].

In adults and children, common causes of convulsive status epilepticus (CSE) are withdrawal from or sub-therapeutic doses of anti-epileptic drugs. In children, the most common cause is febrile illness, whereas in adults, stroke is the most common cause. Approximately 16–38% of children diagnosed with CSE are known to have epilepsy. In adults, this figure increases to 42–50% [Chin, 2004; Neligan, 2010].

3.3.3 Post-ictal phase

For patients who have a generalised tonic–clonic convulsion, they typically enter a post-ictal phase, which is characterised by a period of unresponsiveness and then a gradual return of consciousness. The patient is likely to be drowsy and disorientated, which can last 15 minutes to an hour (and in some cases longer). Complaints of a headache are common [Kumar, 2012].

3.3.4 Management of convulsions

As with all patients, start by ensuring they have a patent airway. This can be achieved by a combination of patient positioning (e.g. the recovery position) and airway adjuncts. An OPA can be difficult to insert when patients are convulsing and should not be forced into the patient's mouth. Consider using a NPA instead [JRCALC, 2023].

Administer high-concentration oxygen (as close to 100% as possible) via a non-rebreathe mask (or BVM) at a flow rate of 15 l/min. In adults, once a reliable pulse oximetry reading has been obtained, oxygen administration can be titrated to maintain saturations of 94–98%. Children should continue to receive high concentrations of oxygen irrespective of the pulse oximeter reading [JRCALC, 2023].

3.4 Stroke

Stroke is a syndrome consisting of rapidly developing (usually seconds or minutes) symptoms and/or signs of focal CNS function. The symptoms last more than 24 hours or lead to death. A transient ischaemic attack (TIA) is essentially the same thing as a stroke, with the exception of the duration of symptoms, which last less than 24 hours and are not caused by a haemorrhage [Ginsberg, 2004]. Stroke is a common cause of death in England with around 30,000 stroke-related deaths each year. Around 57,000 people have a stroke for the first time in England every year, a quarter of them in people under 65 years of age [PHE, 2018].

3.4.1 Anatomy and physiology

The brain cannot store oxygen or glucose and so is dependent on a constant supply of blood, which is provided by two pairs of vessels, the vertebral and internal carotid arteries (Figure 13.4). These arteries are interconnected in the cranial cavity to produce an arterial circle (the circle of Willis), which provides an alternative pathway for blood flow should one of the vessels become occluded [Tortora, 2017].

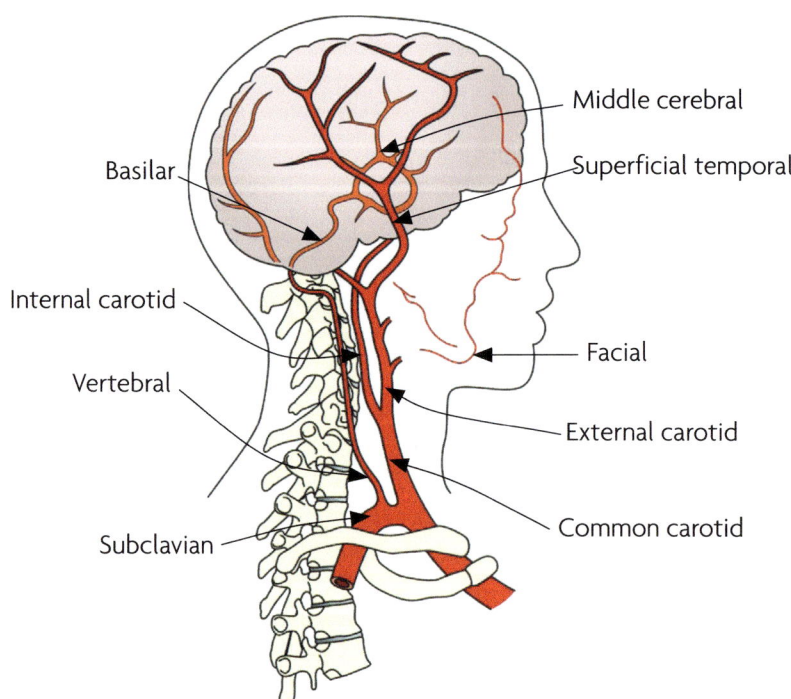

Figure 13.4 Arteries supplying the brain. Note all arteries shown are right-sided except the basilar artery

Disorders of the nervous system

3.4.2 Risk factors

Non-modifiable risk factors for stroke include age, sex, race and family or previous medical history of stroke, TIAs or MI. The chance of having a stroke roughly doubles each decade after the age of 55 years and, although it is more common in men, over half of all stroke deaths occur in women. People of South Asian, African or African-Caribbean origin are more likely to have a stroke [O'Donnell, 2010]. Modifiable risk factors include hypertension, smoking, atrial fibrillation, diabetes, diet, physical activity, alcohol consumption, blood cholesterol and obesity [Rodgers, 2004].

3.4.3 Types of stroke

Strokes can be classified as either ischaemic or haemorrhagic in origin. Ischaemic strokes are the most common and are caused by atherosclerosis or an embolus from the heart, for example. They are responsible for around 85% of all new strokes. Less common are strokes of vascular origin, caused by haemorrhage. Acute stroke is a medical emergency and the treatment to re-open the arteries is time-dependent, so the sooner patients are transported to a dedicated stroke centre, the better [JRCALC, 2023].

3.4.4 Assessment and management of stroke

- Assess ABCDE as for all patients.
- Determining the time of onset in stroke is very important for subsequent treatment. Find out when the patient was last free of stroke-like symptoms.
- Oxygen is not recommended unless the patient is hypoxic.
- Record a blood sugar if trained to do so; hypoglycaemia is a common stroke mimic.

3.5 *Meningococcal disease*

Meningococcal disease is an umbrella term for a systemic bacterial infection caused by *Neisseria meningitidis* (meningococcus). It presents as meningitis (inflammation of the meninges), septicaemia or a combination of both [PHE, 2019].

Although uncommon, 5–10% of those affected will die, and survivors may experience long-term physical, cognitive and psychological consequences. It is most common in infants, followed by children aged 1–4 years of age and a smaller peak in incidence in young adults aged 15–19 years of age [PHE, 2022].

3.5.1 Pathophysiology

Meningococci inhabit the nasopharynx in around 10% of the population, although it is less common in infants (under 5%) and most common in 19-year-olds (over 23%). If the meningococci manage to penetrate the protective mucosa of the nasal passages and enter the bloodstream, they rapidly multiply, doubling in number every 30 minutes.

In some people, meningococci cross the blood–brain barrier, where the bacteria are free to multiply inside the CSF. This leads to inflammation and swelling in the meninges and brain tissue, raising intracranial pressure (ICP), which can result in nervous system damage and even death. Surprisingly, patients with meningococcal meningitis do better than those who go on to develop septicaemia. This is thought to be because the body's immune response has prevented the bacteria from causing an overwhelming sepsis [Ninis, 2010].

3.5.2 Signs and symptoms

A major issue in the recognition of meningococcal disease is the non-specific nature of the signs and symptoms in the initial stages of the disease. These include [NICE, 2015]:

- fever
- nausea/vomiting
- lethargy
- being irritable/unsettled
- ill appearance
- refusing food/drink
- headache
- muscle ache/joint pain
- respiratory signs and symptoms.

However, the diagnosis window is short. Many children will have non-specific signs and symptoms in the first 4–6 hours, but can be close to death

Chapter 13 – Disability

after 24 hours [Thompson, 2006]. Children who show 'classic' signs and symptoms of meningitis or septicaemia are more likely to have the severe disease [NICE, 2015].

3.5.3 Sepsis and shock

The first specific clinical signs to appear are likely to be those of sepsis and shock and include leg pain, abnormal skin colour, cold hands and feet, and, in older children, thirst. Parents of younger children may also report drowsiness and difficulty in breathing (described as rapid or laboured) [Thompson, 2006]. Don't forget to enquire about how much urine a child has been passing or if they have had a wet nappy recently. Oliguria (low output of urine) is an early sign of shock [Ninis, 2010].

3.5.4 Fever

Many children with septicaemia will become acutely ill with a fever. This can be complicated by a trivial viral illness that precedes this, but look for a sudden change in the history. Remember that not all children with meningococcal disease have fever, and you should not dismiss a fever responsive to antipyretics (such as paracetamol and ibuprofen) as being of viral origin [Ninis, 2010]. Rather counter-intuitively, infants can actually develop hypothermia in sepsis [Wells, 2001].

3.5.5 Rash

The classic sign is a petechial non-blanching rash (Figure 13.5). However, only 10% of children presenting with the rash will have meningococcal disease; the remainder will have viral meningitis. On the other hand, febrile and ill children with a purpuric rash (a non-blanching rash of greater than 2 mm in diameter) are very likely to have meningococcal disease [Wells, 2001]. Care needs to be taken with blanching rashes, such as a maculopapular rash, as up to 30% of children may initially present with this, although careful examination will generally yield some non-blanching elements (Figure 13.6) [Hart, 2006]. On dark skin, you may have to check the soles of the feet, palms of the hand, abdomen, or conjunctivae (the thin membrane that covers the inside of the eyelids and white of the eye) and palate. You must fully undress the child and be thorough in your search. Petechial rashes may not be widespread initially and can be easily missed.

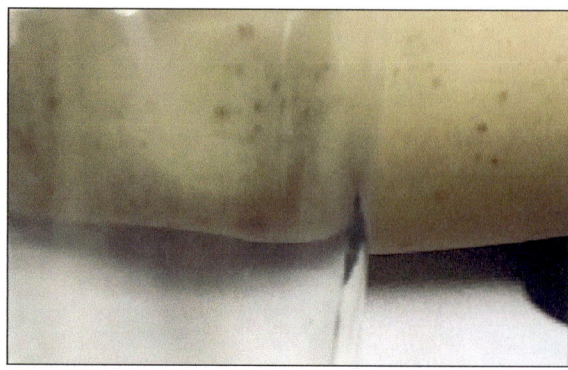

Figure 13.5 Petechial non-blanching rash. Note how this does not blanch under the pressure of a glass
Source: Image reproduced courtesy of Meningitis Research Foundation, www.meningitis.org.

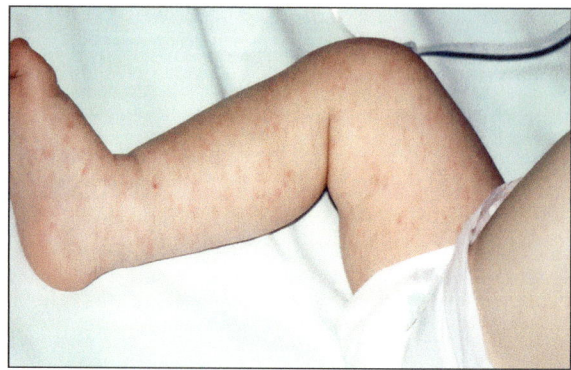

Figure 13.6 Maculopapular rash with scanty petechiae
Source: Image reproduced courtesy of Meningitis Research Foundation, www.meningitis.org.

3.5.6 Management

Patients with meningococcal disease need to be transported to hospital as soon as possible [JRCALC, 2023]. While you wait for an ambulance you should:

- ensure a patent airway
- administer high levels of oxygen to all patients via a non-rebreathe mask
- assist ventilations, if necessary.

3.6 Paralysis

In medical terminology, paralysis is typically represented by the suffix '-plegia'. This is not to be confused with paresis, which is used to refer to muscle weakness, or incomplete loss of muscle function [Porth, 2014]. Four common terms that you will hear used are [Innes, 2018]:
- **Monoplegia:** Paralysis in a single limb.
- **Hemiplegia:** Paralysis of both limbs on the same side of the body.
- **Quadriplegia** (also tetraplegia): Paralysis of all four limbs.
- **Paraplegia:** Paralysis of both the lower limbs.

3.7 Coma

Coma is the absence of consciousness (i.e. unconsciousness) and is often referred to as a loss of consciousness. This presents as a completely unaware patient, unresponsive to external stimuli, with only eye-opening to pain and no eye tracking or fixation, and limb withdrawal to a noxious stimulus (usually pain) at best (often with reflex motor movements) [Wijdicks, 2010].

Full consciousness is an awake state in which one is aware of oneself and the environment, including the ability to perceive and interpret stimuli, and to interact and communicate with others in the absence of motor deficits [Young, 2024].

Common causes of coma include:
- stroke – ischaemic and haemorrhagic
- cardiac arrest
- alcohol abuse
- substance abuse and overdose
- carbon monoxide poisoning
- sepsis
- bacterial meningitis
- syncope (faint)
- convulsions
- traumatic brain injury
- hyper-/hypoglycaemia.

Uncommon causes of coma include:
- subarachnoid haemorrhage
- brain abscess or tumour
- burns
- hypo-/hyperthermia.

It may not always be possible to determine the cause of coma, and the management of the patient may just be supportive. However, for reversible causes, such as hypoglycaemia, convulsions and overdose, it is important to recognise these conditions, as the patient can then receive the appropriate treatment out-of-hospital.

14 Exposure

1 Extremes of temperature

1.1 Learning objectives
By the end of this section you will be able to:
- state the normal temperature range for an adult
- explain the terms 'hypothermia' and 'heat-related illness'
- describe the appropriate management for a patient with signs of hypothermia and heat-related illness.

1.2 Introduction
Despite being exposed to a wide range of environmental temperatures, the human body maintains a stable temperature of around 37°C and is maintained in the range 35.8–38.2°C. Normal fluctuations of about 1°C occur over a 24-hour period, with highest temperatures recorded in the afternoon and early evening, and lowest temperatures in the early morning [Marieb, 2019].

Thermoregulation is primarily the job of the hypothalamus, which receives sensory information from peripheral and central thermoreceptors. This is necessary because the different body regions have differing temperatures [Tortora, 2017]:
- **Core:** Consisting of organs within the skull, thorax and abdomen.
- **Shell:** The skin.

By controlling the flow of blood to the shell, the hypothalamus can control the amount of heat generated and lost.

1.2.1 Heat-promoting mechanisms
When the external temperature falls, the heat-promoting centre is activated. This maintains core body temperature by [Marieb, 2019]:
- constricting peripheral cutaneous blood vessels
- causing shivering – involuntary contractions of skeletal muscle, which generates heat
- increasing the body's metabolic rate.

In addition, there are a number of behavioural changes that can be promoted:
- putting on warmer clothes
- drinking hot fluids
- increasing physical activity.

1.2.2 Heat-loss mechanisms
Most heat loss occurs via the skin by dilation of cutaneous blood vessels and/or enhanced sweating, allowing for heat loss to occur by [Marieb, 2019]:
- **Radiation:** Infrared waves (thermal energy).
- **Conduction:** Direct contact with cooler objects (such as cold water).
- **Convection:** Since warm air expands and rises, warm air around the body is constantly replaced with cooler air, which absorbs heat. This process can be enhanced by moving air more rapidly across the body surface, for example by the use of a fan.
- **Evaporation:** As water absorbs heat from the body, it becomes energetic enough to escape the body as a gas, called water vapour.

1.3 Hypothermia
Hypothermia is defined as a core body temperature of less than 35°C. It is classified into three categories, based on temperature [JRCALC, 2023]:
- **Mild:** 32–35°C.
- **Moderate:** 28–32°C.
- **Severe:** Less than 28°C.

Without a low-reading thermometer, it can be difficult to record accurate core body temperature, so it is important to know the temperature range of the thermometers you use. For example, while consumer tympanic thermometers may have a measurable range of only 34–42.4°C, 'professional' versions can measure down to 20.0°C. Therefore, it is important to suspect that hypothermia might be a factor in the following cases, particularly if

Chapter 14 – Exposure

you cannot get a reading from your thermometer [JRCALC, 2023]:
- older patients (over 80 years of age)
- children
- some medical conditions (for example, hypothyroidism and stroke)
- intoxicated patients (alcohol and/or recreational drugs)
- drowning
- patients suffering from exhaustion
- injured and immobile patients
- decreased level of consciousness.

As patients succumb to hypothermia, they move through five stages [Durrer, 2003]:
1. Conscious and shivering.
2. Decreased level of consciousness and not shivering.
3. Unconscious.
4. Not breathing.
5. Death due to irreversible hypothermia.

1.3.1 Management

The mainstay of pre-hospital treatment is to prevent further heat loss. In the mildly hypothermic patient, this is likely to be enough, but severely hypothermic patients will require active rewarming, which realistically can only be performed in hospital [RCUK, 2021a]. Adopt the following principles when managing a patient with hypothermia [JRCALC, 2023]:
- Move the patient to a warm environment and remove wet clothes.
- If using a foil blanket, ensure that you wrap the patient in a fabric blanket first.
- Give the patient hot drinks if they are conscious, but not alcohol.
- Do not rub the patient's skin – as with alcohol, this leads to peripheral vasodilation, which worsens hypothermia.
- Avoid rough handling as it can cause arrhythmias and cardiac arrest.
- If intravenous fluids are required, ensure they are warmed prior to administration.
- Patients with a decreased LOC should not be encouraged to walk, but managed horizontally.
- If you have access to a heating blanket, place this over the patient.

1.4 Heat-related illness

Heat-related illnesses can occur as a result of external factors, such as the sun, or internal factors, such as drugs and exercise. It presents on a continuum, with heat stress being the least serious heat-related illness, through to multi-organ dysfunction and even death at the other extreme [JRCALC, 2023].

1.4.1 Heat stress

This is a mild form of heat-related illness and is characterised by [JRCALC, 2023]:
- normal temperature or mild temperature elevation
- heat oedema: swelling of feet and ankles
- heat syncope: vasodilation causes hypotension
- heat cramps: depletion of salts leads to muscle cramps.

1.4.2 Heat exhaustion

This is a more severe form of heat-related illness, with symptoms mostly as a result of fluid loss and electrolyte imbalances [Lott, 2021].
- systemic reaction to prolonged heat exposure (hours to days)
- core body temperature over 37°C and less than 40°C
- headache, dizziness, nausea and vomiting, tachycardia, hypotension, sweating, muscle pain, weakness and cramps
- can progress quickly to heat stroke.

1.4.3 Heat stroke

Heat stroke is a systemic inflammatory response to a core body temperature of 40°C or higher, and is associated with altered LOC and organ dysfunction [Lott, 2021]. It comes in two types: non-exertional heat stroke, which is caused by high external temperatures and/or high humidity, and exertional heat stroke, which is caused by excess heat production. Non-exertional heat stroke tends to occur in the elderly, very young and chronically ill, whereas exertional heat stroke is more typical in active groups such as athletes, manual workers and military recruits [JRCALC, 2023].

Clinical features include [JRCALC, 2023]:
- core body temperature of 40°C or more
- hot dry skin (although sweating is present in around half of all cases)
- early signs and symptoms:
  - extreme fatigue
  - headache
  - fainting
  - facial flushing
  - vomiting and diarrhoea
- arrhythmias and hypotension
- respiratory distress
- liver and kidney failure.

1.4.4 Management

Heat stress and exhaustion

The management of patients with heat-related illness broadly consists of cooling the patient and replacing lost fluid and electrolytes. For patients with signs and symptoms of heat stress consider the following [Lipman, 2019]:
- Remove the patient from the heat source.
- Passively cool: move the patient into the shade or an air-conditioned room and loosen or remove tight-fitting clothing.
- Provide oral isotonic fluid replacement.
- Elevate oedematous extremities.

If the patient has developed heat exhaustion, similar management principles apply, except that depending on the patient's LOC, fluid rehydration may have to be intravenous. In addition, cooling should be active, using conductive, evaporative and convective methods. Cold-water immersion is ideal for the ambulant, co-operative patient, but may not be practical otherwise. Alternatives include removing the patient's clothes and spraying or dousing the patient with water. Air movement can be augmented by fanning the patient [Lipman, 2019].

Heat stroke

While supporting the patient's airway, breathing, circulation and disability, begin rapidly cooling the patient [Lott, 2021]. Ice water immersion is useful but not practical, so consider the same techniques as for heat exhaustion to cool the patient. Ice packs are useful if they cover the body, not just the neck, axillae and groin, but should not be applied directly to the skin [Lipman, 2019]. Rehydration is safest intravenously, as an altered LOC increases the chance of aspiration [Lott, 2021].

1.5 Assessment of temperature

There are a range of different thermometers on the market, and you may need to use a different type of thermometer depending on the age of the patient, as shown in Table 14.1 [JRCALC, 2023].

Out-of-hospital, a peripheral temperature is gained to provide an estimation of what the temperature is in the core of the patient.

Table 14.1 Thermometers according to age

Infants under four weeks of age	Electronic thermometer in the axilla
Four weeks and over	Tympanic thermometer Electronic thermometer in axilla

Tympanic temperature readings are broadly accurate, but they can be impacted by factors including:
- build-up of ear wax
- patient lying on one side for a prolonged period
- wearing of ear defenders or muffs prior to temperature being taken
- having been outside for a prolonged period
- water or snow in the ear.

When taking a series of temperature measurements, always use the same site and procedure to try to improve accuracy. For example, if you are using the tympanic thermometer and you take the first reading from the right ear, you should use the right ear for all further temperature assessments.

1.5.1 Axillary temperature measurement

Indications
- Routine physiological assessment.
- Aids recognition of local and systemic infection.

- Guides treatment in cases of hypo- and hyperthermia.

Contra-indications
- None.

Advantages
- Minimally invasive.
- Can be performed even on very small infants.

Disadvantages
- Underestimates core body temperature.
- Left and right axilla temperatures may be different.
- Can take up to 90 seconds to return a reading.

Procedure

Take the following steps to record an axillary temperature [Pilbery & Lethbridge, 2022]:
1. Explain the procedure and obtain consent if appropriate to do so.
2. Don appropriate PPE, and undertake appropriate hand hygiene.
3. Turn on the thermometer, check it is clean and functional, and apply a fresh cover to the probe. Once you have turned it on, the thermometer will be able to perform any self-checks.
4. Place the tip of the thermometer high in the axilla, in the fold where the arm meets the chest. Adduct the patient's arm so it is flush with the side of the chest and ensure the thermometer is covered.
5. Leave in place until the thermometer has finished measuring. Usually there will be a visual or audible indication that this has happened.
6. Remove from the axilla and read the temperature. Check the temperature is recorded in degrees Celsius (°C).
7. Document the procedure.

1.5.2 Tympanic temperature measurement

Indications
- Routine physiological assessment.
- Aids recognition of local and systemic infection.
- Guides treatment in cases of hypo- and hyperthermia.

Contra-indications
- Infants under 4 weeks of age (use electronic axilla thermometer instead).

Advantages
- Quick.
- Minimally invasive.

Disadvantages
- Can give inaccurate results in cases of:
  - excessive ear wax
  - the ears having been covered for any period of time, for example after wearing of ear muffs or lying on one side
  - the patient being susceptible to environmental conditions, for example if they have been outside for a prolonged period of time.
- Temperatures may be different between ears.

Procedure

Take the following steps to record a temperature with a tympanic thermometer [Pilbery & Lethbridge, 2022]:
1. Explain the procedure and obtain consent if appropriate to do so.
2. Don appropriate PPE, and undertake appropriate hand hygiene.
3. Turn on the thermometer, check it is clean and functional, and apply a fresh cover to the probe. Once you have turned it on, the thermometer will perform a self-check.

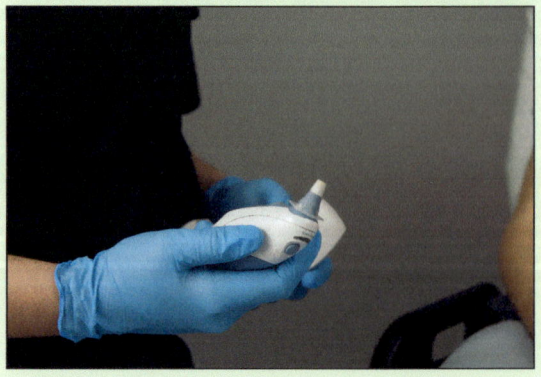

Procedure – *cont*

4. If your model of thermometer has an age setting, select the correct age group.
5. Place the probe into the ear and gently advance until the probe seals the opening. It should be placed straight down the ear canal, so the tip of the device is facing the tympanic membrane. Some thermometers will report if you do not have the thermometer in the correct position.

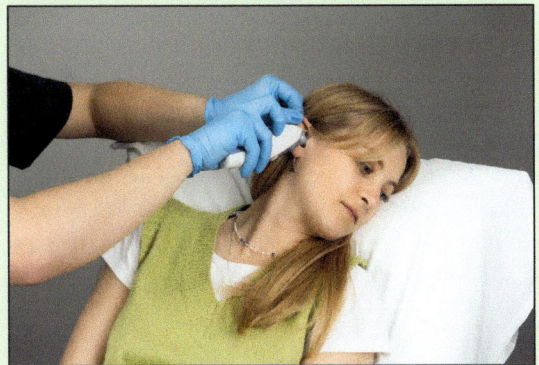

6. Push the button that measures temperature and hold the probe still until it has completed the measurement; this can take a few seconds.
7. Remove from the ear and read the temperature. Check the temperature is recorded in degrees Celsius (°C).

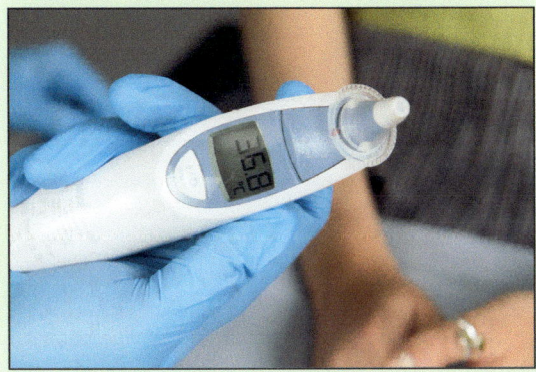

8. Document the procedure.

2 Drowning

2.1 Learning objective

By the end of this section, you will be able to:
- explain the pathophysiology and management of drowning.

2.2 Introduction

The definition of drowning has been complicated in the past and so in 2002 (at the World Congress on Drowning, held in Amsterdam) a single definition was agreed. As a result, drowning is now defined as a process resulting in primary respiratory impairment from submersion/immersion in a liquid [Idris, 2003]. Whether the victim lives or dies after this process is not important, they have still drowned. If they do not survive, then they have fatally drowned [Szpilman, 2012].

2.3 Pathophysiology

When a drowning victim is unable to keep water (the most common liquid in drowning incidents) from their mouth, it is spat out or swallowed. If still conscious, victims will then attempt to hold their breath, but this is likely to continue for less than a minute, depending on levels of panic and the temperature of the water. Once the inspiratory drive is too high to resist, the victim will take a breath and water will be aspirated into the airways [Szpilman, 2012]. Laryngospasm may occur, but this is rapidly terminated by cerebral hypoxia, and active ventilation, with aspiration of water, will resume. With no gas exchange, the victim becomes increasingly hypoxaemic. Unless they are rescued, the victim will succumb to hypoxaemia, leading to loss of consciousness and apnoea [Layon, 2009]. The cardiac rhythm deteriorates, usually following a sequence of tachyarrhythmias, bradyarrhythmias, pulseless electrical activity (PEA) and asystole [Szpilman, 2012].

2.4 Management

Try to avoid getting wet. You should only go into the water to rescue a drowning victim as a last resort and only if you are adequately trained and equipped. Many victims who are drowning can help themselves with firm coaching, or will have already been rescued by bystanders or professional rescuers, who can have a dramatic impact on the victim's outcome.

If you need to rescue the victim, remember to 'call, reach, throw, wade and row'. Encourage victims to self-rescue first by calling out to them. Next, try to reach them with an object such as a pole, tree branch or even items of clothing. Consider throwing something that is buoyant, ideally a rescue ring with a lifeline attached. Wading into the water is the next possibility as long as someone on the shore has hold of you, the water is shallow enough to stand in and the victim is within reach. Alternatively, use a boat, if available.

Get the victim out of the water as soon as possible and place them supine, with head and torso at the same level, and check for breathing. If they are breathing but unconscious, provide high-flow oxygen via non-rebreathe mask as per clinical guidelines and place them in the recovery position. They are at high risk of gastric regurgitation, so ensure that you have suction available [JRCALC, 2023].

Victims of prolonged immersion in water (typically 30 minutes or more, but less as water temperature decreases) may also suffer the added complication of circum-rescue collapse [Golden, 1997]. This is due to the increased hydrostatic pressure from the water on the victim's legs and torso increasing venous return and cardiac output. Central baroreceptors mistake this for hypervolaemia, resulting in increased diuresis (increased production of urination). In addition, peripheral vasoconstriction will occur as the water is cold relative to the body, which magnifies this response [Lord, 2005]. Once the victim is removed from the water, the hydrostatic pressure is lost, exacerbating the hypovolaemia. This can also be compounded by hypothermia and physical effort (if the victim attempts to remove themselves from the water, for example). The sudden drop in venous return can reduce coronary perfusion enough to induce cardiac arrest. For this reason, it is advised to remove victims horizontally from the water if possible [Szpilman, 2012].

Hypothermia is likely to occur and wet clothes should be cut off to minimise movement. Hypothermic patients are at risk of cardiac arrhythmias, including ventricular fibrillation, even with minor movement [Althaus, 1982]. Get the patient covered with blankets and into a warm environment as soon as possible.

Chapter

15 Medical Emergencies

1 Anaphylaxis

1.1 Learning objectives

By the end of this section you will be able to:
- explain the terms 'allergy' and 'anaphylaxis' and their common causes
- describe the signs and symptoms that a patient with anaphylaxis may present with
- state the management of anaphylaxis, including the administration of adrenaline using the patient's own auto-injector.

1.2 Introduction

People who have an overly reactive immune response to a substance that enters the body via the skin, or is inhaled, injected or ingested, are said to be allergic (or hypersensitive) to that substance. These 'substances' are called allergens and lead to an immune response referred to as an allergic reaction [Tortora, 2017]. Common examples of allergens include [NHS, 2022a]:
- tree and grass pollen (hay fever)
- house dust mites
- foods, such as peanuts, milk and eggs (food allergy)
- animal fur, particularly from pets such as cats and dogs
- insect stings, such as bee and wasp stings
- certain medicines, such as antibiotics.

The World Allergy Organization Anaphylaxis Committees define anaphylaxis as a serious systemic hypersensitivity reaction that is usually rapid in onset and may cause death. Severe cases are characterised by a potentially life-threatening compromise in airway, breathing and/or the circulation, and can occur without typical skin features or circulatory shock being present [Cardona, 2020].

The most common causes (triggers) are food, drugs and venom. Food is the most common cause of allergy in young people, whereas in older adults, it is medication [RCUK, 2021c].

1.3 Signs and symptoms

Typical signs and symptoms of an allergic reaction include [NHS, 2022a]:
- runny nose or sneezing
- coughing, wheezing or breathlessness
- a raised itchy rash (urticaria, also often referred to as hives)
- diarrhoea
- nausea, vomiting and abdominal pain
- swollen eyes, lips, mouth and/or throat (angioedema).

Anaphylaxis is likely when all of the following criteria are met [RCUK, 2021c]:
1. Sudden onset and rapid progression of symptoms, particularly after exposure to a known trigger (allergen).
2. Life-threatening airway and/or breathing and/or circulatory problems.
3. Skin and/or mucosal changes (e.g. generalised urticaria, pruritus or flushing, and swollen lips/tongue/uvula, also known as angioedema).

Note: Up to 20% of anaphylaxis cases do not have skin and/or mucosal changes, particularly reactions that occur intraoperatively in adults, and with food/insect sting-induced reactions in children. Patients with severe anaphylaxis resulting in significant hypotension may not exhibit any cutaneous (skin) symptoms until their blood pressure is restored [Lee, 2011].

1.4 Management

Conduct a standard <C>ABCDE assessment to determine whether your patient is likely to be having an anaphylactic reaction. Try to identify the trigger and remove it if possible (e.g. remove bee stings). However, if this is not possible, then do not delay

Chapter 15 – Medical Emergencies

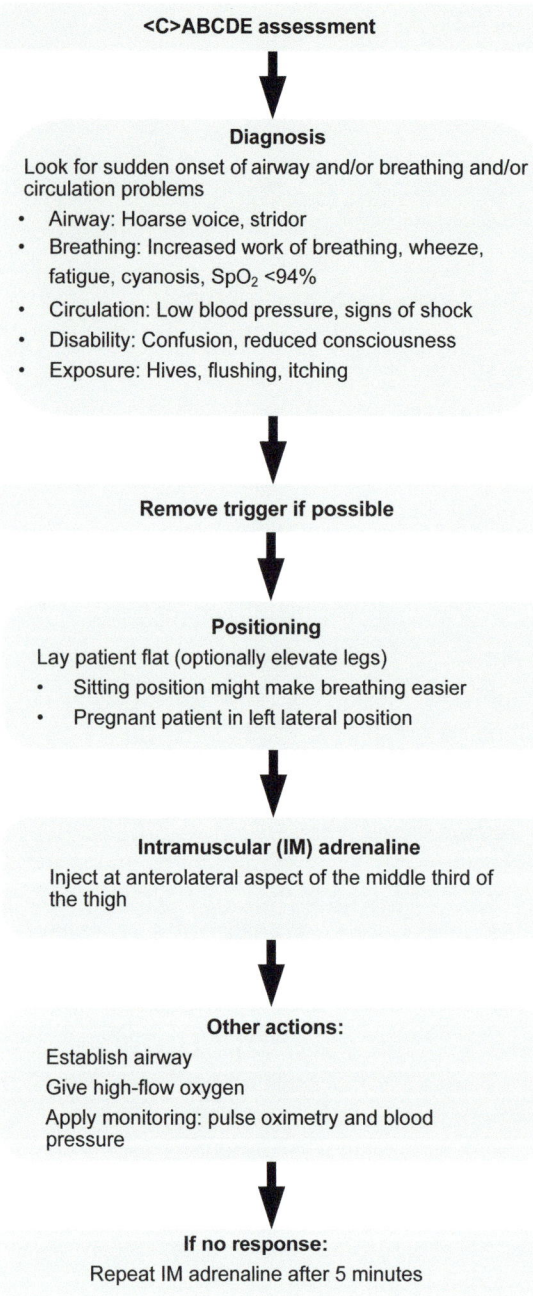

Figure 15.1 Emergency treatment of anaphylaxis

treatment. If you suspect food-induced anaphylaxis, do not try to make the patient vomit [RCUK, 2021c].

Lay the patient flat where possible, with legs raised. Note that patients with A or B problems are likely to be more comfortable sitting up, but do not allow patients to sit or stand if they feel faint as this can cause cardiac arrest.

Intramuscular (IM) adrenaline is the first-line treatment for suspected anaphylaxis [JRCALC, 2023]. Where possible, instruct the patient to administer their adrenaline auto-injector into the middle third of their anterolateral thigh. This site provides a greater margin of safety, it is quick to administer, and the peak plasma concentration is higher when adrenaline is administered in the thigh compared to the deltoid [Simons, 2001]. If the patient cannot administer adrenaline themselves and you have been trained to do so, perform the injection yourself. Follow local guidance.

Once adrenaline has been administered, establish an airway and administer high-flow oxygen until you can obtain a reliable pulse oximetry reading, after which you can titrate oxygen to 94–98%. Obtain a set of observations and continue to closely monitor the patient's condition (Figure 15.1).

If there is no improvement after 5 minutes, another dose of adrenaline can be administered.

1.4.1 Auto-injectors

Patients who are known to have anaphylactic reactions may have been provided with their own adrenaline auto-injector. Common systems in the UK include Jext and Epipen and are typically available as 300 microgram adult and 150 microgram child doses.

Indications
- Anaphylaxis.

Contra-indications
- None in the emergency situation.

Advantages
- The pre-filled syringe means no need to draw up adrenaline from glass vials.
- No need to calculate dosage regimen for the patient.

Disadvantages
- Incorrect use can result in the rescuer injecting themselves instead of the patient.
- Dosage is lower than that provided by ambulance clinicians.

Anaphylaxis

Procedure

Take the following steps to administer adrenaline with a Jext auto-injector [ALK-Abello, 2023]:

1. Grasp the Jext injector in your dominant hand (the one you use to write with) with your thumb closest to the yellow cap.

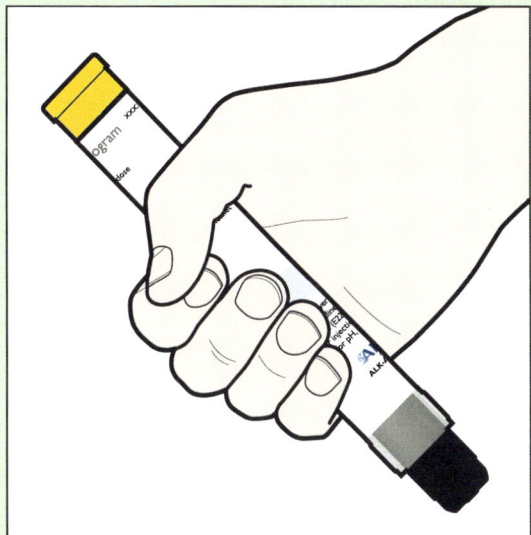

2. Pull off the yellow cap with your other hand.

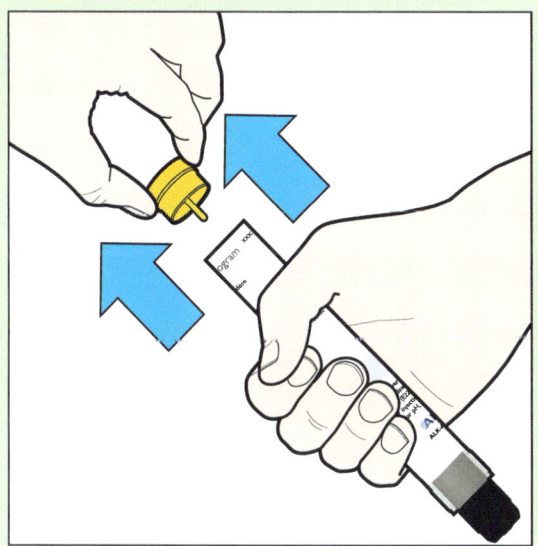

Procedure – *cont*

3. Place the black injector tip against your outer thigh, holding the injector at a right angle (approximately 90°) to the thigh.

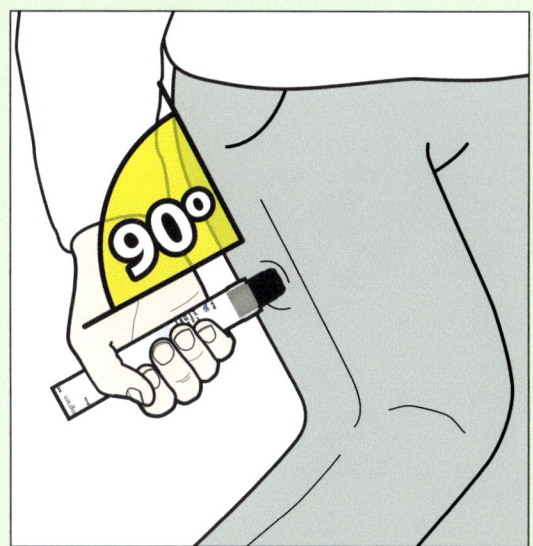

4. Push the black tip firmly into your outer thigh until you hear a 'click' confirming the injection has started, then keep it pushed in. Hold the injector firmly in place against the thigh for 10 seconds (a slow count to 10), then remove. The black tip will extend automatically and hide the needle.

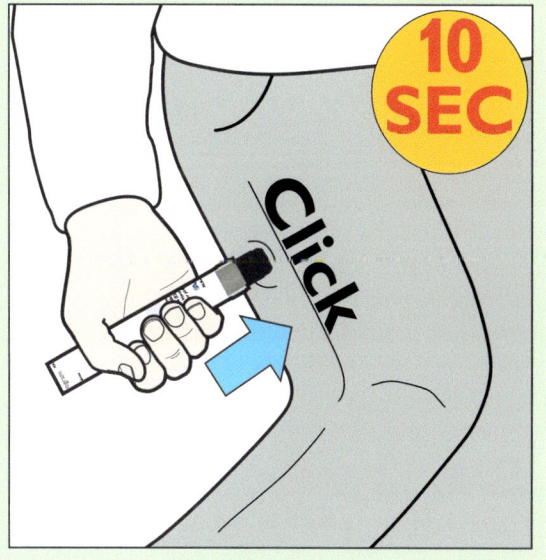

Chapter 15 – *Medical Emergencies*

Procedure – *cont*

5. Massage the injection area for 10 seconds.

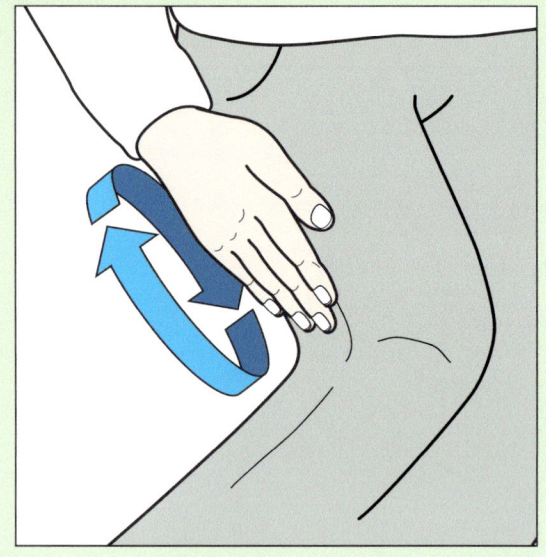

2 Sepsis

2.1 *Learning objectives*

By the end of this section you will be able to:
- explain what sepsis and septic shock are and how they occur
- state how you would recognise a patient with sepsis or septic shock
- describe the out-of-hospital management of sepsis.

2.2 *Introduction*

Sepsis is a life-threatening condition that arises when the body's response to an infection injures its own tissues and organs. It leads to shock, multiple organ failure and death if not recognised early and treated promptly [Czura, 2011]. Around 70% of cases occur in the community meaning that the ambulance service is often the first point of contact for these patients [JRCALC, 2023].

Septic shock is a subset of sepsis that has a higher risk of mortality than sepsis alone [Singer, 2016]. Septic shock causes particularly profound circulatory, cellular and metabolic abnormalities.

Since determining the presence of septic shock can be difficult out-of-hospital, a pragmatic alternative is to treat any patient who is hypotensive despite fluid resuscitation as if they have septic shock. These patients are high risk, as are others with any of the 'red flag' signs/symptoms shown in Figure 15.2. To ensure that these patients receive urgent attention, it is important that the receiving hospital is alerted that the 'patient has suspected sepsis' [JRCALC, 2023].

2.3 *Risk factors for sepsis*

Certain groups of patients are at higher risk of developing sepsis [JRCALC, 2023]:
- infants and older people (over 75 years or very frail)
- patients with impaired immune systems, for example:
  - cancer patients receiving chemotherapy
  - patients without a spleen (due to splenectomy)
  - patients with sickle cell disease
  - patients taking long-term steroid or immunosuppressant drugs for conditions such as rheumatoid arthritis
  - patients who have had recent surgery (in the previous 6 weeks)
  - intravenous drug users
  - pregnant patients, or those who have given birth, or had a termination of pregnancy or miscarriage in the past 6 weeks.

2.4 *Recognition and management*

To simplify the identification of sepsis (particularly red-flag sepsis), a screening tool has been developed for pre-hospital use (Figure 15.2) [JRCALC, 2023]. You should suspect sepsis in any patient who presents with fever and/or is feeling unwell, and who has a National Early Warning Score (NEWS) 2 of five or more and/or looks unwell with a history of infection. A history of infection might be indicated by the presence of [UKST, 2024]:
- pneumonia
- UTI
- abdominal pain/distension
- cellulitis/septic arthritis/infected wound

Sepsis

- device-related infection
- meningitis.

Next, look for the presence of any red-flag signs/symptoms that may indicate the presence of red-flag sepsis (Figure 15.2). Patients who do not meet the criteria for red-flag sepsis but have sepsis still require further assessment and appropriate management to prevent their clinical condition from deteriorating. You can contribute to the patient's care by administering oxygen therapy as per your local guidelines and passing on your clinical assessment findings to the ambulance crew when they arrive.

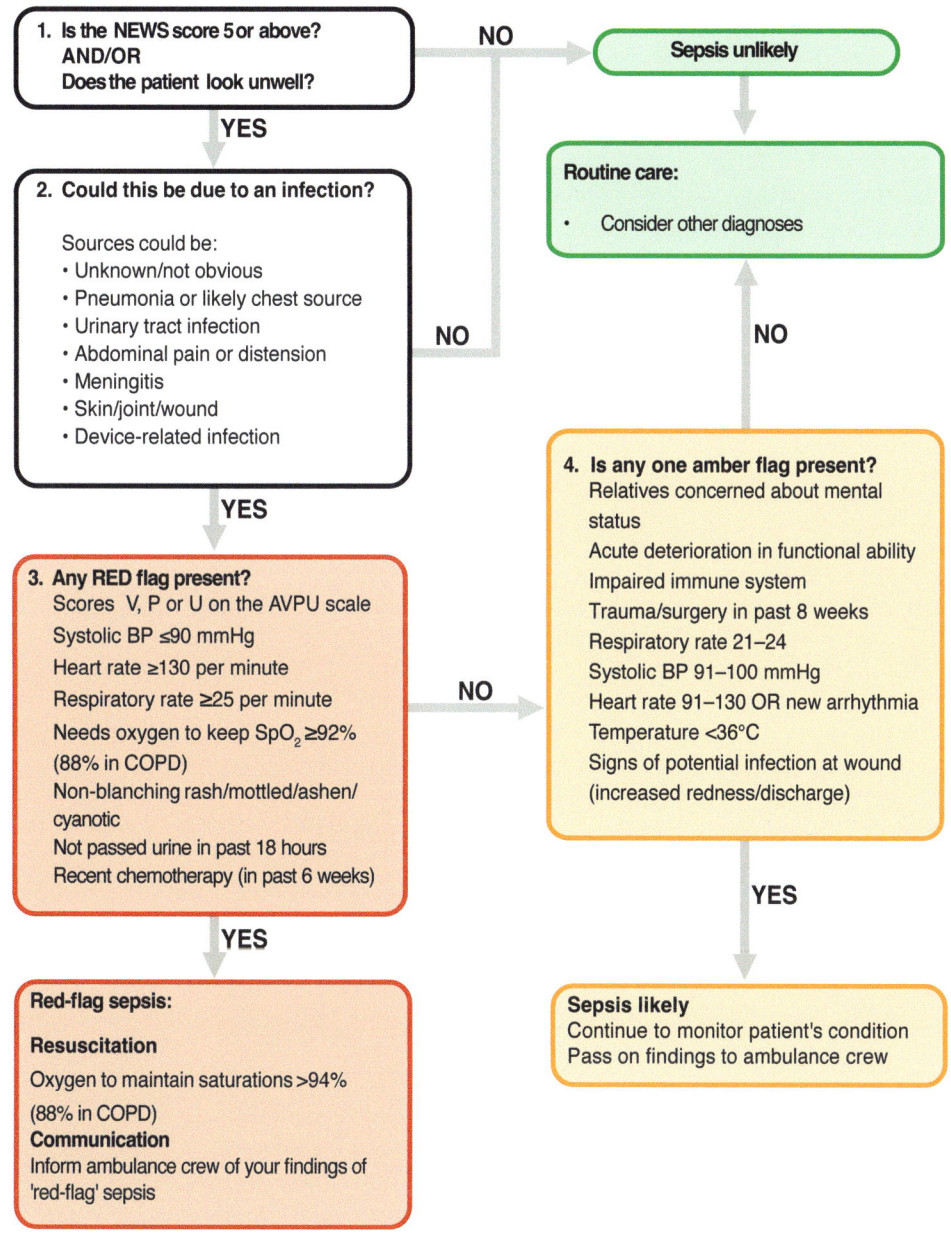

Figure 15.2 Pre-hospital screening tool

3 Endocrine system disorders

3.1 Learning objectives

By the end of this section you will be able to:
- describe the relevant anatomy and physiology of the endocrine system
- describe the types and causes of diabetes
- describe two diabetic emergencies
- explain how to record a blood sugar measurement.

3.2 Introduction

The endocrine system consists of a collection of glands located throughout the body (Figure 15.3) that are responsible for the secretion of hormones, molecules that are released from endocrine glands and regulate the activity of cells in other parts of the body. The endocrine system works alongside the nervous system to help co-ordinate the function of all of the body's systems [Tortora, 2017].

The endocrine system consists of the pineal, pituitary, thyroid, parathyroid and adrenal glands. In addition, there are a number of organs and tissues that are not strictly endocrine glands, but do secrete hormones. These include the pancreas, ovaries, testes, liver and heart.

3.3 Anatomy and physiology of the pancreas

The pancreas is a mixed endocrine and exocrine gland, situated posterior to the stomach, and extends across the posterior abdominal wall from the duodenum on the right to the spleen on the left (Figure 15.4). It is retroperitoneal, apart from its tail [Tortora, 2017].

Around 99% of the cells in the pancreas are involved in the production of pancreatic enzymes. The cells are organised into clusters called acini. Among the acini are collections of endocrine tissue called pancreatic islets, or islets of Langerhans after the German scientist Paul Langerhans, who first described them [Jolles, 2002].

There are five types of cells in the pancreatic islets, which have a range of functions, including regulation of blood glucose (Table 15.1).

Table 15.1 Cells of the pancreatic islets

Cell	Hormone	Action
Alpha	Glucagon	Increases blood glucose
Beta	Insulin, amylin	Insulin: reduces blood glucose Amylin: delays gastric emptying, inhibits insulin
Delta	Somatostatin	Inhibits glucagon and insulin release
PP (or F)	Pancreatic polypeptide	Inhibits somatostatin secretion, gallbladder contraction and secretion of pancreatic digestive enzymes
Epsilon	Ghrelin	Stimulates hunger

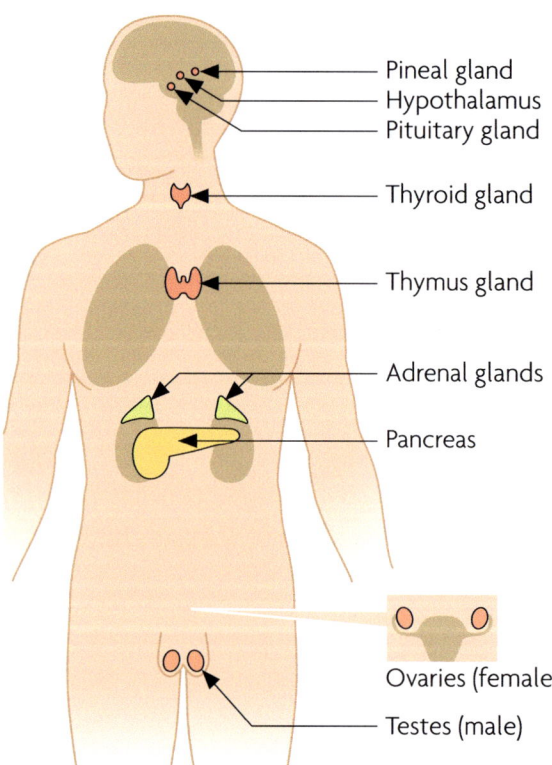

Figure 15.3 The endocrine system

Endocrine system disorders

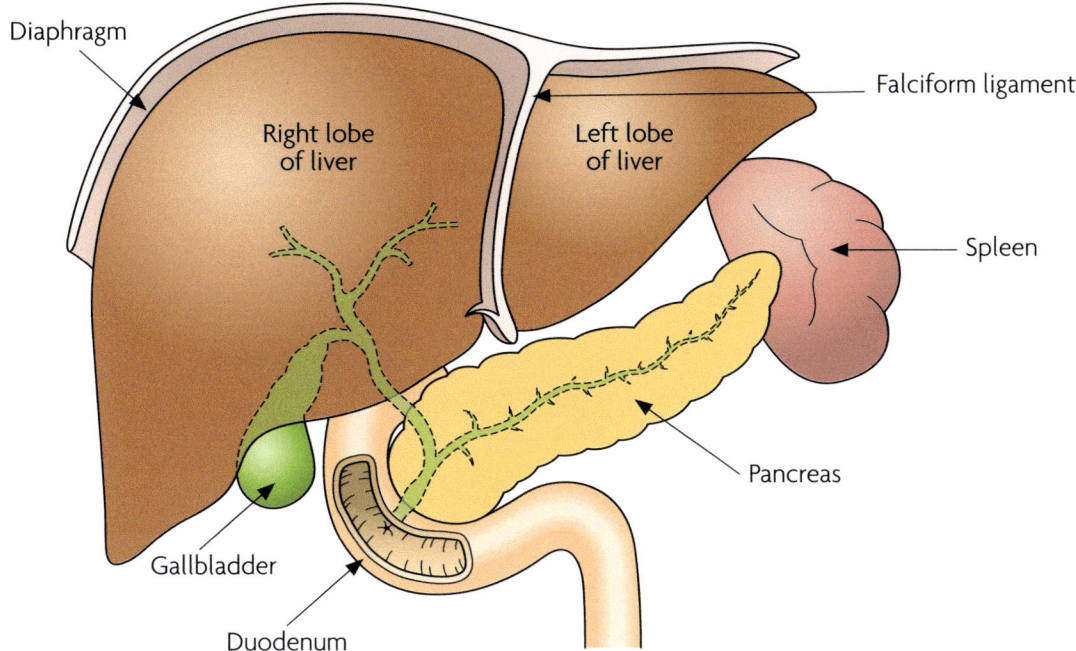

Figure 15.4 The pancreas

3.3.1 Blood sugar regulation

Falling blood glucose levels normally activate a series of glucose counter-regulatory processes to prevent, or quickly correct, hypoglycaemia. This is crucial, given that the brain's demand for glucose is fairly constant and the intake of external (exogenous) glucose from eating is intermittent. This is accomplished by the dynamic control of internal (endogenous) production of glucose by the liver (and to a lesser extent the kidneys) and reduction of glucose consumption by non-neural tissue, such as muscle [Briscoe, 2006].

Hormonal control of blood glucose is largely dependent on the endocrine pancreas via the hormones insulin and glucagon. Insulin increases transport of glucose across cell membranes and is released by the beta cells. It targets the muscle and fat cells to take in glucose, and liver cells to stop gluconeogenesis (glucose creation) and facilitate synthesis of triglycerides, fatty acids and proteins [Tortora, 2017].

Glucagon targets the liver, promoting conversion of glycogen into glucose and the creation of glucose from lactic and amino acids. This results in increased glucose release by the liver, into the blood. Glucagon release is inhibited by insulin and increased by falling blood glucose levels.

Defence against hypoglycaemia (also called glucose counter-regulation) can be broadly classified into physiological and behavioural responses [Briscoe, 2006]. As blood glucose falls (although still within 'normal' limits), insulin secretion from the beta cells is reduced, leading to increased glucose production by the liver and virtual cessation of glucose use by tissue sensitive to insulin.

When blood glucose falls below 4 mmol/l, glucagon release is increased from the alpha cells, further increasing glucose production and decreasing insulin release. In addition, adrenaline release from the adrenal medulla is increased by the sympathetic nervous system (SNS). Adrenaline has similar effects on the liver as glucagon, but can also stimulate renal production of glucose and plays a role in reducing insulin-stimulated glucose uptake [Elliott, 2011].

If blood glucose continues to fall, a more intense sympathetic-mediated adrenaline release causes a behavioural response in the form of hunger, as well as other autonomic symptoms, such as palpitations, sweating and pallor [Graveling, 2009].

3.4 Diabetes

Diabetes mellitus is a common metabolic disorder typified by chronic high blood sugar (hyperglycaemia). It is a major cause of morbidity and premature death due to long-term complications, such as heart attacks, stroke, kidney failure and blindness [Holt, 2010].

- **Type 1:** Previously referred to as insulin-dependent diabetes (IDDM). Patients with type 1 diabetes are unable to produce any insulin, usually due to an autoimmune disease which destroys the insulin-producing beta cells in the pancreas [Holt, 2010].
- **Type 2:** Previously referred to as non-insulin dependent diabetes (NIDDM). Patients with type 2 diabetes have a relative insulin deficiency due to varying degrees of insulin resistance. This is by far the more common type of diabetes, accounting for around 90% of all people with diabetes in the UK.

3.4.1 Causes/risk of diabetes

Underlying causes of diabetes generally fall into four categories (Holt, 2010):

- **Genetic:** A family history of type 1 diabetes or other autoimmune disease is linked to a higher risk of developing type 1 diabetes in the family. Likewise, type 2 diabetes also has a familial component, although this connection is rather more complicated.
- **Obesity:** This increases the risk of developing type 2 diabetes, particularly in people with a body mass index over 25 kg/m^2 or large waist circumference.
- **Age:** People are living longer and beta cell function declines with age, leading to the possibility of developing diabetes in old age.
- **Ethnicity:** Some ethnic groups are at higher risk of developing diabetes, particularly those of South Asian and Afro-Caribbean origin.

3.5 Glycaemic emergencies

Blood sugar is typically maintained within a narrow range. Patients with diabetes are generally encouraged to keep their blood sugar at 4.0 mmol/l or higher, with a target range of 4.0–8.0 mmol/l for children and 4.0–7.0 mmol/l for adults [NICE, 2022a, 2023].

There are two main types of glycaemic emergency that you will encounter:
- hypoglycaemia
- severe hyperglycaemia, which can be further divided into diabetic ketoacidosis (DKA) and hyperosmolar hyperglycaemic state (HHS).

3.6 Hypoglycaemia

Hypoglycaemia in patients with diabetes commonly occurs due to a relative excess of insulin in the blood and a compromised physiological and behavioural response to falling blood glucose levels. Since injected insulin and hypoglycaemic drugs, such as sulphonylureas, are not perfect pharmacokinetically, there are typically periods where there is an excess of insulin in the blood and falling blood glucose levels. The performance of the counter-regulatory defences is crucial in determining whether the patient will develop significant hypoglycaemia.

3.6.1 Signs and symptoms

Although patients with diabetes are generally encouraged to keep their blood sugar at 4.0 mmol/l or higher, some will experience symptoms of hypoglycaemia at blood sugar levels higher than this, making recognition important. Some signs and symptoms of hypoglycaemia include [Deary, 1993]:
- sweating
- palpitations
- shaking
- hunger
- confusion
- drowsiness
- odd/aggressive behaviour
- speech problems
- headache
- nausea.

3.6.2 Management

If the patient is still conscious and able to take oral glucose, administer 15–20 g of glucose. You can find 10 g of glucose in [JRCALC, 2023]:
- 5–7 Dextrosol tablets (or 4–5 Glucotabs) or
- 1 bottle (60 ml) Glucojuice or
- 150–200 ml pure fruit juice, e.g. orange (avoid pure fruit juice for renal dialysis patients because of potassium content) or
- 1–2 tubes of 40% glucose gel or
- 3–4 heaped teaspoons of sugar dissolved in water (NB this is not an effective treatment for patients taking acarbose, as it prevents the breakdown of sucrose to glucose).

Administration of oral glucose can be repeated after 10–15 minutes, if required. If the patient is unable to take oral glucose due to impaired consciousness, is unco-operative or there is a risk of aspiration, then either IM glucagon or IV glucose is usually administered by ambulance staff.

3.7 Severe hyperglycaemia

Severe hyperglycaemia (sometimes referred to as hyperglycaemic crisis) manifests as two conditions: DKA and HHS (previously known as hyperosmolar non-ketotic coma, HONK) [Van Ness-Otunnu, 2013].

3.7.1 Diabetic ketoacidosis (DKA)

DKA is a complex metabolic state characterised by:
- hyperglycaemia
- acidosis
- ketonaemia (high levels of ketones in the blood).

It is a common and potentially life-threatening complication of mainly type 1 diabetes mellitus (T1DM), compared to HHS, which typically affects only patients with type 2 diabetes mellitus (T2DM).

3.7.2 Hyperosmolar hyperglycaemic state (HHS)

HHS does not have a universally agreed definition, but it is generally accepted that the following must be present for the patient to be diagnosed with HHS [Scott, 2015]:

- hypovolaemia (secondary to severe dehydration)
- blood sugar ≥30 mmol/l without signs of hyperketonaemia or acidosis
- hyperosmolality.

3.7.3 Pathophysiology

DKA

DKA and HHS share the complications of severe hyperglycaemia, but early mechanisms are different. In DKA, insulin production is absent or severely reduced. This, coupled with increased levels of insulin counter-regulatory hormones (e.g. cortisol, glucagon, growth hormone and catecholamines), enhances hepatic gluconeogenesis and glycogenolysis (breakdown of stored glucose in the form of glycogen). This leads to severe hyperglycaemia that is exacerbated by simultaneous reduction in glucose take-up by the peripheral tissues because of the lack of insulin. Although blood glucose is high, there is a glucose famine inside the cells, so body fat (adipose tissue) is used to create energy by increasing lipolysis and decreasing lipogenesis.

HHS

Although HHS is also caused by a decrease in insulin and increase in counter-regulatory hormones, the fundamental difference between HHS and DKA is that there is still sufficient insulin production to prevent significant ketosis (a process where the body breaks down fat for energy instead of glucose) but not the severe hyperglycaemia that is a key feature of the condition. As before, hyperglycaemia is caused by increased gluconeogenesis, accelerated conversion of glycogen to glucose, and inadequate utilisation of glucose by the peripheral tissues, particularly muscle.

3.7.4 Signs and symptoms

DKA and HHS typically present in different groups of patients and over differing time periods. DKA most commonly occurs in T1DM (although advanced/severe T2DM patients are also at risk). HHS on the other hand is almost exclusively seen in T2DM and is more common in the elderly [Lupsa, 2014], although its incidence in teenagers and young adults is on the rise [Scott, 2015]. DKA typically presents within hours to days of onset, whereas HHS does not occur for many days to weeks, which explains why the metabolic derangement and dehydration in HHS are so much more severe than in DKA [Savage, 2011].

Typical signs and symptoms of severe hyperglycaemia are common to both DKA and HHS (except where highlighted in the list below) [Corwell, 2014; Lupsa, 2014]:
- polyuria (excessive urination)
- polydipsia (excessive thirst)
- blurred vision
- fatigue
- weakness
- weight loss
- vomiting and abdominal pain (DKA)
- fruity breath odour (DKA)
- Kussmaul breathing (DKA)
- focal neurological signs such as hemiparesis (HHS)
- altered mental state, although this can range from confusion to coma
- signs of dehydration such as dry mucous membranes, poor skin turgor, long furrows on tongue.

3.7.5 Management

Out-of-hospital management of hyperglycaemic crisis is limited and consists of assessing and managing ABCD problems [JRCALC, 2023; RCUK, 2021a]:
- Ensure airway patency, with patient positioning, suction and adjuncts, as required, particularly in patients with a reduced LOC.
- Adults need supplemental oxygen if the patient's SpO_2 is < 94%. Children should receive high-flow oxygen titrated to a target range of 94–98%. Patients can expire CO_2 with spontaneous breathing far more effectively than with artificial ventilation, so avoid assisting/interfering unless the patient is in respiratory failure or arrest.

⚠ 3.8 Blood sugar measurement

You will obtain blood glucose measurements as part of your clinical assessment, but as with all diagnostic tests, they are not perfect and are prone to error if the correct technique is not used. Common causes of error include [Lunt, 2010]:
- Incorrect calibration chip used to read the test strips.
- Contamination of the test finger with glucose-rich foods or dilutional error due to inadequate hand drying or the patient licking their finger clean.
- Expired strips or strips stored in adverse environmental conditions such as heat, humidity or extreme cold.
- Patient conditions such as anaemia and hypoxia. Shocked patients may have a reduced capillary blood glucose reading compared to a venous blood sample.
- Aspirin, paracetamol and vitamin C can all raise blood glucose, although this may not be clinically significant.

3.8.1 Procedure

Indications
- Patients with acute illness.
- Patients suspected of having hypo- or hyperglycaemia.
- As part of reassessment following treatment for hypoglycaemia.
- Any patient with confusion or reduced LOC.

Contra-indications
- None in the emergency setting, but see cautions.

Cautions
The following conditions can adversely affect the accuracy of capillary blood glucose measurement. A laboratory-analysed venous sample is preferable in the following presentations:
- patients on home dialysis
- peripheral circulatory failure, for example shock (venous sample from a cannula probably suitable)
- severe dehydration
- extremes of haematocrit (can be seen in neonates and pregnant patients)
- hyperlipidaemia.

Endocrine system disorders

Advantages
- Can be performed at the patient's side.
- Easy to perform.

Disadvantages
- Not as accurate as a laboratory-analysed blood sample.
- Painful.
- Invasive; infection prevention and control measures must be in place

Procedure

Take the following steps to measure a patient's blood sugar [Pilbery & Lethbridge, 2022]:

Note: The SD Codefree monitor is used here, but the steps are likely to be the same for most other devices. However, make sure you are familiar with the blood glucose meters you will be using.

1. Explain the procedure to the patient and obtain consent if appropriate to do so.
2. Don appropriate PPE, and undertake appropriate hand hygiene.
3. Select an appropriate site, which is typically the side of a finger in an adult or older child (the non-dominant hand, if possible) and the heel of the foot in a younger child or infant. Clean the area with water or water-soaked gauze and dry thoroughly.

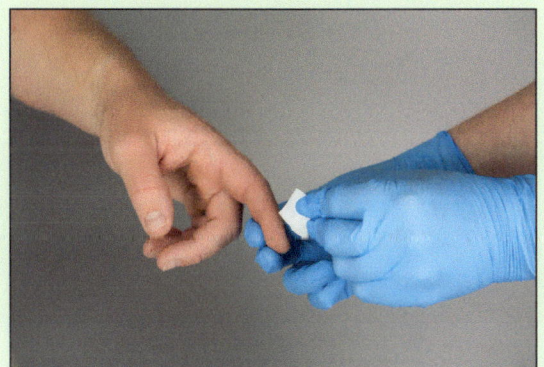

Procedure – *cont*

4. Check the use-by date on the test strip container. Do not use test strips past their use-by date.

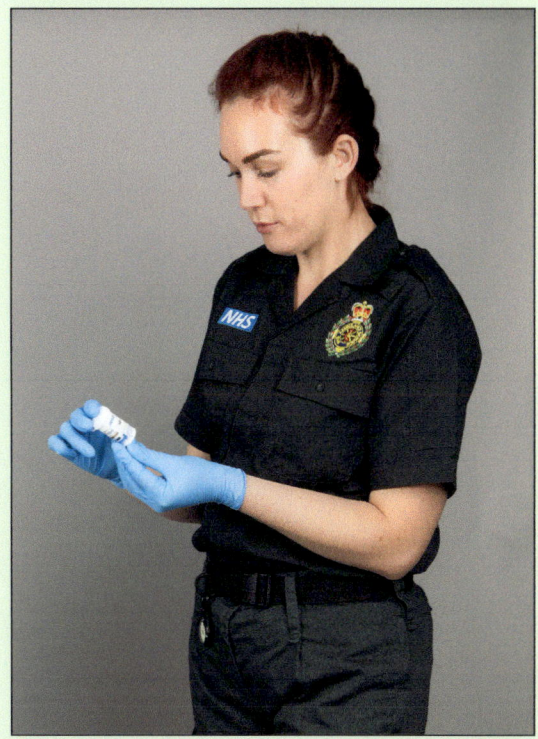

5. Insert a test strip into the bottom of the meter. This will turn it on (some models will beep too).

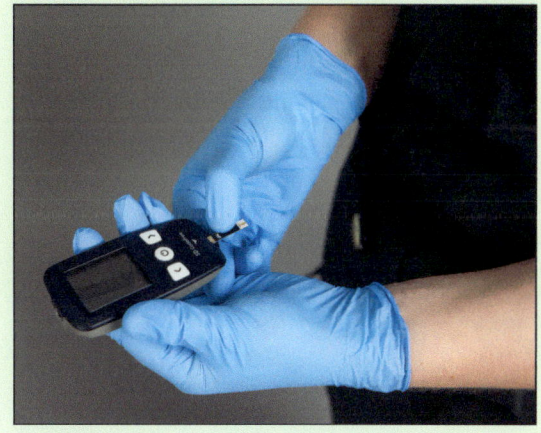

Chapter 15 – *Medical Emergencies*

Procedure – *cont*

6. On the screen, an icon showing the test strip and a flashing blood drop will appear. Ask the patient to dangle their arm down at their side to encourage blood flow to their fingertips.

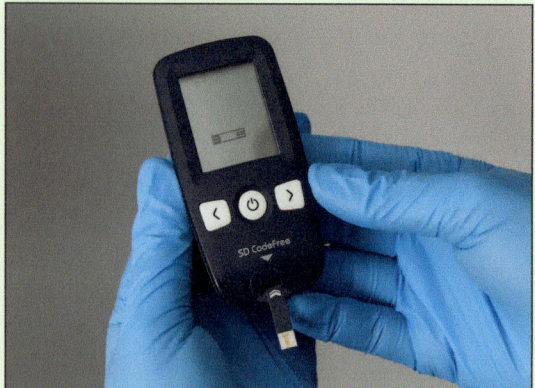

7. Prick the target area with a lancet, disposing of it immediately in a sharps bin after use.

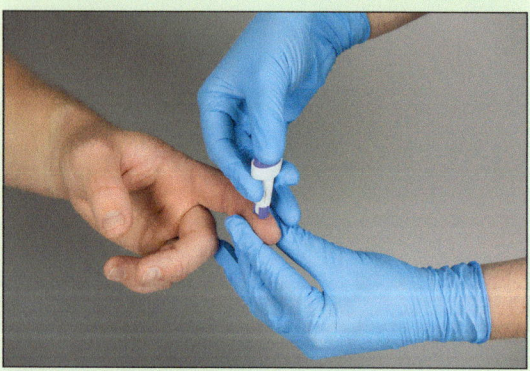

8. Wait a couple of seconds and then, with the patient's hand facing downwards, gently squeeze their finger to assist the flow of blood.

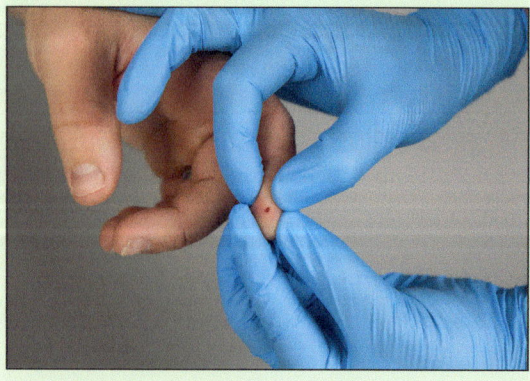

Procedure – *cont*

9. Touch the blood drop to the front edge of the yellow window of the test strip. When you have enough blood, you will see a countdown timer.

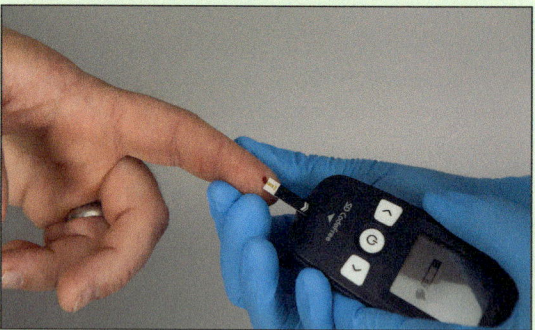

10. Ask the patient to apply pressure to the puncture site with gauze until bleeding has stopped.

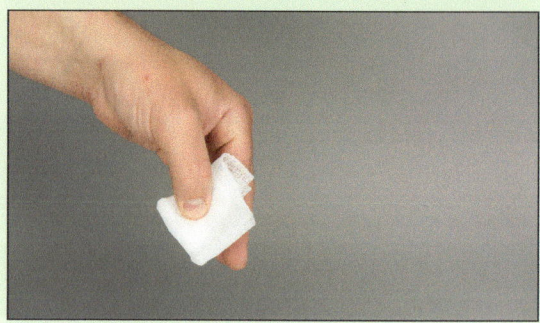

11. The blood sugar result will appear on the display.
    Check that the unit of measure is mmol/l and not mg/dl.

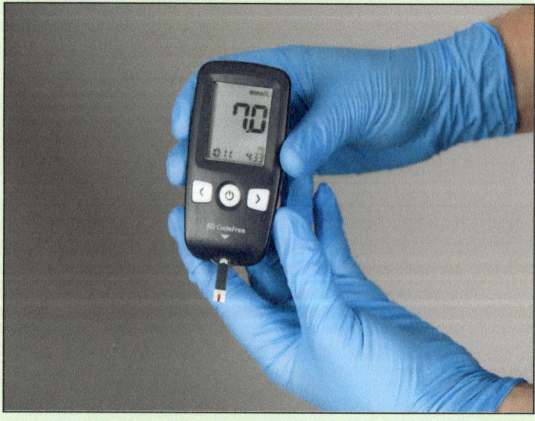

12. Document the procedure.

4 Poisoning

4.1 Learning objectives

By the end of this section you will be able to:
- state the routes by which poisons can enter the body
- describe the signs and symptoms of poisoning
- explain the management of a poisoned patient.

Common toxidromes are summarised in Table 15.2 and Figure 15.5.

4.2 Introduction

Poisoning is the exposure by ingestion, inhalation, absorption or injection to a quantity of a substance or substances that may result in illness or death. In children, poisoning is typically accidental, whereas in adults the majority of cases are caused by drug overdose secondary to self-harm [NPIS, 2022].

4.3 Toxidromes

A toxidrome is a collection of signs and symptoms associated with a particular class of toxins. Substances are grouped together based on these signs and symptoms, which provides some indication as to which substances have been taken and helps guide management of the poisoning. It is not perfect, as not all signs and symptoms will be present in your patient, and overdoses of multiple types of substance are common, leading to variable signs and symptoms [Boyle, 2009].

Table 15.2 Common toxidromes

Toxidrome	Signs/symptoms	Example causes
Sympathomimetic	<ul><li>Tachycardia, hypertension</li><li>Mydriasis (dilated pupils)</li><li>Diaphoresis (sweating)</li><li>Piloerection ('goose bumps')</li><li>Hyperthermia convulsions</li></ul>	Caffeine, cocaine, amphetamines, Ritalin, MDMA (ecstasy) Alcohol/drug withdrawal
Anticholinergic	<ul><li>Confusion</li><li>Mydriasis and blurring of vision</li><li>Decreased salivation, dry mouth, intense thirst and difficulty swallowing</li><li>Marked flushing of face and chest, elevated body temperature, blockade of sweat glands</li><li>Urinary retention</li><li>Absent bowel sounds</li></ul>**NOTE:** Children are especially at risk due to receptor sensitivity, particularly children with Down's syndrome	<ul><li>Anticholinergics, e.g. atropine</li><li>Antihistamines, e.g. chlorphenamine, hydroxyzine, diphenhydramine</li><li>Antipsychotics, e.g. chlorpromazine, olanzapine, thioridazine</li><li>Antispasmodics, e.g. clidinium, hyoscyamine, oxybutynin</li></ul>

continued

Table 15.2 Common toxidromes *continued*

Toxidrome	Signs/symptoms	Example causes
Cholinergic	• Sweating • Lacrimation (crying) • Miosis (pinpoint pupils) • Rhinorrhoea (runny nose) • Frothing at mouth due to excessive salivation • Vomiting • Bradycardia • Urinary incontinence • Diarrhoea	• Nicotine • Nerve agents, e.g. sarin • Organophosphates
Opioid	• Miosis, altered LOC, decreased bowel sounds and respiratory depression (rate and depth) • Nausea and vomiting can occur	Morphine, codeine, tramadol, heroin, fentanyl, methadone, oxycodone, hydrocodone
Sedative-hypnotic	• Altered LOC • Slurred speech • Ataxia (poor muscle co-ordination) • Amnesia • Cardiovascular and respiratory depression • Decreased bowel sounds	• Barbiturates, e.g. thiopental, phenobarbital • Benzodiazepines, e.g. diazepam, lorazepam • Z-drugs, e.g. zopiclone, zolpidem • Drugs of abuse, e.g. GHB
Serotonin syndrome	• Delirium • Mydriasis • Sweating • Tachycardia • Clonus, myoclonus, hyperreflexia, increased limb tone • Increased bowel sounds • Nausea	• Drugs of abuse, e.g. MDMA, amphetamines • Antidepressants, e.g. tricyclics, citalopram, fluoxetine, sertraline • Monoamine oxidase inhibitors • Novel psychoactive substances: synthetic cathinones such as mephedrone
Alcohol	• Vomiting • Slurred speech • Confusion • Convulsions • Unconsciousness • Change in rational thinking • Hypoglycaemia	Alcohol-containing product or a mixture of alcohol-containing products

Poisoning

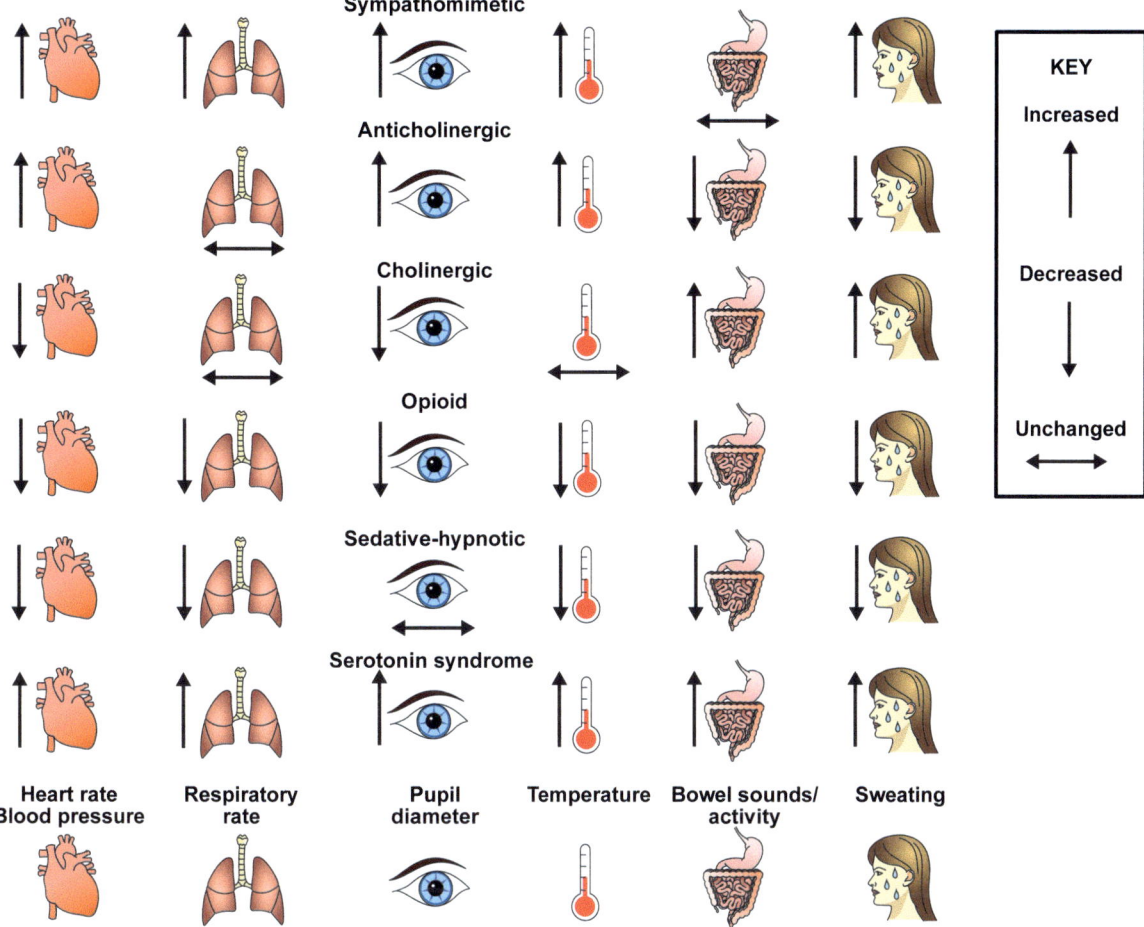

Figure 15.5 Toxidrome signs

4.4 *Management*

Acute poisoning is a dynamic medical illness and patients can quickly deteriorate. Altered LOC, decreased airway reflexes and hypotension are common problems. Despite the time-sensitive nature of poisoning episodes, it is important that prior to approaching the patient(s) you make a dynamic risk assessment to avoid becoming poisoned yourself.

The assessment and management of poisoning patients follows the same ‹C›ABCDE approach explained in Chapter 9, 'Patient assessment'. Correct any life-threatening signs and symptoms where you can, and alert the EOC early on with your findings. The UK Ambulance Services Clinical Practice Guidelines provide some useful advice for poisoning, but tailor your assessment and management to the patient [JRCALC, 2023]:

- Establish the event, drug or substance involved, the quantity, mode of poisoning and any alcohol consumed.
- NEVER induce vomiting.
- After confirmed exposure to a low-toxicity substance, some patients may be considered for home management by ambulance crews.
- Consider exposure to carbon monoxide (CO).

Chapter 16 Trauma

1 Mechanism of injury (MOI)

1.1 Learning objectives
By the end of this section you will be able to:
- define MOI and outline the different types
- explain the kinetics associated with trauma
- describe the mechanisms that can cause injury to the head, spine, chest, abdomen and pelvis.

1.2 Introduction
Trauma is the acute physiological and structural change (injury) that occurs in a patient's body when an external source of energy transfers to the body faster than the body's ability to sustain and dissipate it. The MOI can be defined as the sum of all physical forces that result in the patient's injury, and is primarily concerned with the transfer of energy. Since human tissue, organs and systems can only withstand a limited range of physical, environmental and physiological stresses, injury occurs when the energy delivery to the body exceeds these limits. The tolerance to external energy delivery is dependent on which type of tissue(s) has been targeted; the age and physical health of the patient; and the type, magnitude and duration of the energy that has been transferred [Greaves, 2008].

1.2.1 Types of trauma
Trauma is generally divided into two types [NAEMT, 2020]:
- **Blunt:** Injuries that do not cause penetration of the skin by an external object. Typical mechanisms of blunt trauma include road traffic collisions (RTCs) involving vehicles, pedestrians and motorcyclists, for example; falls from a height; serious sports injuries; and blast injuries (although this mechanism often also causes penetrating trauma). Blunt trauma is the most common type of trauma in the UK [Kehoe, 2015].
- **Penetrating:** Injuries caused by projectiles penetrating the skin. Examples include stab and gunshot wounds, and blast injuries involving shrapnel and secondary projectiles. In the UK the most common form of penetrating trauma is knife injuries.

1.2.2 Elderly patients and pre-existing disease
The Trauma Audit Research Network (TARN) collects data on patients experiencing major trauma in the UK. A review of this data showed that over the past few decades the demographic of people experiencing major trauma and the causes of it are rapidly changing. In 1990, the mean age of patients was 36.1 years and the most common cause of major trauma was an RTC. By 2013, this had changed, with the mean age rising to 53.8 years and the most common cause of major trauma being a fall from less than 2 metres [Kehoe, 2015].

Older adults are suffering more major trauma, so the age of the patient should be a consideration when assessing the severity of traumatic injuries. For example, it is unlikely that a fall from standing height will be fatal to a young healthy person, whereas for an elderly patient who may have a pre-existing disease, such as osteoporosis, such a fall has a far greater chance of causing fatal injury [TARN, 2017]. This recognition of major trauma in older people is now the focus of a lot of work, and you may hear the phrase 'silver trauma' when referring to trauma in the elderly [Wallace, 2018].

1.3 Mechanisms that cause injury
There are many mechanisms that can result in a host of both isolated and multiple injuries to the human body. Some of the more common mechanisms and the injuries they cause to the head, spine, thorax, abdomen and pelvis are covered in this section.

1.3.1 Head

If the head is travelling ahead of the body, such as during a head-first fall, it is the first structure to receive the force of the impact and energy transference. The continued movement of the rest of the body results in compression, which can damage the scalp and skull. If the skull fractures, bony fractures can end up damaging the brain. The same damage can also be caused by the application of an external force, such as occurs as a result of a blow to the head during an assault [NAEMT, 2020].

The brain is soft and compressible and can move following the application of external forces. This can lead to shearing of brain tissue and the rupture of the blood vessels surrounding the brain, leading to intracranial haemorrhage.

If a projectile penetrates the skull, the damage can be very severe, as the kinetic energy is distributed within the confines of the skull. Small-calibre bullets, for example, may not have enough energy to exit the skull, but instead contour around it, leading to extensive damage [NAEMT, 2020].

1.3.2 Spine

The main mechanisms that cause spinal injury can be divided into abnormal flexion, extension, rotation and compression. Extension or flexion with rotation are the main causes of injury to the cervical spine [NAEMT, 2020].

Flexion

Hyperflexion injuries are typically caused by RTCs where lap-belts (rather than three-point belts) are used, direct blows to the occiput, and rapid deceleration in flexed positions, such as diving and contact sports like rugby. Hyperflexion on its own is uncommon in the cervical spine, since the chin abutting the chest limits flexion (Figure 16.1).

Flexion with rotation

The design of the first two cervical vertebrae allows for significant rotation. Injuries due to this mechanism are considered unstable, as there is little in the way of bony or soft-tissue support. Not surprisingly, this mechanism is much more likely to produce significant cervical injury and is often caused by lateral impact RTCs or direct trauma. Note that rotation rarely occurs in isolation (Figure 16.2).

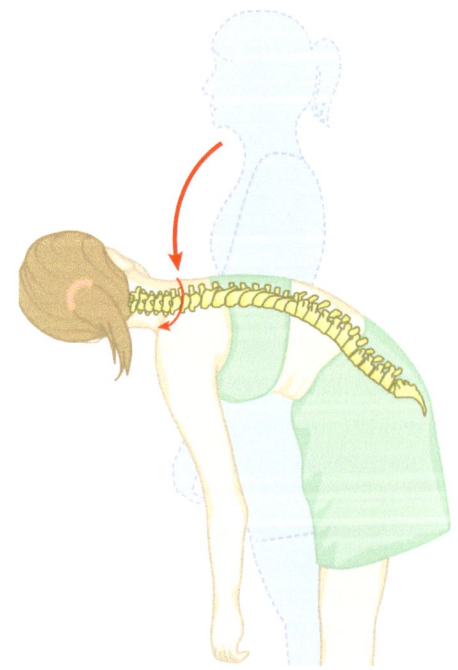

Figure 16.1 Flexion

Figure 16.2 Flexion with rotation

Mechanism of injury (MOI)

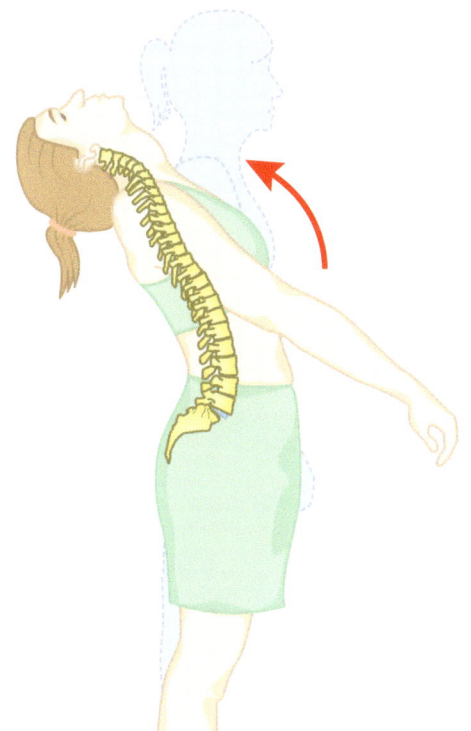

Figure 16.3 Extension

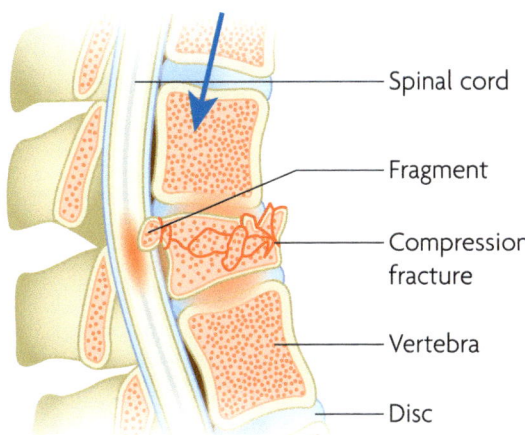

Figure 16.4 Compression

Extension
These injuries are generally found only in cervical and lumbar regions and can be caused by hanging, striking the chin on the steering wheel during a collision or a rear-impact collision where the headrest is improperly positioned [NAEMT, 2020] (Figure 16.3).

Compression
Wedge fractures are the most common type of fracture of the lumbar and thoracic spines, but if a weight falls on the head or if the patient lands on their head after a fall, then the cervical vertebrae can be fractured and/or ligaments ruptured. Most fractures caused by compression are stable, but spinal cord injury can occur if the vertebral body is shattered and fragments of bone become embedded in the cord (Figure 16.4).

1.3.3 Thorax
Severe blunt thoracic trauma most commonly occurs as a result of RTCs (about 70–80%) where high speeds are involved, leading to rapid deceleration. This causes shearing forces that can rupture large blood vessels, tear the bronchial airways and damage the lungs, causing a pneumothorax, for example. Even with lower-velocity mechanisms, such as direct blows to the chest, fractures of the rib cage and sternum, as well as bruising to the underlying structures including the heart and lungs, can occur [NAEMT, 2020]. It is common for elderly patients to receive significant chest wall injuries from a fall from standing height.

In penetrating trauma, the most serious consequences arise as a result of rupture of the major blood vessels, which can lead to serious haemorrhage. In the UK, knife crime is the most common form of penetrating chest trauma [Greaves, 2018]. Projectiles penetrating the chest wall can also cause an open pneumothorax.

1.3.4 Abdomen
Abdominal injury is most commonly caused by blunt trauma, usually due to RTCs, and often as part of a multi-system pattern of injuries. If the abdomen comes into contact with the steering wheel during rapid deceleration, crush injuries can occur. Compression of the abdominal organs increases the intra-abdominal pressure, which in turn can rupture the hollow organs and/or the diaphragm. Penetrating trauma is less common, and

in the UK is more likely to be the result of a stab wound than a gunshot. Fortunately, less than half of all stab wounds actually penetrate the peritoneum (the lining of the abdominal cavity) [Greaves, 2018].

1.3.5 Pelvis

As with any trauma patient, you should consider the MOI to provide an indication as to possible underlying injuries. Pelvic ring fractures usually require high forces, so it is no surprise that the most common cause is RTCs. This injury is most commonly seen in front-seat passengers in head-on collisions and those on the side of impact in T-bone-type collisions. These are closely followed by motorcyclists, pedestrians and people falling from heights [Gabbe, 2011; Papadopoulos, 2006]. However, a significant sub-group are the elderly, who will typically fall from standing and may have osteoporosis [Garlapati, 2012].

2 Integumentary system anatomy and physiology

2.1 Learning objective

By the end of this section you will be able to:
- describe the anatomy and physiology of the integumentary system.

2.2 Introduction

The integumentary system (or skin) is the largest organ in the human body, in terms of both surface area and weight. In adults, skin has a surface area of 2 m^2 and weighs 5 kg [Tortora, 2017]. It is composed of two main layers, the epidermis and dermis. Under the skin is a supportive subcutaneous layer, known as the hypodermis or superficial fascia (Figure 16.5) [Dykes, 2002].

2.3 Epidermis

This is the outermost layer and consists of five sublayers. Most of the cells (90%) are keratinocytes, which produce a tough, fibrous protein (keratin). This helps protect the skin and tissues from heat and microbes. Keratinocytes also produce lamellar granules, which decrease water entry and loss, and

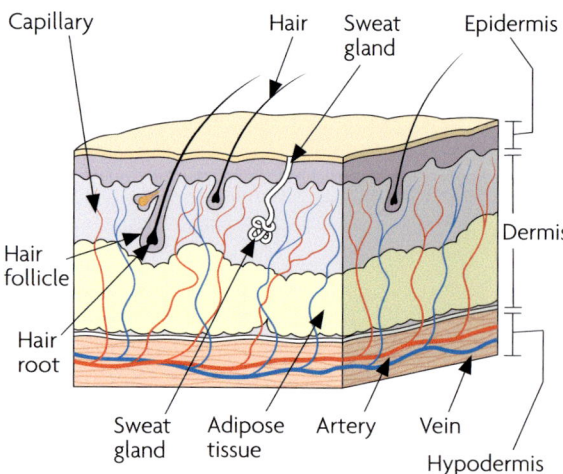

Figure 16.5 Cross-section of the skin

prevent entry of foreign material. Around 8% of the cells are melanocytes, which produce melanin. This is taken up by keratinocytes, protecting the cell's nucleus from the harmful effects of ultraviolet (UV) light. Keratin is either a yellow-red or brown-black pigment and contributes to skin colour. The remaining cells consist of Langerhans cells, which help in the body's immune response, and Merkel cells, which are involved in touch perception [Tortora, 2017].

It takes around 2–4 weeks for a cell starting at the lowest layer of the epidermis to become a keratinocyte and migrate up to the top layer (stratum corneum) and slough off (Paxton, 2003).

2.4 Dermis

This deeper layer of skin mostly consists of connective tissue, elastin and an extracellular matrix, which provides strength and pliability. However, it also contains blood and lymphatic vessels, nerve fibres, hair follicles, and sebaceous and sweat glands. The dermis is divided into two regions, the papillary and the reticular. The papillary region consists of connective tissue that anchors the epidermis and a dense network of capillaries and small blood vessels, in nipple-like projections called dermal papillae. These play an important part in temperature regulation. In addition, the dermal papillae also contain free nerve endings, which act as pain and fine touch receptors (Meissner corpuscles) [Tortora, 2017].

The reticular region makes up 80% of the dermis and consists of dense, irregular connective tissue. Interlocking collagen fibres run in various planes, forming 'lines of cleavage'. Surgeons try to make incisions parallel to these lines, since the skin does not gape as much, resulting in less scarring [Thompson, 2008].

2.5 Hypodermis

Also known as the superficial fascia, this layer contains subcutaneous fat, connective tissue, sweat glands, muscle and bone. It helps to insulate the body, absorbs shocks to the skeletal system, and enables the skin to move easily over underlying structures [AAOS, 2011].

2.6 Physiology

The skin provides a range of functions, which any damage can impair [Thompson, 2008; Tortora, 2017]:
- protection against infection by forming a physical barrier to microbes and foreign material
- sensory perception of pain, pressure, heat and cold
- thermoregulation using nerves, blood vessels and sweat glands to control body temperature
- excretion of trace amounts of water and body waste, while helping to prevent dehydration
- maintenance of mineralisation of bones and teeth, and synthesis of vitamin D
- absorption of lipid-soluble substances, such as fat-soluble vitamins and drugs, through the skin.

3 Wounds and bleeding

3.1 Learning objectives

By the end of this section you will be able to:
- describe the types of bleeding
- explain how to appropriately assess and manage bleeding
- explain how to detect concealed bleeding
- describe various types of wounds and how to manage them
- discuss the implications of foreign objects in wounds
- explain complications associated with bleeding and wounds.

3.2 Introduction

Wounds and bleeding are a common reason for an emergency call. Even in the emergency ambulance service, these calls will vary in their severity, from wounds and bleeding that require basic first aid only, through to life-threatening wounds and bleeding that require prompt and more advanced intervention in order to prevent death.

3.3 Bleeding

Bleeding is the loss of blood from a damaged blood vessel. You will often hear the term 'haemorrhage' used, which is bleeding, but in medical circles is usually reserved for severe bleeding. Bleeding is often classified by the type of vessel involved (i.e. artery, vein or capillary) or whether it is external or internal.

3.3.1 Assessment

Sources of bleeding

Bleeding can be defined by whether it is visible on the outside of the body and/or which type of vessel is responsible [NAEMT, 2020; SJA, 2021]:
- **Internal:** This bleeding is concealed within the body and can be hard to detect. The thorax, abdomen, pelvis and long bones provide good hiding places for significant volumes of blood. The MOI and the presence of shock without signs of external haemorrhage can help with diagnosis. These patients need to be in hospital to stop the bleeding.
- **External:** This bleeding is visible and should be detected during your primary and/or secondary survey. This bleeding can usually be controlled.
- **Arterial:** Blood inside the arteries is under relatively high pressure and so bleeding from these vessels can lead to significant blood loss. It is characterised by bright red (oxygenated) spurting, in time with the heartbeat.
- **Venous:** Since veins carry blood back to the heart, they typically carry deoxygenated blood and so bleeding is a darker red. Since the pressure is lower, blood does not spurt but flows freely. However, blood loss can still be severe, particularly from veins in the neck and legs.

Chapter 16 – Trauma

- **Capillary:** These are the smallest blood vessels in the body and carry a mixture of oxygenated and deoxygenated blood, so the colour of bleeding will vary. Blood loss tends to be small as blood oozes from wounds.

Estimating blood loss

Estimating blood loss accurately is very difficult and ambulance staff (and doctors/nurses/midwives) generally do not do this well [Bose, 2006; Frank, 2010; Rothermel, 2016]. Figure 16.6 provides examples of what a small and large volume of blood loss looks like [JRCALC, 2023]. Fractures can cause significant blood loss, depending on the bone(s) affected and whether the fracture is open or closed (Table 16.1) [NAEMT, 2020].

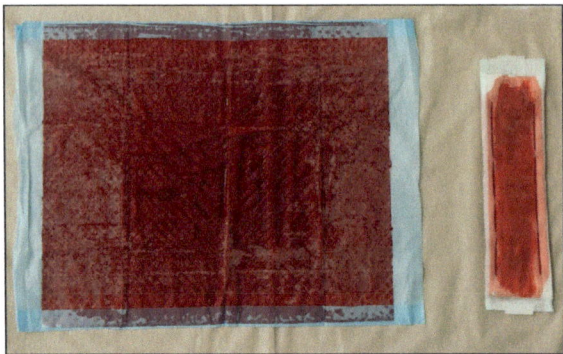

Figure 16.6 Maternity pad with 500 ml blood and sanitary pad with 50 ml blood

Table 16.1 Approximate internal blood loss due to fractures

Fracture	Blood loss (ml)
Rib	125
Radius or ulna	250–500
Humerus	500–750
Tibia	500–1,000
Femur	1,000–2,000
Pelvis	1,000–entire circulating volume; in adults that can be 5,000–6,000 ml

3.3.2 Management

The ‹C› in ‹C›ABCDE highlights the importance of recognising and managing catastrophic bleeding immediately in the primary survey, even before airway management if the two cannot be managed simultaneously [Nutbeam, 2013]. Once the scene assessment has been completed, you need to check for, and manage, any actual or potential catastrophic haemorrhage. Only once this has been completed can you continue with the remainder of the primary survey.

During the assessment of circulation (the second C), any interventions to manage catastrophic haemorrhage must be reassessed to ensure that bleeding is being controlled appropriately. Don't forget the bleeding you cannot see. 'Blood on the floor plus four more' is a good way to remember the areas where significant blood loss can accumulate, i.e. the thorax, abdomen, pelvis and long bones [Greaves, 2010].

Most external haemorrhage can be controlled with simple first-aid measures, such as direct pressure and elevation of the bleeding extremity. In some cases, additional interventions are required, but these should be introduced in an incremental fashion, as shown in the haemostasis escalator (Figure 16.7) [Lee, 2007b; Moorhouse, 2007].

Catastrophic haemorrhage management

If you suspect the bleeding is likely to cause death in minutes (i.e. is a catastrophic haemorrhage),

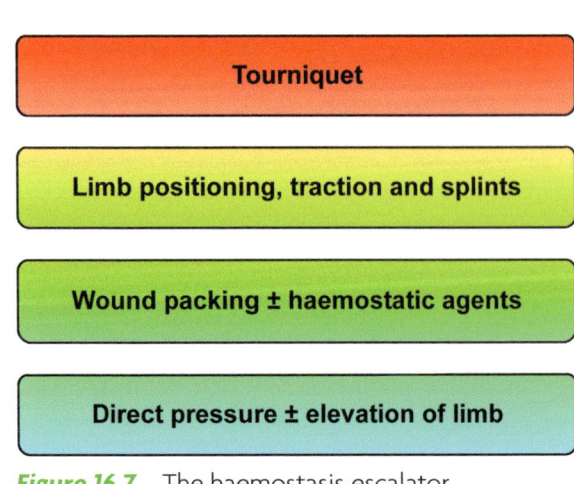

Figure 16.7 The haemostasis escalator

you are likely to ascend the haemostasis escalator rather faster than for non-catastrophic haemorrhage. If the haemorrhage involves a limb distal to a junctional area, a tourniquet should be immediately applied. Should the first tourniquet not adequately control the bleeding, a second tourniquet should be applied above the first. If bleeding continues, pack the wound with a haemostatic gauze and apply a fresh dressing. Apply firm direct pressure [JRCALC, 2023].

In other body areas, such as the head, neck, torso and junction regions (i.e., groin and armpit), it will not be possible to use a tourniquet. In this instance, you should apply a wound dressing to the site of bleeding and apply firm pressure directly over the wound. Elevation is unlikely to be appropriate with these types of bleeds. If direct pressure fails to stem the bleeding, then wound packing should be undertaken and may be supplemented with haemostatic agents. This is achieved by inserting a sufficient quantity of gauze into the wound to create mechanical pressure on the injured vessel and provide a structure for coagulation. Where available, haemostatic agents should be used and placed as close to the bleeding point as possible, and then direct pressure should be applied for at least 3 minutes over the top. Following this, constant pressure should be applied with a suitable elastic bandage holding the haemostatic dressing in place. If this fails to control the bleeding, add more direct pressure and consider adding a further dressing.

Assess limb positioning and consider whether the use of splinting may help to reduce bleeding. Straightening angulated fractures and applying a pelvic binder may help to reduce blood loss [NICE, 2016].

Non-catastrophic haemorrhage management
For other, non-catastrophic external haemorrhage, you can move up the haemorrhage escalator. Start by applying direct pressure, with or without a dressing and, if the injury is below the knee or elbow, consider elevating the affected limb above the level of the heart, if practicable. If this does not control the bleeding, consider applying a further dressing while continuing to apply firm direct pressure [JRCALC, 2023].

If bleeding continues despite sustained direct pressure and dressing, you should treat the haemorrhage as a potential catastrophic bleeding event. For limbs, this means applying a tourniquet, and in the case of head, neck, torso or junction wounds, packing with haemostatic dressing. As with catastrophic haemorrhage, consider whether splinting a limb or applying a pelvic binder would help reduce blood loss.

3.3.3 Tourniquets

While the use of arterial tourniquets (Figure 16.8) originated on the battlefield, they do have a place in civilian ambulance services for use in specific circumstances.

Indications
- Life-threatening limb haemorrhage unable to be controlled by simple techniques alone.

Contra-indications
- Absence of bone inside the limb in cases of extreme trauma (tourniquet requires a bone to compress against).

Advantages
- Can be rapidly applied.
- Improves survival from peripheral vascular injury when applied early [Teixeira, 2018].

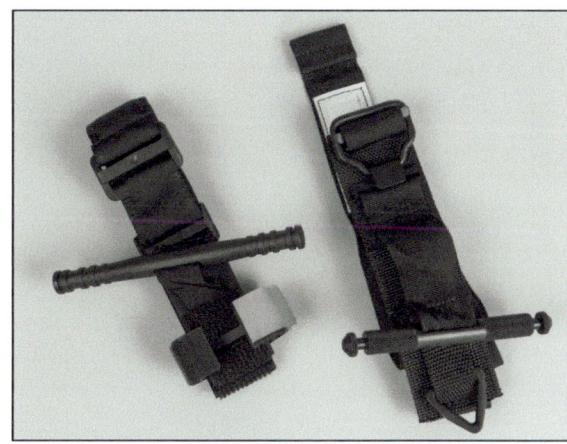

Figure 16.8 Two tourniquets: a Combat Application Tourniquet (CAT) on the left and a SOF® Tourniquet on the right

Chapter 16 – *Trauma*

Disadvantages
- Causes significant pain; strong analgesia is likely to be required [Greaves, 2018].
- Can worsen bleeding if applied incorrectly (increases venous bleeding if not applied tightly enough) [FPHC, 2017].
- Can cause soft-tissue injury around the site of application.

Procedure – CAT application

Take the following steps to apply a CAT [Pilbery & Lethbridge, 2022]:

1. Explain the procedure to the patient (including that the procedure may be painful) and obtain consent if appropriate to do so.
   If possible, arrange for analgesia to be administered.
2. Don appropriate PPE, and undertake appropriate hand hygiene.
3. Place the tourniquet around the limb about 5–8 cm above the site of bleeding and directly on to the skin.
   This can be on a single- or double-bone limb but should not be immediately over a joint.

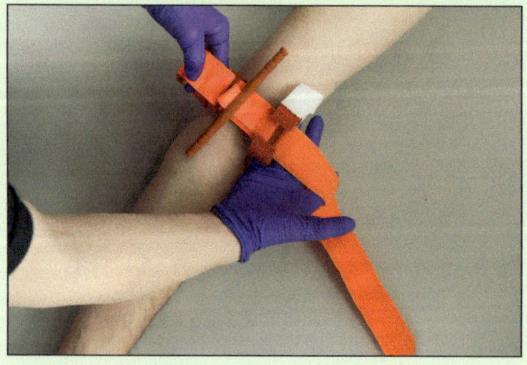

Procedure – *cont*

4. Pull the band of material so it pulls through the buckle and becomes tight on the limb. Once tight, stick it back to itself around the limb. It may help to hold the body of the tourniquet in place while you do this.
   The band should be tight enough that three fingers cannot be slid between the band and the limb.

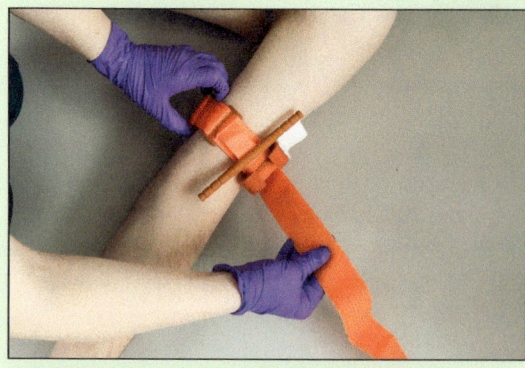

5. Turn the rod until the bleeding stops.

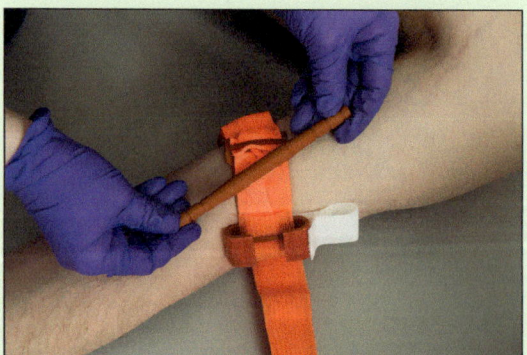

6. Once bleeding has ceased, keep turning the rod until it can be clipped into the holder.

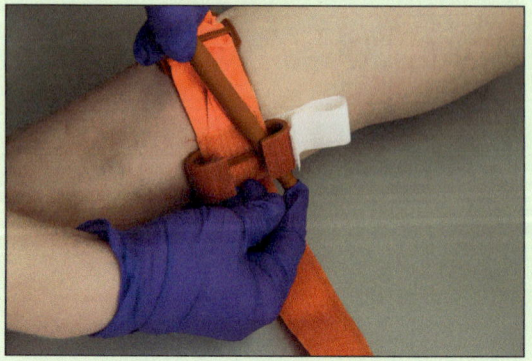

Wounds and bleeding

Procedure – *cont*

7. Wrap the remaining strap between the clips and then place the time strap over the top to secure the rod.

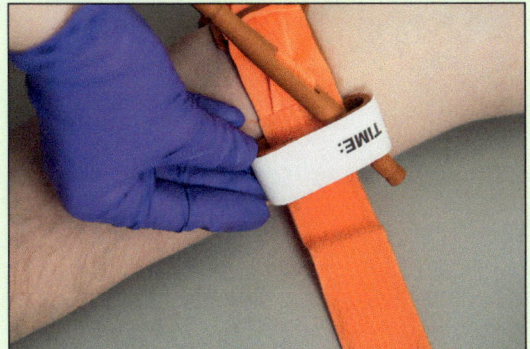

8. Document the procedure, including the time it was undertaken and any complications.
9. Continually reassess the tourniquet. If necessary, re-tighten it or add another tourniquet proximal to the first.

Procedure – SOF® Tourniquet application

Take the following steps to apply a SOF® Tourniquet [Pilbery & Lethbridge, 2022]:

1. Explain the procedure to the patient (including that the procedure may be painful) and obtain consent if appropriate to do so. If possible, arrange for analgesia to be administered.
2. Don appropriate PPE, and undertake appropriate hand hygiene.
3. Place the tourniquet around the limb, around 5–8 cm above the site of bleeding and directly on to the skin.
   This can be on a single- or double-bone limb but should not be immediately over a joint.

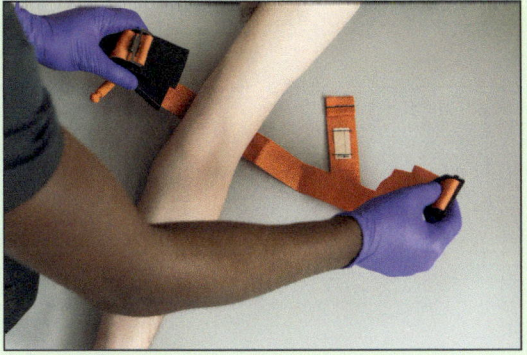

Procedure – *cont*

4. Clip the buckle on the strap to the body of the tourniquet. Ensure it is properly clipped into place.

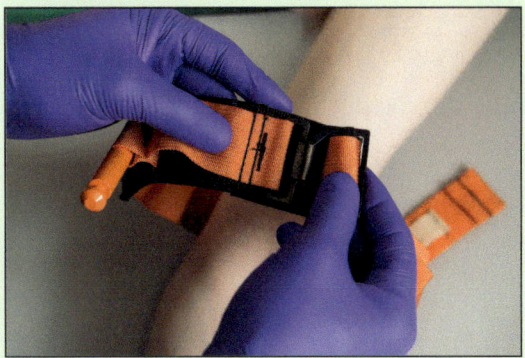

5. While stabilising the body of the tourniquet with one hand, pull the strap until the slack has been taken out.
   The band should be tight enough that three fingers cannot be slid between the band and the limb.

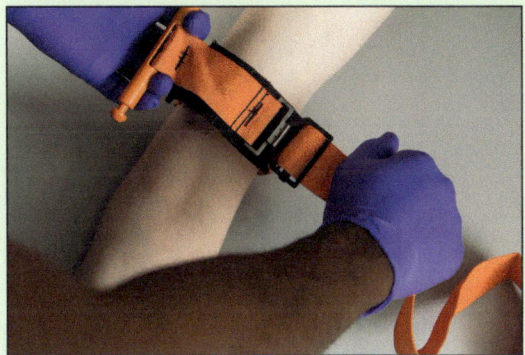

6. Turn the windlass rod until the bleeding stops.

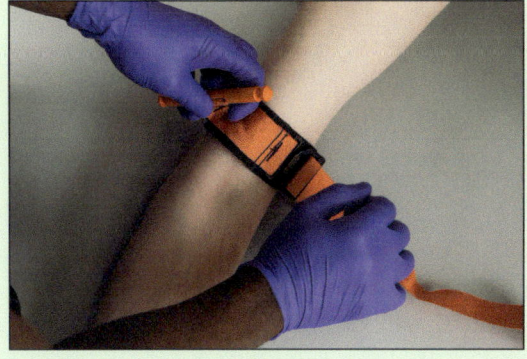

Chapter 16 – *Trauma*

Procedure – *cont*

7. Once bleeding has ceased, keep turning the windlass until it can be clipped into the holder.

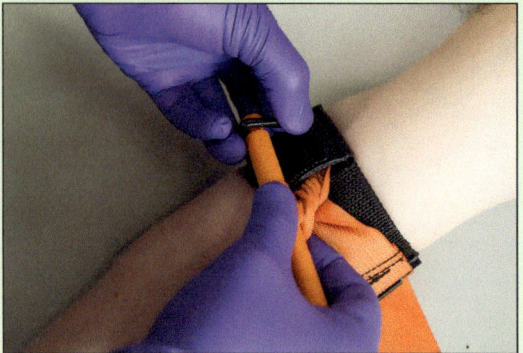

8. Wrap the remaining strap neatly round the windlass.
9. Document the procedure, including the time it was undertaken and any complications.

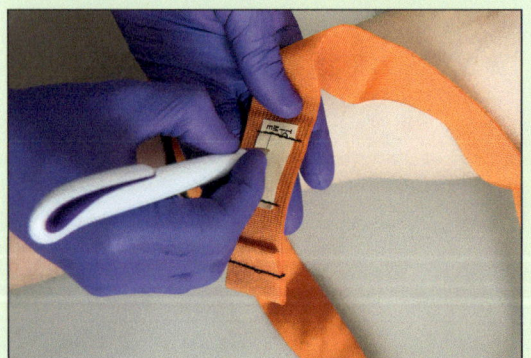

10. Continually reassess the tourniquet. If necessary, re-tighten it or add another tourniquet proximal to the first.

3.3.4 Haemostatic dressings

Where direct pressure and wound packing are ineffective, and in areas such as the groin, neck and axilla, where tourniquet application is not possible, haemostatic agents can be used to control haemorrhage [Boulton, 2018; JRCALC, 2023]. Modern haemostatic agents usually come as dressings, whereby the dressings have been impregnated with the active ingredients. They work by either concentrating clotting factors or acting as a precursor to coagulation, or are mucoadhesive [Boulton, 2018].

Indications
- Life-threatening haemorrhage from wounds which can be packed with a dressing. Haemostatic dressings are of particular value in areas that are hard to compress, including the thorax and junctional areas around the groin, arms and neck.

Contra-indications
- Do not apply over the eyes.
- Do not apply close to the spine.

Advantages
- The clotting mechanism works independently of clotting factors in the blood so is not impacted by coagulopathy or use of anticoagulants [Greaves, 2018].

Disadvantages
- Commonly misapplied, due to not being packed deeply enough into the wound.

Procedure

Follow the procedure below to apply HemCon ChitoGauze XR Pro [Pilbery & Lethbridge, 2022]:

Note: While this procedure is specific for HemCon ChitoGauze XR Pro, it is likely that other haemostatic agents will be applied using similar principles.

1. Explain the procedure to the patient and obtain consent if appropriate to do so.
2. Don appropriate PPE, and undertake appropriate hand hygiene.
3. Open the packet and remove the ChitoGauze, keeping it folded up. Take care not to drop the gauze or allow it to become contaminated prior to use.

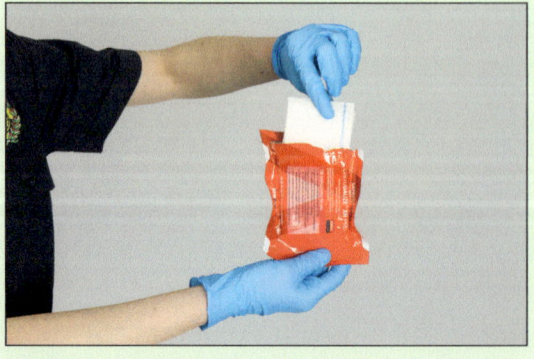

Wounds and bleeding

Procedure – *cont*

4. Pack the gauze deep into the wound.
   Note: This should not be laid over a wound as it will not work if used like this – it must be packed deep into a wound.
   More than one pack of gauze may be required.

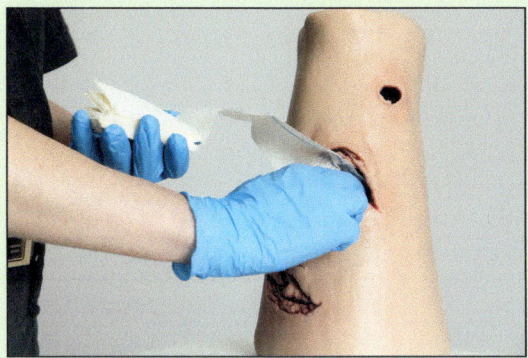

5. If there is excess dressing after packing the wound, cut off the remaining dressing, ensuring that what remains includes some X-ray-translucent strip (the thin blue line).
6. Maintain direct pressure until bleeding is controlled.

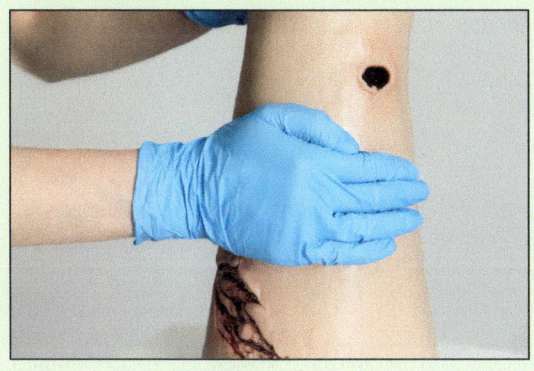

Procedure – *cont*

7. Dress the wound, ensuring that the dressing continues to apply pressure.

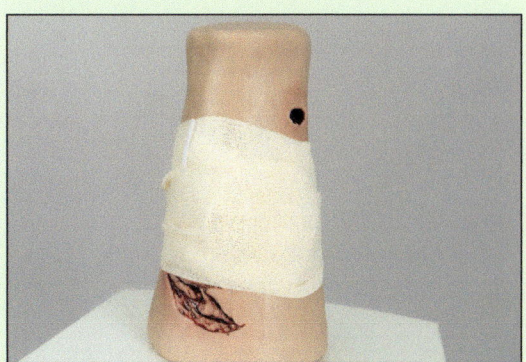

8. Continually reassess the wound area and dressing.
9. Document the procedure, including the time it was undertaken and any complications.

3.4 *Wounds*

A wound is an injury to living tissue, breaking its continuity. There are seven basic categories [Purcell, 2016]:

- **Contusion (bruises):** Caused by bleeding from damaged blood vessels under the skin. They cause a bluish/purple discolouration beneath the skin and are typically caused by blunt trauma.
- **Abrasion (grazes):** Injuries caused by friction shearing the skin away. These usually involve the superficial layers of the skin, but can go much deeper. They can be very painful and are often dirty, with embedded grit and mud.
- **Laceration (tear):** Tearing or splitting of the skin due to blunt trauma. These cause a ragged wound, which can extend through the skin surface to the underlying structures.
- **Incision (cut):** A break in the continuity of the skin by a sharp implement, such as broken glass or a knife. These are usually clean wounds (unless the implement is dirty) with neat edges.

Chapter 16 – Trauma

- **Puncture (stab):** A penetrating wound caused by an object that is pointed and narrow, such as a nail or knife. Although these wounds are typically small, they can be deep, causing serious damage to vessels and other body structures below the skin.
- **Burn:** An injury caused by energy transfer to the body's tissues, causing necrosis and an associated inflammatory reaction (covered in section 6, 'Burns', later in this chapter).
- **Gunshot:** A complicated wound caused by a projectile moving at speed. The wound consists of an entry point, with varying amounts of tissue destruction and cavitation underneath the skin, and, if there is sufficient energy left, an exit wound.

There are a range of external and internal factors that can lead to wound formation [Thompson, 2008]:
- **External:** Mechanical (friction), chemical, electrical, temperature extremes, radiation and micro-organisms.
- **Internal:** Circulatory system failure, endocrine (e.g. diabetes), neuropathy, haematological, malignancy (cancer).

3.4.1 Management

Wound management will be determined by the size and nature of the wound and the presence of complicating factors. The main initial problems are bleeding, pain and the risk of infection [Purcell, 2016]. Always enquire about tetanus immunisation in any patient who has a wound with a higher risk of infection, such as a dirty wound, a wound caused by a bite (human or animal) or involving a puncture by a dirty object [SJA, 2021]. In addition, consider whether there has been damage to other structures, such as blood vessels, nerves, tendons and ligaments, which can have life-changing consequences if not managed appropriately. For example, consider a pianist who injures their hand, causing damage to ligaments. Although the external wound may be minor, without prompt management of the ligamentous injury, their fingers may not function properly in the future.

If the wound is small and bleeding easily controlled, clean the wound:

- Use a wet gauze to clean the edges of open wounds, wiping away from the wound to avoid contaminating it further. Continue until all visible dirt and blood has been removed.
- Irrigate wounds with tap water, as rubbing or scrubbing can cause tissue damage and swabs or cotton wool can leave fibres in the wound.

Once cleaning is complete, cover with a sterile, non-adherent dressing.

If there is a foreign object in the wound, it may be possible to remove it if it is small (e.g. grit) by irrigating the wound with water or using tweezers. However, larger objects or those that appear firmly embedded should not be removed but left in place and a sterile, non-adherent dressing be applied.

Larger wounds are going to require closure by someone trained in wound care. This may be in hospital, but it might also be possible for a specialist paramedic or minor injuries unit to manage the closure, helping to avoid the need to take the patient to the ED.

4 Assessment and management of the trauma patient

4.1 *Learning objectives*

By the end of this section you will be able to:
- explain the assessment and management of patients with a range of traumatic injuries
- describe the complications associated with a range of traumatic injuries.

4.2 *Introduction*

The approach to the trauma patient is similar to that of all patients, with an initial scene assessment followed by a primary survey. However, there are some aspects of this process that are specific to trauma and they are going to be covered in this section. In addition, there are a range of complications that can arise as a result of traumatic injury to specific regions, and a number of these are going to be covered in this section, specifically injuries to the head, spine, thorax, abdomen and pelvis.

4.3 Scene assessment

The SCENE mnemonic can be used to ensure that you cover all aspects of an initial trauma scene assessment [JRCALC, 2023]:

- **S:** Safety. A dynamic risk assessment should highlight current as well as potential dangers. If you are not equipped in terms of kit and expertise to deal with the scene, withdraw and request specialist help, for example from the HART. Remember to continually reassess safety as the situation can change quickly. Make sure you are wearing appropriate PPE.
- **C:** Cause, including MOI. Finding out what happened is important in order to appreciate likely injuries and energy transfer. However, ensure that the scene matches the story you are being told, as you may have come across a crime scene or case of abuse.
- **E:** Environment. Consider whether there are any environmental factors that need to be taken into account. These may complicate your extrication by affecting access to and from the scene and/or increase the risk of harm to the patient, due to increased risk of hypothermia, for example.
- **N:** Number of patients. Determine the number of patients early on in your assessment to help you decide whether you can manage the scene on your own. It may also help to identify patients who have either wandered off from the scene or who have been ejected from a vehicle, for example, and are currently hidden from view.
- **E:** Extra resources needed. Depending on the number of patients, the severity of their injuries and the nature of the incident, you may need additional help from other emergency services, such as the police to keep a scene safe, or additional ambulances, including the air ambulance, for patient transport.

4.4 Primary survey

The aim of the primary survey is to identify threats to life promptly and intervene as soon as they are found. The steps of the primary survey should be undertaken sequentially, unless there are enough personnel to allow for simultaneous assessment and treatment [Halliwell, 2011].

4.4.1 Procedure

Take the following steps to undertake a primary survey in the trauma patient [Greaves, 2010, 2018; JRCALC, 2023; NAEMT, 2020; Nutbeam, 2013]:

1. **General impression:** As you approach the patient, perform a global assessment. Are they sitting up and watching you approach, with well-perfused skin, or are they lying unresponsive, pale and clammy with an expanding pool of blood leaking from a wound?
2. **Catastrophic haemorrhage:** This is bleeding that is likely to cause death within minutes, so cannot wait until airway and breathing have been addressed. Typically, bleeding can be controlled with direct pressure and elevation of the bleeding site, but may require the use of haemostatic agents or tourniquets.
3. **Airway with cervical spine consideration:** If a patient has suffered significant blunt trauma or the MOI suggests that the cervical spine may have been damaged, provide prompt manual in-line stabilisation (MILS). This should be applied as soon as there are sufficient personnel at scene to do so, but should not commit a member of the team if more important treatments are required. Assess the airway by looking for obvious obstruction, listening for noisy airflow (snoring or gurgling) and feeling for air movement.
4. Manage the airway using appropriate airway manoeuvres, such as:
   - Jaw thrust–chin lift
   - Suction
   - Naso- and oropharyngeal airways.
5. **Breathing:** Administer high-flow oxygen to patients to obtain a target saturation of 94–98%, even if they have COPD.
6. Examine the neck for:
   - **T**racheal deviation
   - **W**ounds and swellings
   - **E**mphysema (surgical/subcutaneous)
   - **L**aryngeal crepitus
   - **V**eins.

Procedure – *cont*

7. Look for obvious chest injuries, wounds, bruising, flail segments and equal rise and fall on both sides of the chest. Assess the rate, depth and quality of respiration:
    - Ventilate with a BVM if respirations are absent or fewer than 10 breaths/min.
    - If respirations are greater than 30 breaths/min, it may also be clinically appropriate to support the patient's ventilations.
    - Monitor closely if respirations are in the range of 10–30 breaths/min.
8. Listen (auscultate) over both axillae for air entry. If bilateral air entry is not heard, use percussion to indicate the underlying problem.
9. Feel for equality of chest movement and note any instability or crepitus.
10. Manage breathing problems as you find them. This may include:
    - applying an appropriate dressing to sucking chest wounds
    - a clinician inserting a cannula into the chest to decompress a tension pneumothorax
    - positioning to support a patient with a flail segment (not possible if the patient has a suspected spinal injury).
11. **Circulation:** If a catastrophic haemorrhage was encountered at the start of the primary survey, reassess this now.
12. Assess both central and distal pulses if confident in doing so (carotid and radial, typically), noting rate, rhythm and volume. Note the skin colour, temperature and the presence of clamminess. If additional personnel are available, the blood pressure can also be measured.
13. Assess for signs of blood loss, remembering the phrase 'blood on the floor plus four more':
    - Externally: Don't forget to consider bleeding into clothing, splints and dressings.

Procedure – *cont*

- Chest: Completed during assessment of breathing.
- Abdomen: Look for bruising or external marks and feel for rigidity and to elicit tenderness.
- Pelvis: Examine the pelvis for obvious deformity or bruising. The pelvis should not be manipulated or 'sprung' to assess for instability. A suggestive MOI is often sufficient to immobilise the pelvis, especially if it is accompanied by haemodynamic instability.
- Long bones: Assess long bones, particularly the femurs, but do not be distracted by fractures that are more peripheral and not likely to cause sufficient bleeding to endanger life at this stage of the primary survey.

14. Manage bleeding appropriately (see section 3, 'Wounds and bleeding', earlier in this chapter).
15. A clinician on scene may wish to gain intravenous access now if fluids and/or tranexamic acid (TXA) are required.
16. To minimise clot disruption, patient movement should be kept to a minimum.
17. **Disability:** Assess LOC with AVPU, and pupil size, equality and reaction to light. Don't forget to check the blood glucose if authorised.
18. **Exposure:** To identify all injuries, it is necessary to remove the patient's clothing. In cases of severe injury or suspected spinal injury, clothes should be cut off the patient to minimise movement. Take care to prevent hypothermia, as this can dramatically increase the patient's chances of dying (up to three times higher if core body temperature drops below 35°C [Balvers, 2016]). It may be more appropriate to remove patients to a heated ambulance before completing this step.

4.5 Head injuries

Common causes of traumatic brain injury (TBI) include RTCs, falls, assault and direct blows to the head [Shivaji, 2014]. The worst outcomes are associated with [Moppett, 2007]:
- penetrating injuries
- non-accidental injury in children aged under 5 years
- pedestrians and pedal cyclists
- ejection from a vehicle.

4.5.1 Recognition

Suggestive signs and symptoms of TBI include [NAEMT, 2020]:
- lacerations, contusions or haematomas to the scalp
- boggy areas when palpating the scalp
- visible fractures or deformity of the skull
- Battle's sign or 'panda eyes' (not apparent for several hours)
- CSF and/or blood leaking from the nose or ears
- Cushing's triad: rising blood pressure, reducing heart rate and irregular respirations
- dizziness
- nausea and vomiting
- abnormal pupils and/or pupil reaction
- visual disturbances (double or blurred vision, seeing 'stars')
- severe headache
- altered LOC
- perseveration (repeatedly asking the same questions)
- amnesia
- paraesthesia/paralysis of the extremities
- convulsions
- posturing
- abnormal respirations.

4.6 Spinal injuries

Spinal injuries, or more specifically spinal cord injuries (SCIs), are rare, with around 2,500 new cases per year [SIA, 2020]. In adult major trauma, approximately 10% of patients will sustain a spinal fracture/dislocation, but less than 2% will sustain an SCI. The most common cause is a fall (46%), although, significantly, a third of these are falls of LESS than 2 m in height. Falls are closely followed by RTCs (40%) and other, much rarer, causes, such as sports injuries (under 3%), stabbings (1%) and shootings (0.6%). SCIs most commonly occur at the cervical level (45%), followed by thoracic (29%), lumbar (24%) and multi-level injuries (2%) [Hasler, 2011].

Risk factors for SCI include [Hasler, 2011]:
- male sex
- under 45 years of age
- reduced Glasgow Coma Scale score
- accompanying chest injury
- dangerous MOI (falls greater than 2 m, sports injury, RTC, shooting).

4.6.1 Management

All patients who are suspected of having a spinal injury should be immobilised as soon as possible. Patients with isolated penetrating trauma to the head or limbs do not require immobilisation, but if, in torso or neck trauma, it is possible that the projectile could have passed near or through the spinal cord and there are signs of SCI, then immobilisation is appropriate.

In blunt trauma, there are guidelines that allow clinicians to discontinue immobilisation, so you may on occasion be asked to stop immobilising a patient once a thorough assessment has been completed [JRCALC, 2023].

4.7 Thoracic injuries

Thoracic trauma accounts directly for 25% of all trauma deaths and is a contributing factor to around another 50% [Greaves, 2018]. Major causes are RTCs, industrial accidents and domestic and sporting injuries [Greaves, 2008]. The most common problem associated with severe thoracic injury is hypoxia [JRCALC, 2023].

4.7.1 Pneumothorax

The lungs are surrounded by a pleural membrane. The outer layer (parietal pleura) lines the chest wall, and the inner layer (visceral pleura) covers the lungs. Between them is the pleural space, which is lubricated to ensure that the surfaces glide smoothly over one another as well as creating surface tension that results in the surfaces 'sticking together'.

Pneumothorax, or air in the pleural space, is generally classified as being spontaneous, if there is no obvious causal factor, or traumatic, if there is an external cause [Noppen, 2010]. In the event that air within the alveoli can escape into the pleural space, or there is an external breach of the thoracic cavity allowing atmospheric air to enter the pleural space, the normal physiology of ventilation is disrupted and the lung collapses [Yarmus, 2023]. Spontaneous pneumothorax is regarded as common and normally benign so long as it does not progress to a tension pneumothorax [Yoon, 2013].

A traumatic pneumothorax is caused by penetrating trauma, such as stab and gunshot wounds or impalements; blunt trauma that leads to rib fractures and increased intrathoracic pressure; and bronchial rupture and barotrauma, where changes in pressure of the air delivered to the lungs lead to expansion. This phenomenon has been reported in air crew and scuba divers [Sharma, 2008].

Assessment
Arguably, the most important type of pneumothorax to recognise is one under tension. However, the clinical course of a tension pneumothorax is not the same for all patients, with the progression of clinical deterioration for an awake, spontaneously breathing patient likely to be considerably longer than for those who are being ventilated with PPV [Leigh-Smith, 2005].

Signs and symptoms of a tension pneumothorax in awake patients include:
- pleuritic chest pain (sharp pain, worse on breathing in and out)
- air hunger
- respiratory distress
- tachypnoea (rapid breathing rate)
- tachycardia (rapid heart rate)
- falling SpO_2
- agitation
- on the same side as the injury:
  - hyper-expansion
  - hypomobility
  - decreased breath sounds
- pre-terminal (near death):
  - decreasing respiratory rate
  - hypotension
  - decreasing LOC.

Management
Patients with a simple pneumothorax with no signs of cardiovascular compromise, suggesting tension, will be closely monitored en route to hospital, but are typically managed conservatively [Lee, 2007a]. All patients with a pneumothorax should receive oxygen at the appropriate target range (usually 94–98%, except for patients with COPD, who should be managed at either 88–92% or their usual range [JRCALC, 2023]). If the patient maintains saturations of 94–98% without oxygen, it may not be required.

If there is an open pneumothorax, the clinician may choose to cover it with a commercial chest seal [Leech, 2017]. Patients with signs of a tension pneumothorax require prompt decompression by needle thoracentesis, which involves inserting a large-bore cannula into the patient's chest and should only be performed by a clinician.

4.7.2 Haemothorax

Haemothorax, or blood in the thoracic cavity, usually occurs as a result of penetrating trauma. Life-threatening haemorrhage can occur in cases of severe lacerations of the lung, large vessels in the mediastinum and the heart. Each hemithorax (literally: half of the chest) can easily accommodate half of the patient's circulating blood volume before the physical signs are obvious [Greaves, 2008].

However, this amount of bleeding will lead to the signs and symptoms of shock. Since blood occupies space usually reserved for the lung, lung collapse occurs, leading to absent or decreased lung sounds, reduced chest wall expansion on the injured side and dullness on percussion [Leech, 2017].

There are few treatment options available outside of hospital; usually, expedient transport to the nearest major trauma centre is indicated.

4.7.3 Flail chest

Blunt chest trauma can lead to multiple rib and sternal fractures. In the event that two or more ribs are broken in two or more places, a flail segment will be created, allowing that section of the chest wall to move more freely. This will result in a paradoxical movement of this chest segment, that is, it will move inwards during inspiration and outwards on expiration [Athanassiadi, 2010]. If this area is large enough, it results in compromised ventilation. However, it is usually bruising of the underlying lung that leads to hypoxia and there can also be significant blood loss, with each rib fracture causing around 100 ml of blood loss or more [Greaves, 2008].

The flail segment is not always obvious, as muscular spasm can support the segment until the muscles are exhausted. However, these injuries are painful and the ambulance clinician is likely to want to provide intravenous analgesia [JRCALC, 2023]. Do not attempt to splint the flail segment as this is likely to further impair ventilation [NAEMT, 2020].

4.8 Abdominal injuries

The abdominal cavity extends from the diaphragm to the pelvic bones and from the vertebral column to the muscles of the abdomen and flanks (Figure 16.9). Organs are classed as peritoneal if they are covered by a lining called the peritoneum. These include the spleen, liver, stomach, gallbladder, the tail of the pancreas, parts of the large intestine and most of the small intestine, and the female reproductive organs [Tortora, 2017]. The retroperitoneal space is the area behind the peritoneum. This area contains the kidneys, ureters, pancreas (except the tail), parts of the small and large intestines, and the aorta and inferior vena cava.

In blunt trauma, the spleen, liver and structures that are firmly fixed, such as the retroperitoneal organs, are most commonly injured due to shearing forces associated with rapid deceleration. Penetrating trauma can also cause serious damage and severe bleeding. Depending on the angle at which the penetrating object enters, thoracic injury is also possible, particularly in upper abdominal stab injuries [NAEMT, 2020].

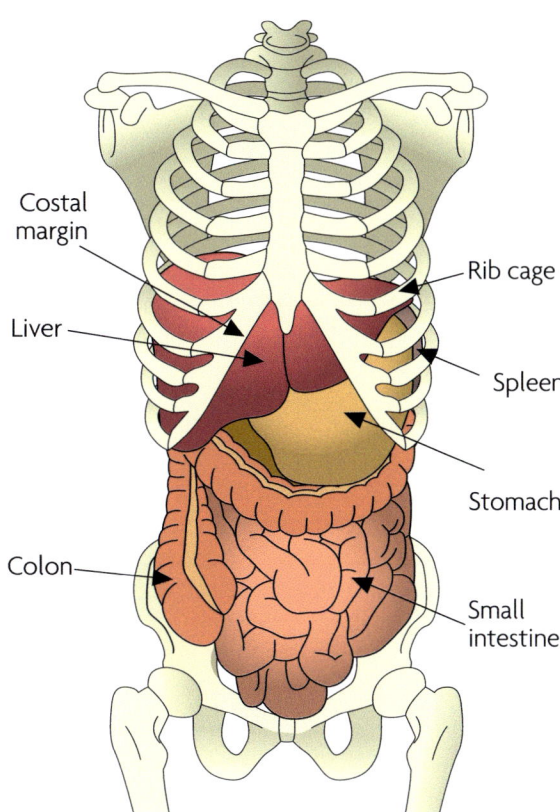

Figure 16.9 The abdominal cavity

Patients suffering from abdominal trauma may not exhibit many symptoms initially, although you should suspect internal injury in any shocked patient with a suggestive MOI. Look at the abdomen for signs of injury, such as bruising, abrasions and seat-belt marks. Gently feel the abdomen for signs of tenderness, but don't be reassured by a normal examination [JRCALC, 2023].

There is no specific management of blunt abdominal trauma, but in penetrating trauma, if the injury has caused the bowel to protrude out of the abdomen, you should not push it back in. Instead, cover it with a dressing soaked in warm saline [NAEMT, 2020].

If the penetrating object is still in place in the patient's abdomen, do not attempt to remove it. Instead, secure it appropriately, although if it is pulsating, allow some movement of the object, but not its removal [JRCALC, 2023].

4.9 Pelvic injuries

Fractures of the pelvic ring are uncommon, with around 20–37 per 100,000 people suffering a fracture, about 2–8% of all skeletal injuries [Garlapati, 2012; McCormack, 2010]. However, where the patient has experienced a significant MOI that results in multiple injuries, a pelvic fracture is much more likely to occur. The major cause in the younger population is RTCs, with around 44–64% of pelvic ring fractures due to the patient being involved in an RTC.

All pelvic fractures cause some bleeding, although the source can vary. Bleeding from cancellous bone (usually found at the ends of long bones) that has been fractured is common, but bleeding can also occur from lacerations to retroperitoneal veins and the internal iliac arteries. Arterial bleeding accounts for up to 25% of haemodynamically unstable pelvic ring fractures [McCormack, 2010], but most bleeding is actually low-pressure bleeding (i.e., not arterial) and usually responds well to appropriate stabilisation (such as with a pelvic binder or external fixator) and tamponade [Abrassart, 2013].

4.9.1 Associated abdominal injuries

As well as the potential vascular damage that pelvic ring fractures can cause, the soft tissues are also vulnerable, and injuries to the anorectum, vagina, urethra and nerves can occur. The most common is bladder injury, typically caused by compression or tearing of the bladder wall. Urethral and anorectal injuries are more common with straddle injuries, for example when a motorcyclist straddles the fuel tank during an RTC, resulting in the separation of the two pelvic bones and severe tearing of the pelvic floor [Leenen, 2010].

4.10 Musculoskeletal injuries

Musculoskeletal injuries are very common, and you are likely to see the whole spectrum of injuries from sprains to fractures. Joint injuries can be particularly debilitating, so it is important that you have a low threshold for referring or transporting patients to ensure that they can receive a thorough assessment and appropriate management. Although the principles here mainly apply to limb injuries, they can be applied to other musculoskeletal injuries.

Adopt a methodical assessment and always obtain a good history before you start examining the patient:
- history
  - MOI
  - symptoms and any change over time
  - previous injuries/past medical history
- examination
  - joint above/below
  - look
  - feel
  - move
  - nerves and vessels.

4.10.1 History

It is important that you determine the exact MOI. A good way to do this is to produce a mental image of the direction, magnitude and duration of the force that was applied to the injured limb or joint. For example, in ankle injuries it can be useful for the patient to show you the position of the ankle at the time of injury (although do get them to use the uninjured ankle to do this) [Wardrope, 2008]. In lower limb injuries, check whether the patient could weight bear immediately after injury occurred and be alert for any repeated 'giving way' of knee or ankle joints and past injuries.

Ask about symptoms and their progress over time. For example, swelling that developed within minutes of the injury is more likely to be due to bleeding in the joint space. In patients with knee injuries, make sure you enquire about weight-bearing immediately following the injury, as a complete loss of function (e.g. being stretchered off the field) following injury is not a good sign. Common symptoms of knee injuries are generally pain, swelling and loss of function, but ask about paraesthesia (pins and needles) and additional injuries.

Finally, enquire about the patient's past medical history, and note any joint conditions, such as arthritis, as patients such as haemophiliacs and those taking anti-coagulant medication are at an increased risk of bleeding.

4.10.2 Examination

In lower limb injuries, observe the patient walking and standing, if they are able. In knee injuries, for example, patients who cannot straighten their injured knee might walk on the ball of their foot. In upper limb injuries, patients may be cradling an injured arm or, in the case of a dislocated shoulder, dangling the affected limb and holding it to the body with their uninjured arm [Purcell, 2016].

Joint above/below

Depending on the mechanism, forces can be transmitted along limbs, resulting in injuries elsewhere, for example a knee or hip injury following a fall, or a proximal humerus injury when falling on an outstretched hand.

Look

Check for swelling, erythema (redness), bruising and/or deformity. If the injury is to a limb, compare with the uninjured side. Limbs that are clearly abnormally angled are almost certainly broken (fractured). Do not attempt to realign the bones unless the fracture is causing severe bleeding (although follow local guidance), but splint in the position you find them. If the bone is protruding through an open wound (an open fracture), cover with a sterile dressing to prevent further contamination.

Feel

Gently palpate the area surrounding the injury in a systematic fashion. It is not necessary to directly palpate the most tender area of an injury, but instead note its location.

Move

If the injured area or limb is not obviously fractured, ask the patient if they can slowly move it. Note whether the range of movement of a joint is reduced by comparing it with the other limb. Instruct the patient to stop the movement if it is painful and splint the joint to prevent further movement.

Nerves and vessels

Check sensation below the injury and compare it with the other side. Note reduced or absent sensation and paraesthesia. In limbs, check for a pulse below the level of an injury. In the case of an obvious deformity of a limb, an absent pulse below the level of an injury should be treated as an emergency.

4.10.3 Fractures and dislocations

A fracture is a break (or breaks) in a bone. There are a number of types [Tortora, 2017] (Figure 16.10):

- **Transverse:** A single horizontal break through the bone, splitting it into two parts.
- **Comminuted:** A fracture that results in the bone being split into more than two parts.
- **Oblique:** The bone is broken diagonally along its shaft.
- **Spiral:** Caused by a twisting force.
- **Open:** Sometimes called a compound fracture. A fracture with a wound at the site of the injury caused by bone pushing through the skin.
- **Closed:** Sometimes called simple fracture. A fracture where no puncturing of the skin has occurred.
- **Greenstick:** An incomplete fracture where only one side of the periosteum fractures. This fracture is common in children because their bones are soft and porous.

A dislocation is an abnormal separation of joint surfaces. They can occur in isolation, or be associated with a fracture (or fractures). Since joints are kept in place by soft tissues such as ligaments, these will have been injured for a dislocation to have occurred. Prompt reduction of the dislocation to its original anatomical position is required, following analgesia and/or a local anaesthetic. A competent clinician is required for this procedure.

The management of fractures and dislocations follows the standard primary and secondary surveys for the trauma patient, but specifically consider:
- splinting the affected limb
- providing analgesia: these injuries can be very painful
- covering open fractures with a sterile dressing.

Chapter 16 – *Trauma*

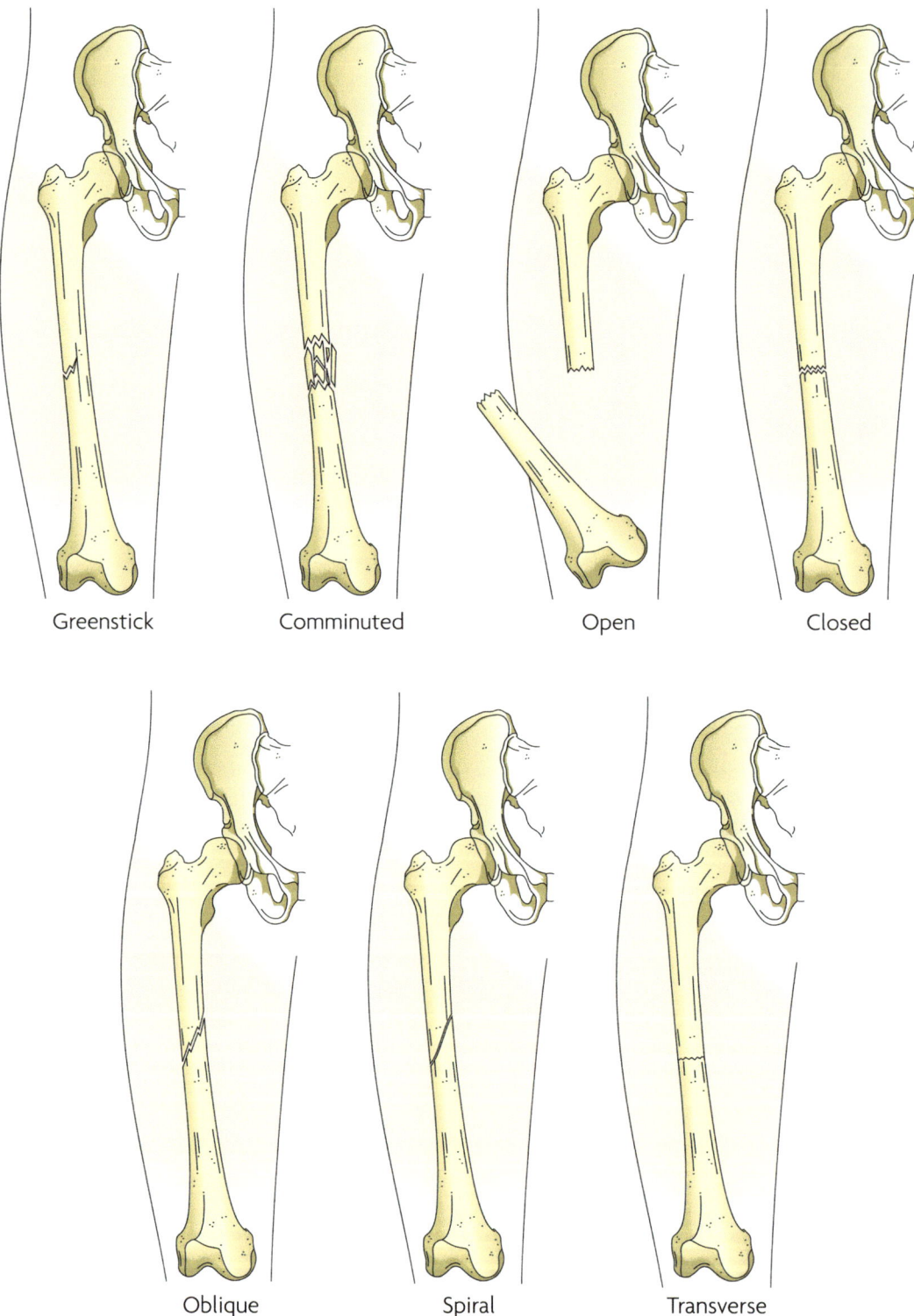

Figure 16.10 Types of fracture

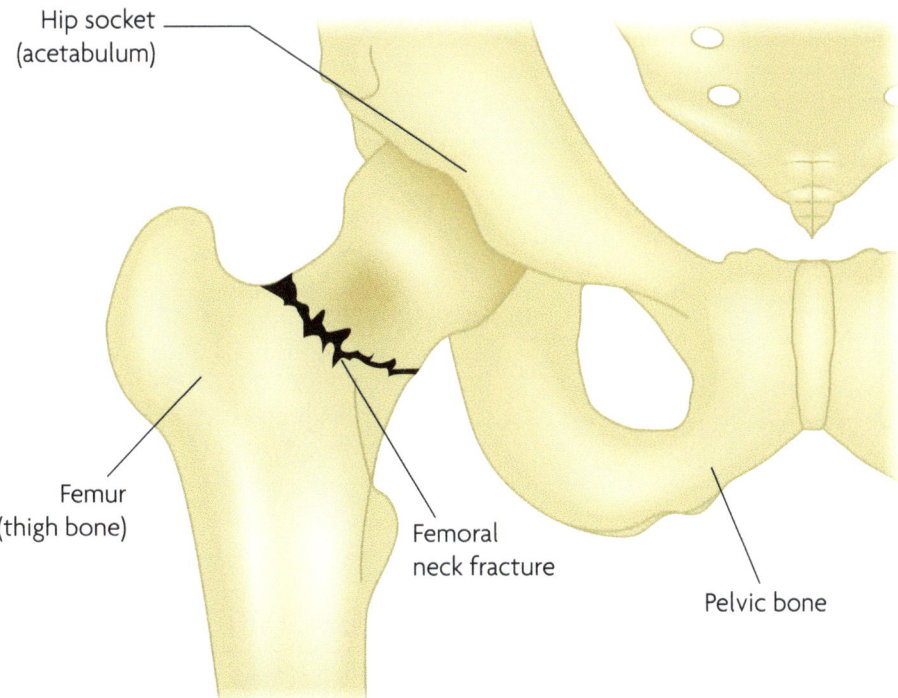

Figure 16.11 Fractured neck of femur

4.10.4 Neck of femur (NOF) fractures

Commonly referred to as an 'NOF', a fractured neck of femur, also known as a fractured hip, is a very common injury in those aged over 65 years (Figure 16.11). The most common cause of a fractured hip is a fall from standing height, and conditions that make the bones weaker, such as osteoporosis, make it more likely for the injury to occur.

Signs and symptoms of a hip fracture include [NHS, 2023b]:
- pain
- inability to lift, move or rotate the leg
- inability to stand or put weight on the leg
- a shorter leg on the injured side
- foot turning outwards on the injured side.

Treatment is the same as for most other fractures including analgesia, immobilisation and conveying to hospital. Several hospitals now have direct 'NOF' pathways designed to support patients with hip fracture from the point they arrive and to provide rapid diagnosis and treatment.

4.10.5 Sprains and strains

Sprains are ligamental injuries, that involve a partial or complete (depending on severity) tear of the ligament, whereas strains are tears in muscles. Their management is essentially the same, and consists of the following actions [NICE, 2020]:
- **P**rotect from further injury.
- **R**est the injured limb.
- **I**ce wrapped in a damp towel should be applied to the injury for 15–20 minutes.
- **C**ompress with a simple elastic bandage or elasticated tubular bandage, which should be snug, but not tight.
- **E**levate the limb above the level of the heart.

5 Skeletal immobilisation

5.1 *Learning objective*

By the end of this section you will be able to:
- describe how to perform a range of skeletal immobilisation techniques.

Chapter 16 – *Trauma*

5.2 Introduction

Skeletal immobilisation is an important skill to learn and remains a core concept in managing a large number of trauma patients. It has the following benefits when performed correctly [Greaves, 2018; NAEMT, 2020]:
- reduces pain
- reduces risk of further damage to soft tissues, nerves and blood vessels
- helps to control bleeding
- reduces risk of fat embolus.

In this section you will learn how to perform the following techniques and/or use the equipment listed:
- first-aid techniques
  - triangular bandages
- using splints
  - box splint
  - vacuum splint
  - pelvic splint
  - traction splint
- spinal immobilisation
  - manual methods
  - cervical collar application
  - helmet removal
  - scoop stretcher.

5.3 First-aid techniques

Effective splinting does not have to require expensive equipment, which may or may not be available. Sometimes it is preferable to use basic first-aid methods, such as triangular bandaging for the management of upper limb injuries.

5.3.1 Broad arm sling

Indications
- To provide support to an injury of the arm.

Contra-indications
- None – though consider whether other forms of splinting or immobilisation may be more appropriate, for example a vacuum splint.

Advantages
- Simple to apply.
- Minimal equipment required.
- Can provide effective analgesia by supporting the weight of the limb.

Disadvantages
- Does not provide complete immobilisation of the limb.

Procedure

Take the following steps to apply a broad arm sling [Pilbery & Lethbridge, 2022]:
1. Explain the procedure and obtain consent if appropriate to do so.
2. Don appropriate PPE, and undertake appropriate hand hygiene.
3. Ensure that all clothing is removed from the injured limb and a full neurovascular assessment has been completed. Any wounds should be dressed.
4. Ensure the patient has adequate analgesia.
5. Ask the patient to support their injured arm with the uninjured arm and to flex the elbow to 90°.

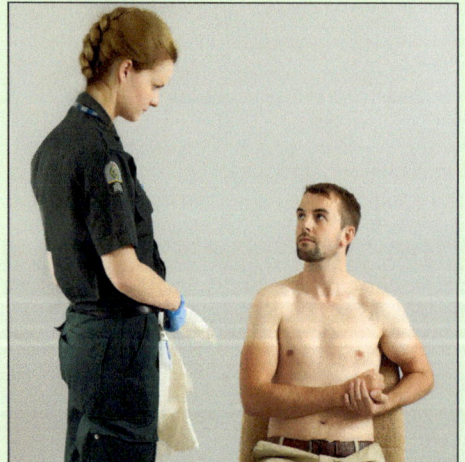

6. Open the triangular bandage and gently pass it under the injured arm with the point under the elbow of the injured arm.

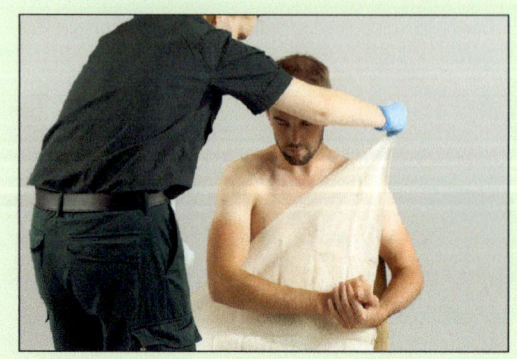

Skeletal immobilisation

Procedure – *cont*

7. Slide the upper end of the triangular bandage around the back of the neck towards the shoulder on the injured side.

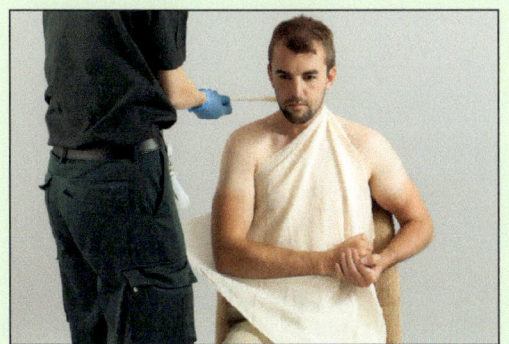

8. Lift the other end of the triangular bandage up over the forearm.

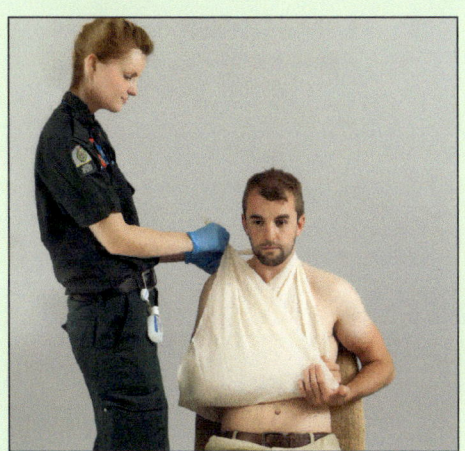

9. Tie the two ends together, preferably using a reef knot, to the side of the neck. Consider using a piece of gauze padding under the knot if it sits directly on skin.

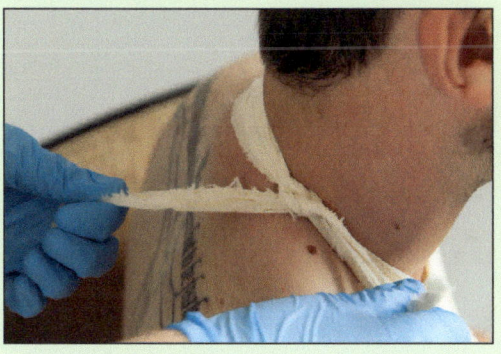

Procedure – *cont*

10. Take hold of the point of the bandage beyond the elbow and twist until the fabric is snug to the elbow. Then fold the excess into the bandage or tape it to the outside.

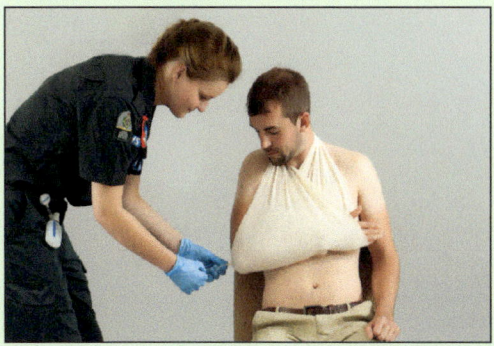

11. Recheck the limb distally for any change in neurovascular status.

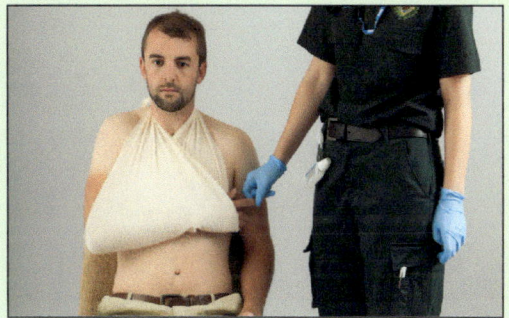

12. Document the procedure.

5.3.2 Elevated arm sling

Indications
- To provide support to an injury of the arm.

Contra-indications
- None – though consider whether other forms of splinting or immobilisation may be more appropriate, for example a vacuum splint.

Advantages
- Simple to apply.
- Minimal equipment required.
- Can provide effective analgesia by supporting the weight of the limb.
- Elevation may help to control bleeding or minimise swelling to hand.

Chapter 16 – *Trauma*

Disadvantages
- Does not provide complete immobilisation of the limb.

Procedure
Take the following steps to apply an elevated arm sling [Pilbery & Lethbridge, 2022]:
1. If the patient is conscious, explain the procedure and obtain consent if appropriate to do so.
2. Don appropriate PPE, and undertake appropriate hand hygiene.
3. Ensure that all clothing is removed from the injured limb and a full neurovascular assessment has been completed. Any wounds should be dressed.
4. Ensure the patient has adequate analgesia.
5. Ask the patient to support their injured arm with the uninjured arm. The injured arm should be placed across their chest with the fingers of the injured arm resting on the opposite shoulder.

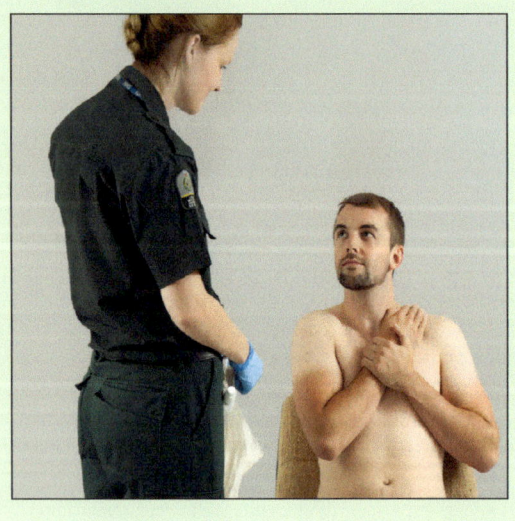

Procedure – *cont*
6. Place the triangular bandage over the injured arm with the point of the bandage just beyond the elbow of the injured arm.

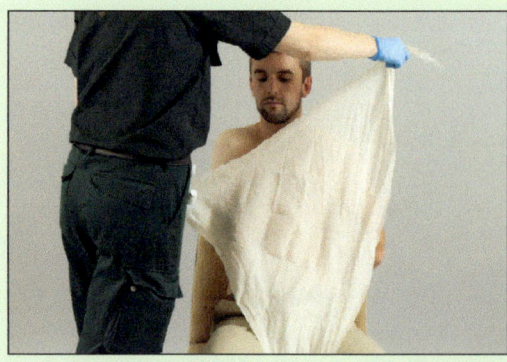

7. Ask the patient to let go of the injured arm and tuck the bandage under the injured arm and bring it around to their back.

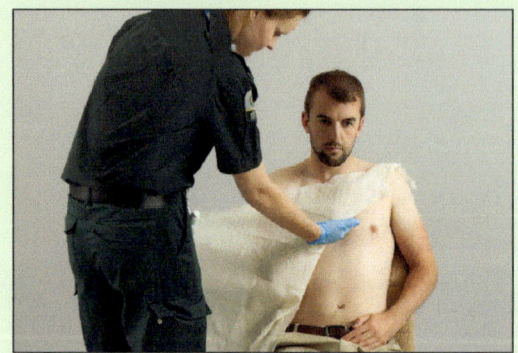

8. Bring the bandage up across the patient's back to meet the other end at the shoulder on the uninjured side.

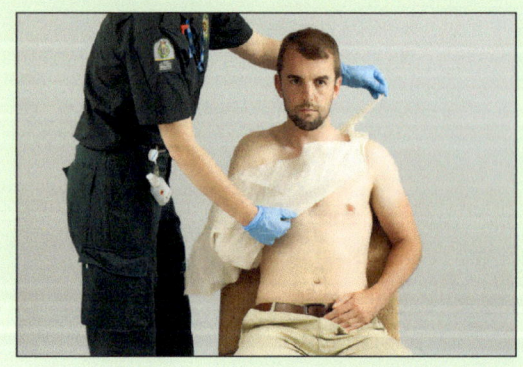

Skeletal immobilisation

Procedure – *cont*

9. Tie the two ends together, preferably using a reef knot, to the side of the neck. Consider using a piece of gauze padding under the knot if it sits directly on skin.

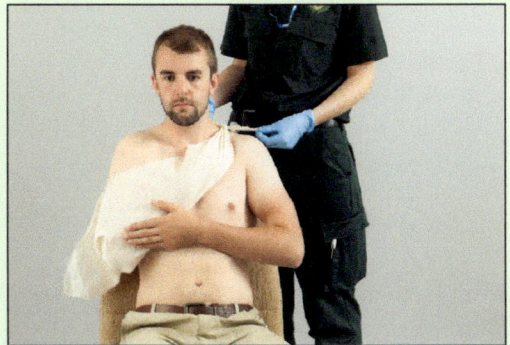

10. Take hold of the point of the bandage beyond the elbow and twist until the fabric is snug to the elbow. Then fold the excess into the bandage or tape it to the outside.

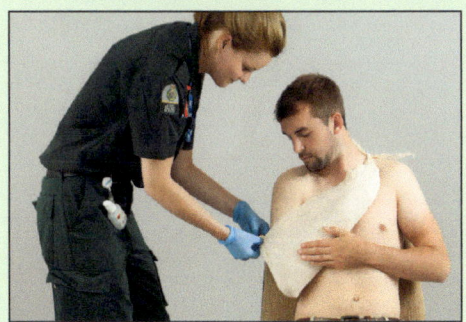

11. Recheck the limb distally for any change in neurovascular status.

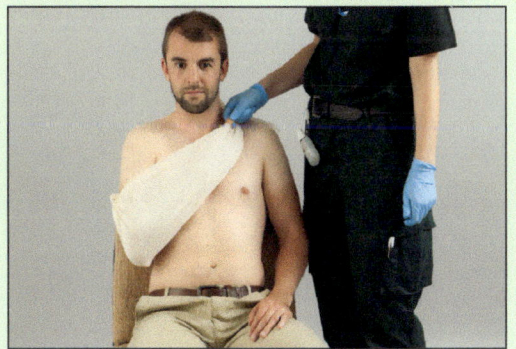

12. Document the procedure.

5.4 Splints

Splinting forms an important part of fracture management, particularly in the lower limbs. The benefits of splintage include reducing [Greaves, 2018]:
- pain
- blood loss
- pressure on skin
- pressure on adjacent neurovascular structures
- risk of fat embolism
- risk of further damage
- risk of infection if the fracture is open.

Basic principles of immobilisation should consist of assessment and reassessment of the neurovascular status before and after any manipulation or handling of the fracture, and immobilisation of the joints above and below it.

Note: It is not possible to show the application of every type of splinting device in this text. Instead, a selection of commonly used devices is explained. This is not a substitute for hands-on training.

5.4.1 Box splints

Box splints are simple devices that are most commonly used for lower leg fractures (Figure 16.12).

Indications
- To immobilise a limb, typically due to a suspected fracture or dislocation.

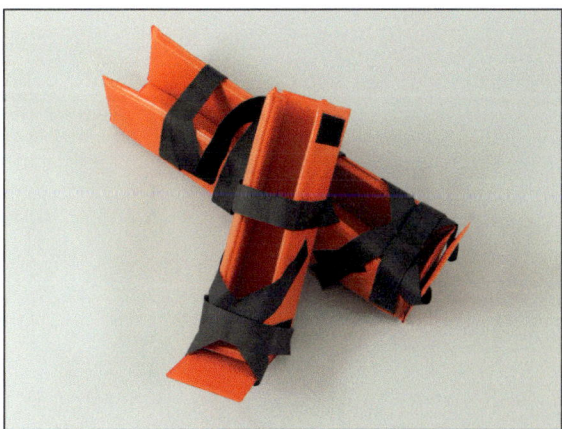

Figure 16.12 A box splint

Chapter 16 – *Trauma*

Contra-indications
- None – though consider whether other forms of immobilisation may be more appropriate, for example a traction splint for an isolated mid-shaft femur fracture.

Advantages
- Unlike vacuum splints, box splints are not easily damaged and will continue to work if minor damage is caused to the coverings.

Disadvantages
- Does not conform to the patient's limb, so may provide less effective immobilisation.
- Can only be used on straight limbs without significant deformity.

Procedure

Take the following steps to apply a box splint (Pilbery & Lethbridge, 2022):

1. If the patient is conscious, explain the procedure and obtain consent if appropriate to do so.
2. Don appropriate PPE, and undertake appropriate hand hygiene.
3. Ensure that all clothing is removed from the injured limb and a full neurovascular assessment has been completed. Any wounds should be dressed.
4. Choose an appropriately sized splint.
5. Ensure the patient has received adequate analgesia.

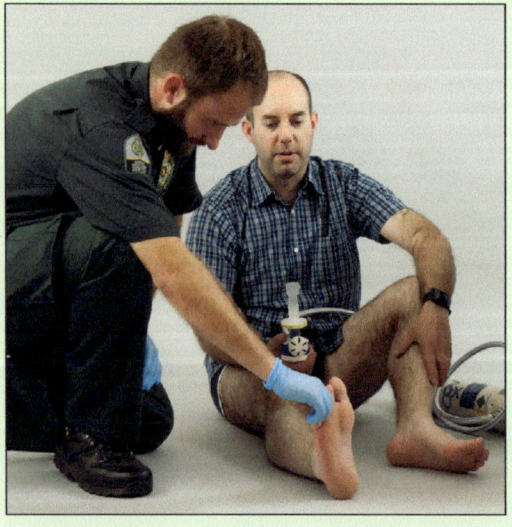

Procedure – *cont*

6. Open the splint and place it next to, or in line with, the injured limb with the Velcro pointing out towards you.
Prepare additional padding in the form of a sheet, blanket or incontinence sheets, which may be required.
7. In a co-ordinated move with other team members, lift the limb just enough to move the splint into position. Warn the patient in advance.

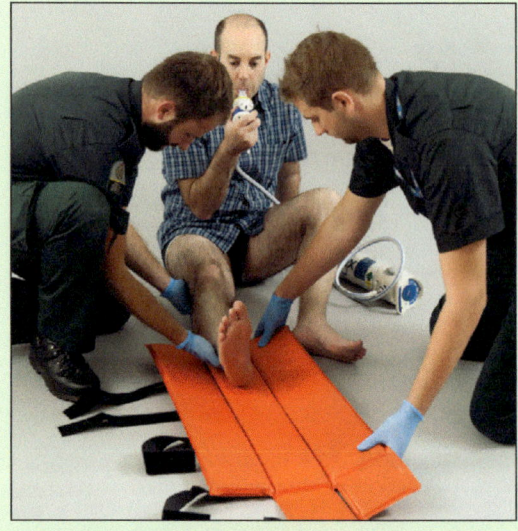

8. Once the splint is in position, lower the limb back on to the splint.
9. Lift the two side pieces to create an open box shape around the limb. If the splint is being applied to a lower limb, there may be a foot plate. This should be lifted so that it sits against the sole of the foot.
All of these pieces should be firm but not tight against the skin of the limb.

Skeletal immobilisation

Procedure – *cont*

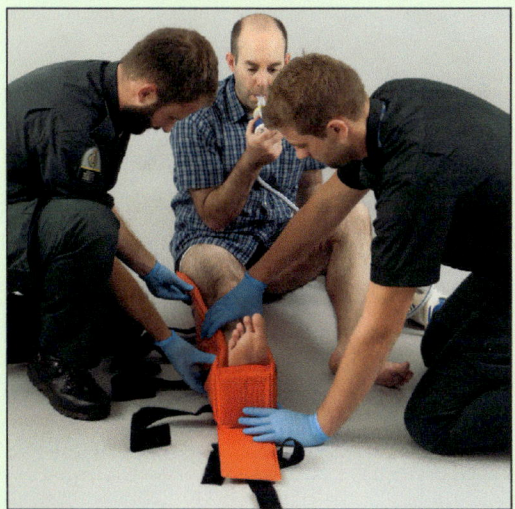

10. Gently fasten the Velcro straps to the opposite side of the splint, taking care to avoid placing straps directly over the site of the injury.
Straps from the foot plate should cross over the top of the foot to provide additional lateral strength to the splint.

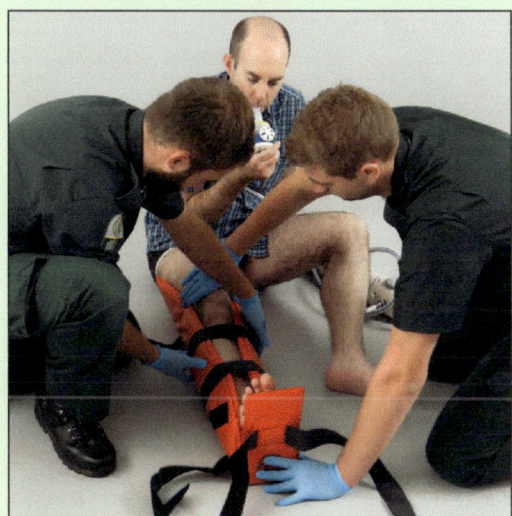

11. If there are large gaps around the limb inside the splint, consider padding the voids with soft items, such as incontinence sheets, for transport.

Procedure – *cont*

12. Recheck distal pulse and sensation for any change in neurovascular status now the limb has been immobilised. You may need to reposition the limb if neurovascular status has been compromised during immobilisation.

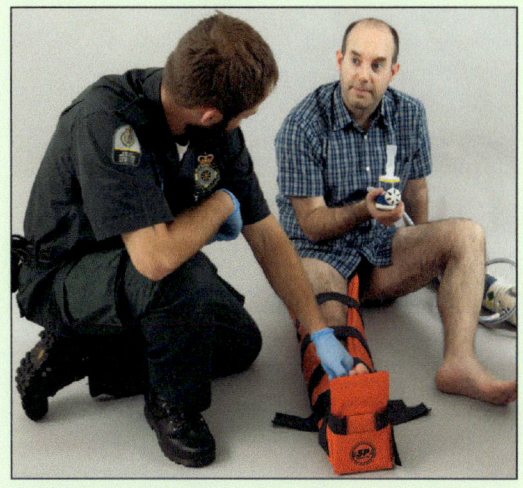

13. Document the procedure.

5.4.2 Vacuum splints

Vacuum splints are made from a case of conformable plastic filled with small polystyrene beads. When air is in the splint, these beads are free to move around, but once the air has been vacuumed out the splint becomes hard and stays in the shape it has created. The advantage of vacuum splints is that they can be conformed to the shape of the patient's limb, which makes them more comfortable for the patient and results in less movement.

Indications
- To immobilise a limb, typically due to a suspected fracture or dislocation.

Contra-indications
- None – though consider whether other forms of immobilisation may be more appropriate, for example a traction splint for an isolated mid-shaft femur fracture.

Advantages
- Conforms to the patient's anatomy, resulting in a comfortable and rigid splint.

Chapter 16 – *Trauma*

Disadvantages
- Requires a proprietary hand pump or suction unit to remove air from the splint.
- The splints are easily damaged; when damaged, they do not retain the vacuum and inflate, which results in a loss of immobilisation.

Procedure

Take the following steps to apply a vacuum splint [Pilbery & Lethbridge, 2022]:

1. If the patient is conscious, explain the procedure and obtain consent if appropriate to do so.
2. Don appropriate PPE, and undertake appropriate hand hygiene.
3. Ensure that all clothing is removed from the injured limb and a full neurovascular assessment has been completed. Any wound should be dressed.
4. Choose an appropriately sized splint (generally, the joint above and below the injury should be immobilised too) and check it is working in advance.
5. Ensure the patient has adequate analgesia.
6. Open the splint and place it next to the injured limb with the valve pointing towards you.
   Open the valve to allow air to enter and use your hand to evenly distribute the polystyrene ball bearings inside so that the splint is flat.
   Securely close the valve.
7. In a co-ordinated move with other team members, lift the limb just enough to slip the splint into position. Warn the patient in advance.

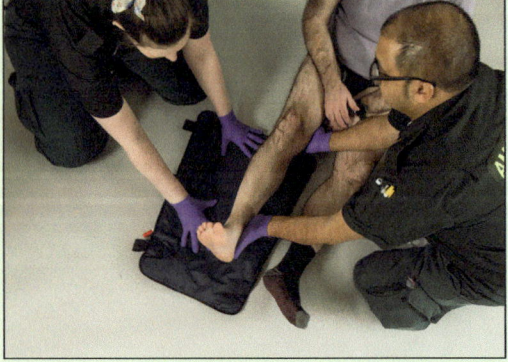

Procedure – *cont*

8. Once the splint is in position, lower the limb on to it.

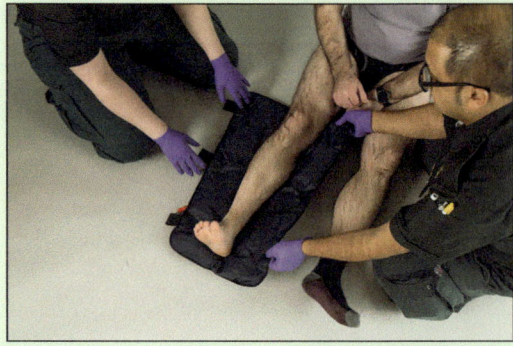

9. Form the splint around the injured limb. Try to leave the end of the splint open and a small gap of approximately 2.5 cm (1 in) along the top of the splint so the limb can still be visualised.
   If required, the straps can be loosely placed at this point to help keep the splint in shape.

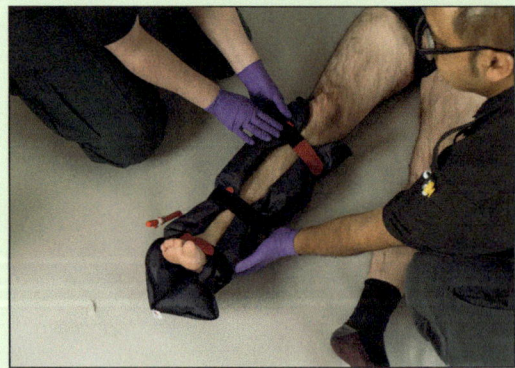

10. Attach the pump to the valve and, while the splint is being held in position, another team member should operate the pump until the splint becomes firm.

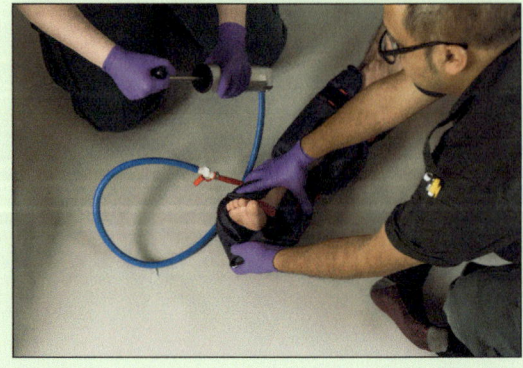

Procedure – cont

11. Once the splint is firm, remove the pump.

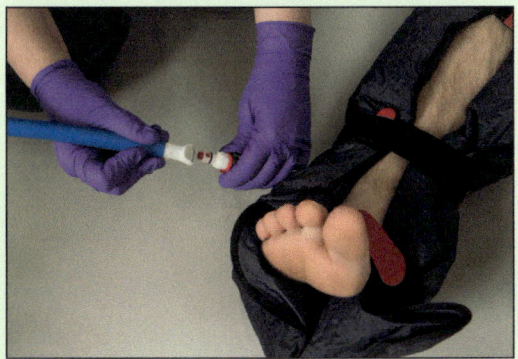

12. Wrap the Velcro straps around the now rigid splint.

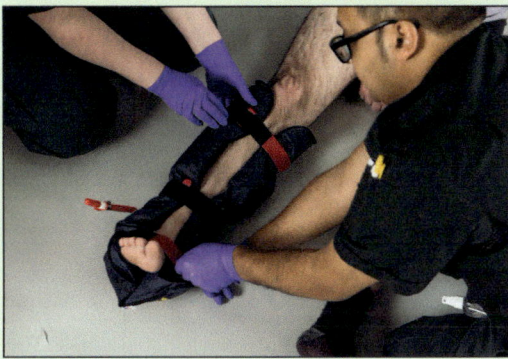

13. Recheck the limb distally for any change in neurovascular status now it has been immobilised. You may need to reposition the limb if neurovascular status has been compromised during immobilisation.
14. Regularly check the splint during transport. If it is becoming loose, use the pump and remove air until it becomes firm again.
15. Document the procedure.

5.4.3 Pelvic splints

Serious pelvic fractures are associated with a high risk of death due to internal bleeding [Vaidya, 2016]. Commercial pelvic splints (commonly called pelvic binders) have been shown to reduce stable 'open book' and rotational and vertically unstable fractures adequately (Figure 16.13), with no significant displacement of fractures, irrespective of device [Knops, 2011]. That said, there is no conclusive evidence that the use of pelvic binders

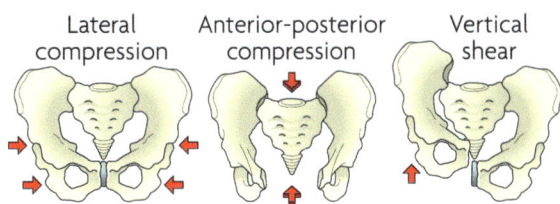

Figure 16.13 Types of pelvic fracture. The red arrows indicate the direction of the force

reduces morbidity or mortality from serious trauma either [Stewart, 2013]. Despite this, their early application in suspected serious pelvic trauma with internal bleeding is recommended as a method for stabilising the fracture and helping to reduce further blood loss [NICE, 2022b]. Ultimately it will be the decision of the ambulance clinician at scene as to whether a patient requires a binder.

There is currently no reason to recommend one device over another, though two devices, the SAM pelvic sling and T-POD device, have the most available evidence [Scott, 2013], both of which are covered below.

SAM pelvic sling
Indications
- Suspected ongoing bleeding due to pelvic fracture.
- Local guidelines indicate application of a pelvic binder. An example of local guidelines for application would be:
- MOI that suggests a pelvic fracture and is accompanied by any of the following:
  - haemodynamic instability or signs of shock
  - deformity on examination
  - suspected open pelvic fracture, including bleeding from the urethra (PU), vagina (PV) or rectum (PR), or scrotal haematoma.

Contra-indications
- Isolated NOF fracture.
- Patient who has an impaled object which would be covered by the binder.

Advantages
- Reduces fractures of the pelvis.
- May help to reduce bleeding associated with pelvic fractures.
- Simple to apply in the pre-hospital setting.

Chapter 16 – *Trauma*

Disadvantages
- Pelvic binders utilise pressure to reduce the fracture. This pressure can be sufficient to cause soft-tissue injury.
- Can cause the pelvis to not align appropriately if applied incorrectly.
- Accurate placement is challenging and binders often end up in the wrong place (typically too high).
- Three sizes exist, which means having to carry multiple devices to accommodate all patients.

Procedure
Take the following steps to apply a SAM pelvic sling [Pilbery & Lethbridge, 2022]:
1. If the patient is conscious, explain the procedure and obtain consent if appropriate to do so.
2. Don appropriate PPE, and undertake appropriate hand hygiene.
3. Check all the patient's clothing (including underwear) has been removed.
4. Choose the correctly sized binder, as there are three sizes available based on patient waist size:
    - small: 27–45 in (69–114 cm)
    - medium: 32–50 in (81–127 cm)
    - large: 36–54 in (91–137 cm).
5. Locate the level of the greater trochanter by identifying the iliac crest and then moving down on the lateral side of the leg to the next obvious underlying bone structure. This is the greater trochanter.

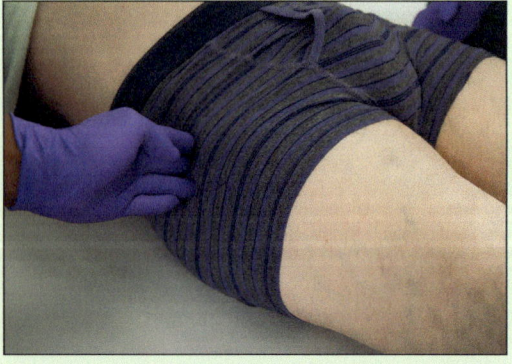

Procedure – *cont*
6. As long as there are no other injuries that may be made worse, strap the feet together using a triangle bandage (or similar) in a figure of eight.

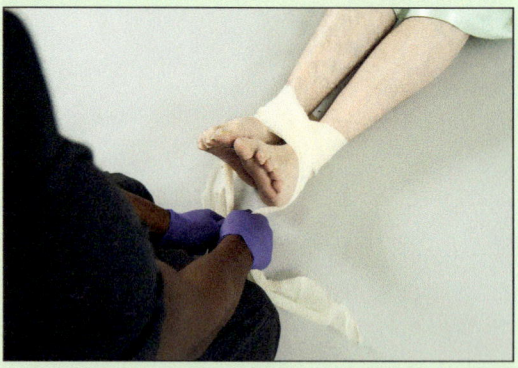

7. Insert the binder under the legs.

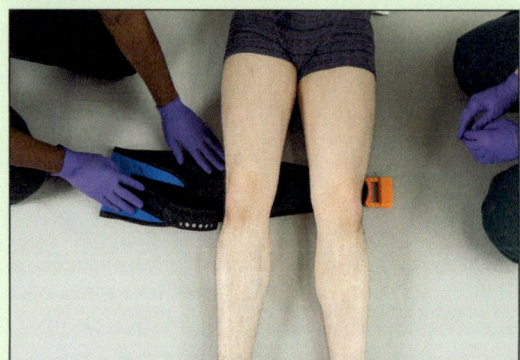

8. Slide the binder up into position and confirm the centre of the binder is in line with the greater trochanters.
   You may need to just 'lift' the hips a very small amount to help the binder get to the correct position.

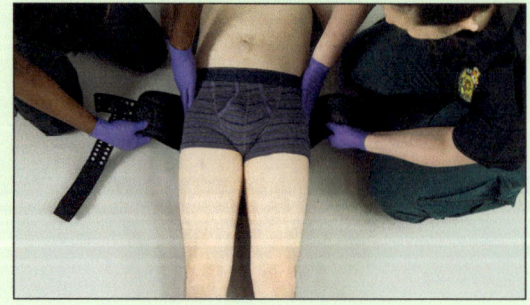

Skeletal immobilisation

Procedure – *cont*

9. Pull the strap through the orange buckle, and ensure that there is an equal amount of binder on each side of the patient.

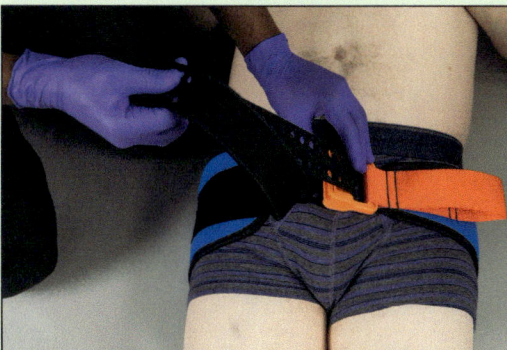

10. With one person on each side, pull the black strap and orange handle in opposite directions until the buckle clicks. Maintain tension and secure the Velcro of the black strap to the splint. Do not be concerned if the buckle clicks again during this manoeuvre.

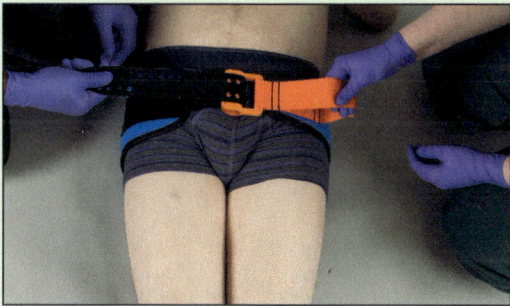

11. Document the time of application and ensure this is communicated at handover.

T-POD stabilisation device

Indications
- Suspected ongoing bleeding due to pelvic fracture.
- Local guidelines indicate application of a pelvic binder. An example of local guidelines for application would be MOI that suggests a pelvic fracture and is accompanied by any of the following:
  - haemodynamic instability or signs of shock
  - deformity on examination
  - suspected open pelvic fracture, including bleeding from the urethra (PU), vagina (PV) or rectum (PR), or scrotal haematoma.

Contra-indications
- Isolated NOF fracture.
- Patient who has an impaled object which would be covered by the binder.

Advantages
- Reduces fractures of the pelvis.
- May help to reduce bleeding associated with pelvic fractures.
- Simple to apply in the pre-hospital setting.

Disadvantages
- Pelvic binders utilise pressure to reduce the fracture. This pressure can be sufficient to cause soft-tissue injury.
- Can cause pelvis to not align appropriately if applied incorrectly.
- Accurate placement is challenging and binders often end up in the wrong place (typically too high).

Procedure

Take the following steps to apply a T-POD stabilisation device [Pilbery & Lethbridge, 2022]:

1. If the patient is conscious, explain the procedure and obtain consent if appropriate to do so.
2. Don appropriate PPE, and undertake appropriate hand hygiene.
3. Check all the patient's clothing (including underwear) has been removed.
4. Ensure all parts are present and that the pulley system has been fully opened up and is not twisted.

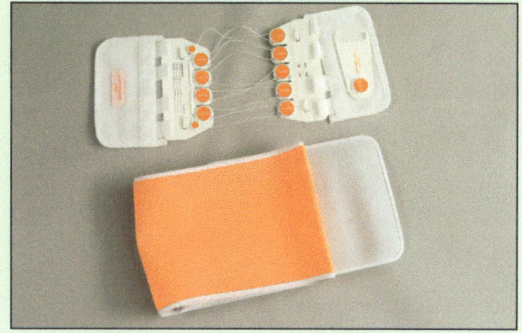

Procedure – *cont*

5. As long as there are no other injuries that may be made worse, strap the feet together using a triangle bandage (or similar) in a figure of eight.

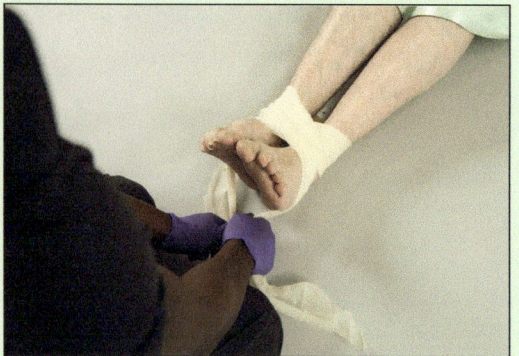

6. Locate the level of the greater trochanter by identifying the iliac crest and then moving down on the lateral side of the leg to the next obvious underlying bone structure. This is the greater trochanter.

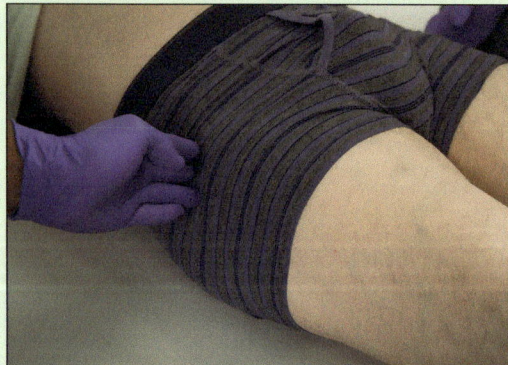

7. Insert the belt under the legs, with the white side facing the patient.

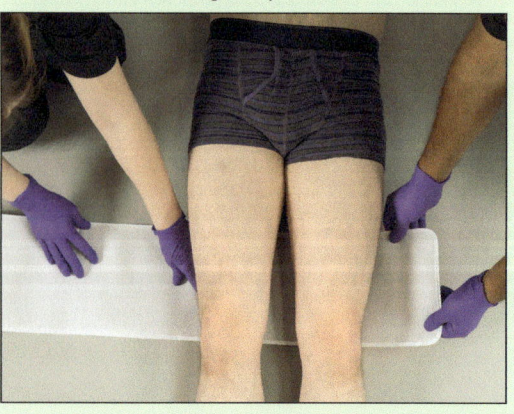

Procedure – *cont*

8. Slide the belt up into position and confirm the centre of the belt is in line with the greater trochanters.
   You may need to just 'lift' the hips a very small amount to help the belt get to the correct position.

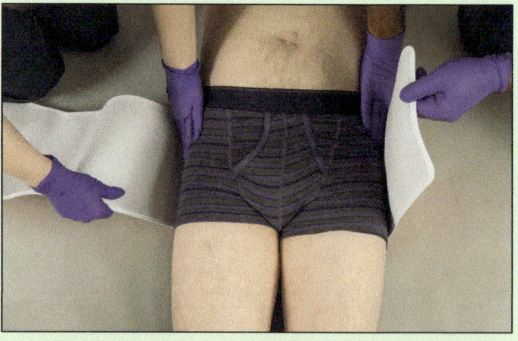

9. Cut the excess belt, so there is a 15–20 cm (6–8 in) gap over the centre of the pelvis. Do not fold the material back on itself.

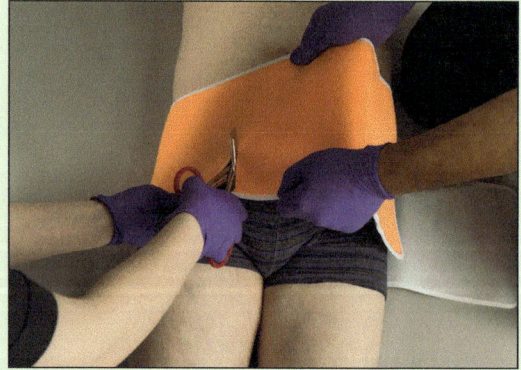

10. Place the pulley system on the belt, ensuring that the Velcro is stuck down well.

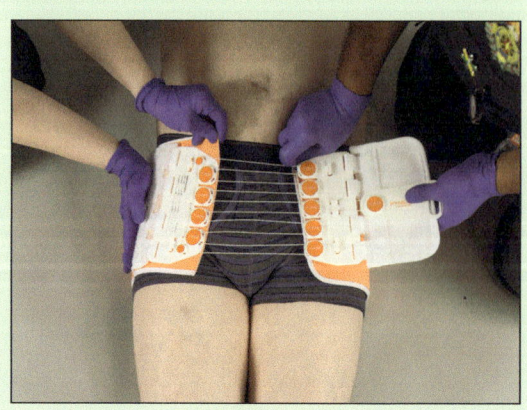

Skeletal immobilisation

Procedure – *cont*

11. Gently apply tension to the pull cord by pulling on the attached tab, which will apply circumferential pressure to the pelvis.

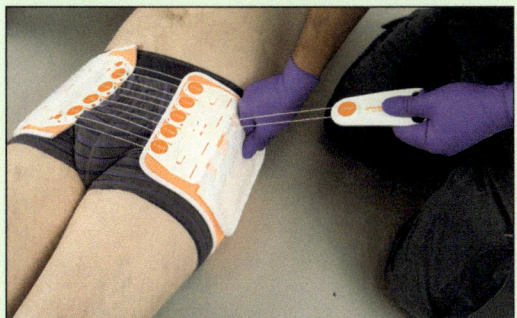

12. Once appropriate tension has been applied, wrap the excess pull cord around the vertical posts located next to the pulleys until the excess cord has been wrapped up sufficiently for the plastic tab to be conveniently stuck to the Velcro.

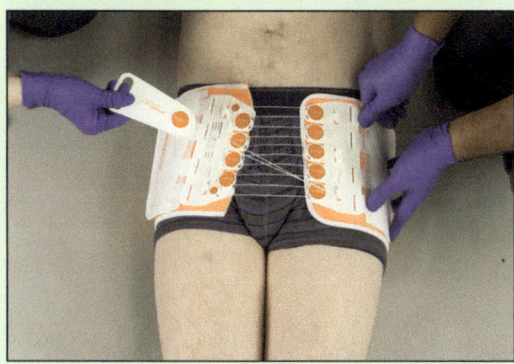

13. Stick the plastic tab down so it is secure. It needs to be in an easily accessible location.

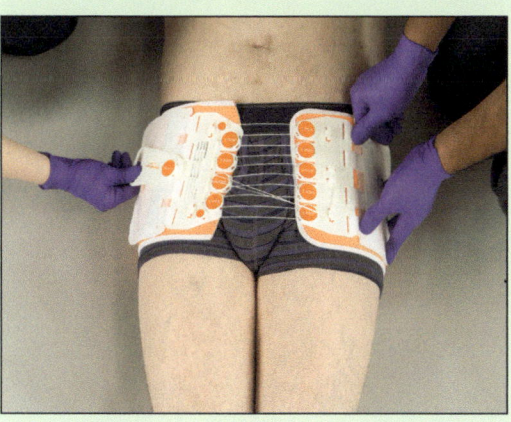

Procedure – *cont*

14. Document the time of application and ensure this is communicated at handover.

5.4.4 Traction splints

Traction splints apply longitudinal force to long bones (normally the femur). Correctly splinting the femur using this method helps to reduce [JRCALC, 2023]:
- pain
- haemorrhage and damage to blood vessels and nerves
- movement of bone fragments and the risk of a closed fracture becoming an open fracture
- the risk of a fat embolus
- muscle spasm.

Kendrick Traction Device

Indications
- Mid-shaft femur fractures.

Contra-indications
- Fractures of the lower limb other than mid-shaft femur.

Advantages
- Can be used where there is suspicion of a co-existing pelvic fracture (apply pelvic binder first).
- Compact, lightweight device.
- Applying traction may help to:
  - reduce discomfort by anatomically realigning the fractured sections
  - reduce ongoing bleeding
  - reduce the risk of fat embolus.

Disadvantages
- Requires training and familiarisation to apply appropriately.
- Once applied, it extends beyond the foot of the patient, which can make moving or conveying in an aircraft challenging.

Procedure

Take the following steps to apply a Kendrick Traction Device [Pilbery & Lethbridge, 2022]:
1. If the patient is conscious, explain the procedure and obtain consent if appropriate to do so.

Chapter 16 – Trauma

Procedure – *cont*

2. Don appropriate PPE, and undertake appropriate hand hygiene.
3. Ensure all the patient's clothing has been removed from the leg.
4. Ensure that all parts are present.

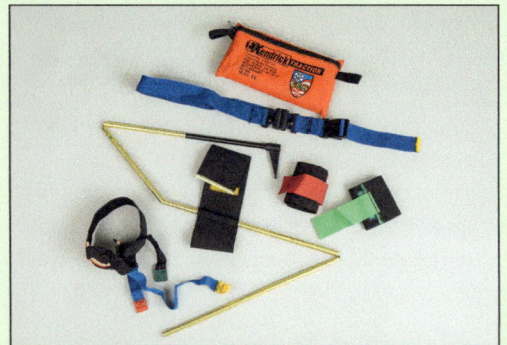

5. Apply the ankle strap by passing the padded part of the strap around the back of the ankle. Secure the strap firmly with the Velcro.

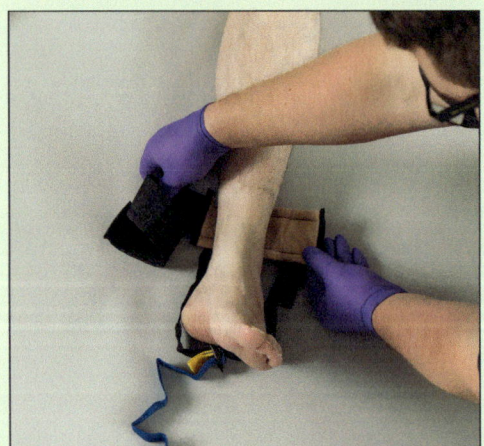

6. Place the thigh strap under the back of the knee.

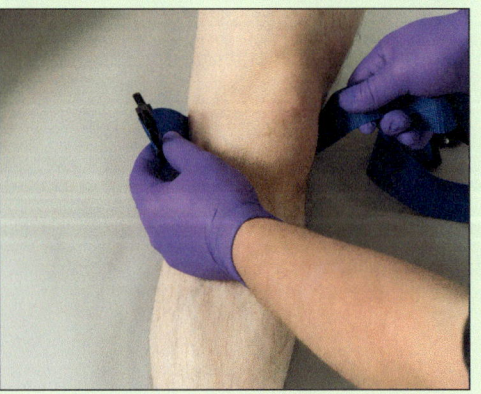

Procedure – *cont*

7. Slide the thigh strap so that it is high in the groin.
   Ensure that genitals are not trapped under the strap.
   Clip the buckle so it is on the superior aspect of the limb.
   Adjust the strap so that the pole receptacle is at the level of the iliac crest.
   Note: While underwear has been left on in these images, it would be more common to perform this at skin level.

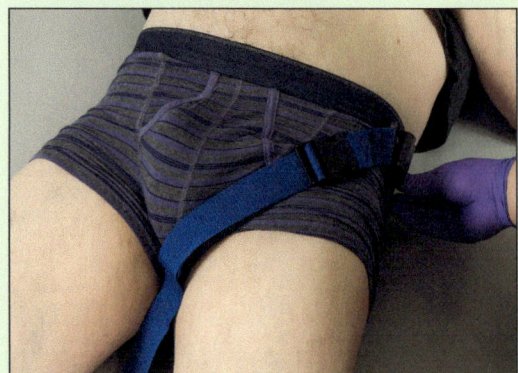

8. Take the pole and straighten it out. Then place it next to the patient and ensure that at least one full section of pole extends beyond the foot.

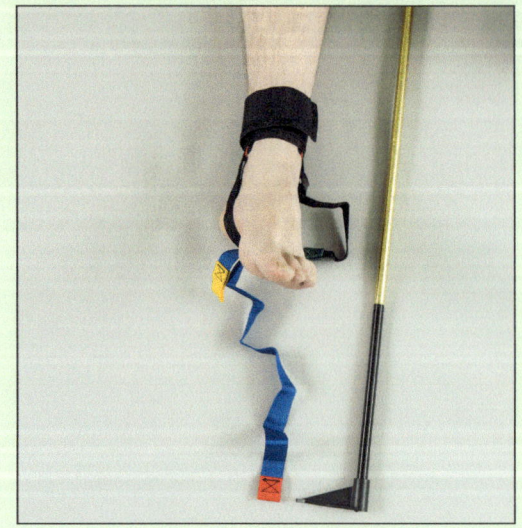

Skeletal immobilisation

Procedure – *cont*

9. Once the pole is in the correct position, the length can be adjusted. Once set to the correct length, it is inserted into the receptacle.

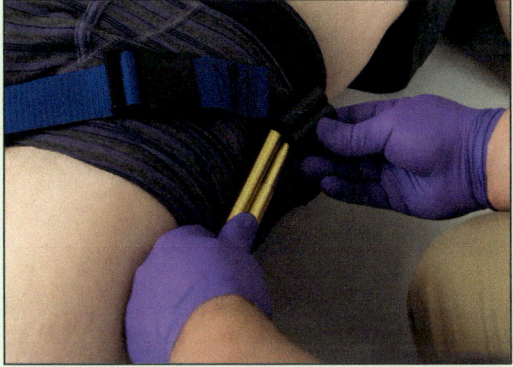

10. Place the yellow strap around the knee and secure – this is the strap that comes pre-attached to the pole.

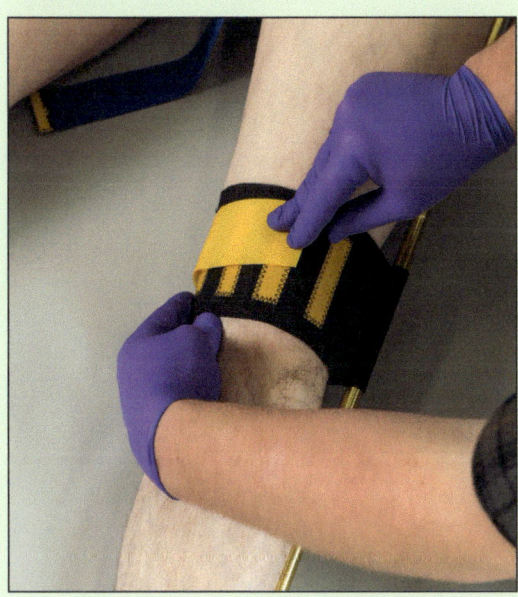

Procedure – *cont*

11. Place the dart at the end of the black pole through the yellow loop on the section of strap that hangs down from the foot.

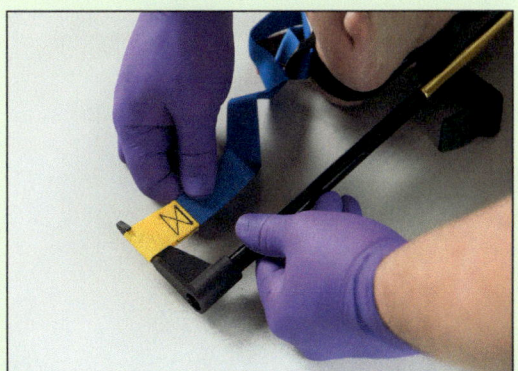

12. Apply traction by simultaneously pulling down on the red tab on the foot strap and feeding the other side of the strap with the yellow tab through the buckle.
    Apply traction until normal anatomical alignment or significant reduction in pain is achieved.

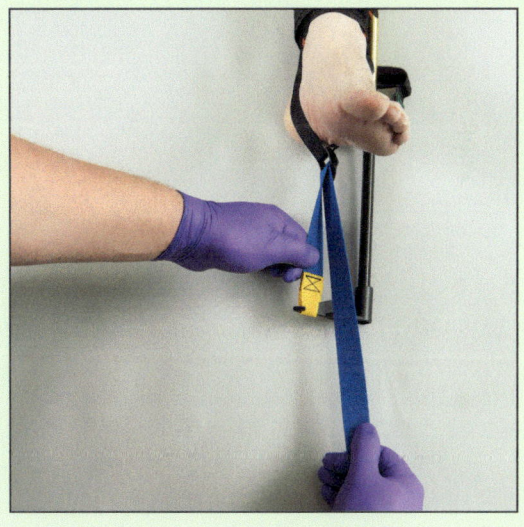

Chapter 16 – Trauma

Procedure – *cont*

13. Apply straps over the thigh and ankle following the traffic light colour system: red at the top and green at the bottom.

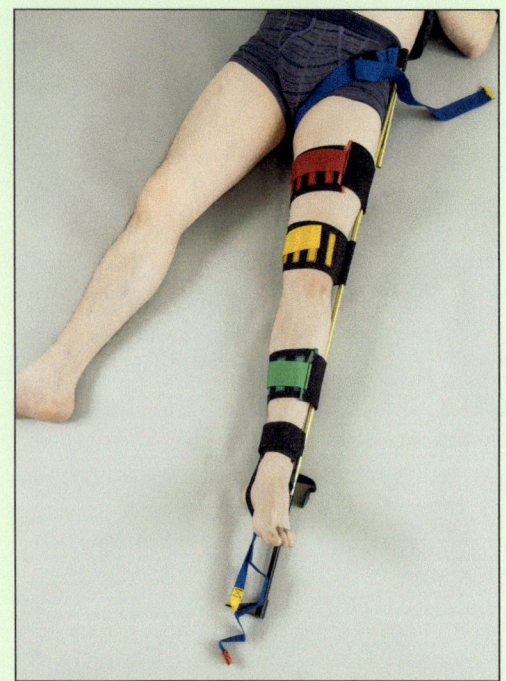

14. Assess the pulse, movement and sensation distally on the limb.
15. Document the procedure and be sure to hand over at the hospital the suspected fracture and application of a traction splint.

5.5 Spinal immobilisation

All patients with the possibility of spinal injury should have manual immobilisation commenced at the earliest opportunity so long as doing so does not delay other life-saving interventions. As part of the assessment of the patient, the senior clinician will consider whether spinal immobilisation is required and, if so, come up with a plan to apply other forms of immobilisation [JRCALC, 2023].

5.5.1 MILS immobilisation

Indications
- Spinal immobilisation is indicated according to local procedure.
- While awaiting definitive cervical spine immobilisation.

Contra-indications
- Distressed and agitated patients where performing MILS may cause further distress and movement.

Advantages
- Rapid technique to immobilise the cervical spine.
- Requires no equipment.

Disadvantages
- Requires a member of the clinical team to be dedicated to the task of providing MILS.
- Can make airway management more challenging.

Procedure

Take the following steps to apply MILS immobilisation [Pilbery & Lethbridge, 2022]:
1. If the patient is conscious, explain the procedure and obtain consent if appropriate to do so.
2. Don appropriate PPE, and undertake appropriate hand hygiene.
3. Advise the patient not to move their head and explain you are going to hold their head to help keep it still.
4. Place yourself in a comfortable position behind the patient; this should be either kneeling behind the patient or lying behind the patient. Rest your arms on the floor, on your knees or other objects that will help to stabilise them.

Procedure – *cont*

5. Place your hands either side of the head and over the mastoid process. This should result in your hands being positioned under the ears, and not covering them. If necessary, move one finger to above the ear, as shown here.

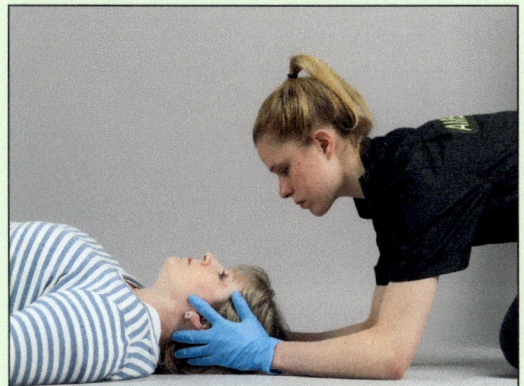

6. If the patient's head is not facing forwards and the patient is conscious, ask them to slowly move their head into a neutral in-line position (eyes looking straight ahead and nose in line with the umbilicus). If the patient is unconscious, gently move the head into a neutral position. Movement to the neutral position should cease if there is:
   - resistance to movement
   - neck muscle spasm
   - increased pain
   - an increase in neurological deficit (numbness, tingling, etc.).

   In any of these cases the neck should be immobilised in the position that it presents in.
7. MILS should be maintained until:
   - The patient is fully immobilised.
   - It is decided that immobilisation is no longer required.
8. Document the procedure, including the time it was undertaken and any complications.

5.5.2 Helmet removal

Patients who are wearing helmets need to have them removed in order to assess and manage their airway and ventilation. In addition, hidden bleeding at the back of the head can be identified and the head moved into a position of neutral alignment. Note that some degree of spinal motion will occur, even in optimal circumstances [NAEMT, 2020].

Indications
- To assess and manage a patient wearing a motorcycle helmet following a traumatic incident.

Contra-indications
- Single rescuers should not attempt this procedure unless immediate interventions which could not be completed with the helmet in situ are required, for example clearing or maintaining an airway.

Advantages
- Removes helmet with minimal movement of the spine.
- Allows for full assessment of the patient's face and airway.

Disadvantages
- Requires two rescuers to complete.

Note: Manufacturers of motorcycle helmets have evolved designs significantly over the years. Many dedicated safety technologies now exist, including helmet airbags and emergency helmet removal systems (EHRSs), which you should ensure you are familiar with.

Another commonly found feature is the emergency quick release system (EQRS), which is typically two red straps built into the padding around the base of the chin. If these are present, pulling on them will easily remove some of the padding around the lower face, making helmet removal simpler. Inspect for these prior to following the procedure below; if they are present, incorporate their removal into step 5.

Chapter 16 – Trauma

Procedure

Take the following steps to remove a motorcycle helmet [Pilbery & Lethbridge, 2022]:

1. If the patient is conscious, explain the procedure and obtain consent if appropriate to do so.
2. Don appropriate PPE, and undertake appropriate hand hygiene.
3. The clinician leading the procedure should verbalise their plan and ensure that others involved are clear on the process and their roles.
4. One rescuer should position themselves at the head end and take a grip of the helmet by placing their hands on either side of the head and curling their fingers under the edges of the helmet.
5. From the side, a second rescuer should remove the face shield if present and release the chin strap or padding where possible. Remove EQRS padding, if present.

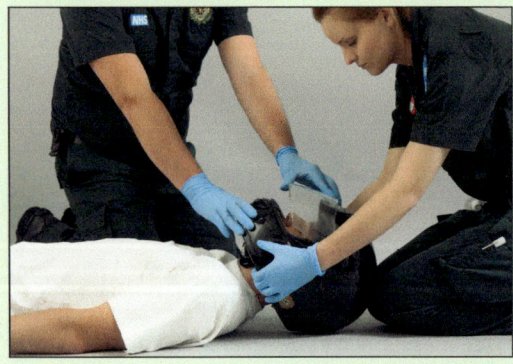

Procedure – *cont*

6. The second rescuer should take control of the head by placing their upper hand around the patient's mandible, in a 'c grip', and the lower hand under the back of the head, reaching up towards the occiput. Once in position with a firm grip, this rescuer should say 'I'm on' to indicate they have a firm grip and are controlling movement of the neck. The other rescuer can now release their grip.

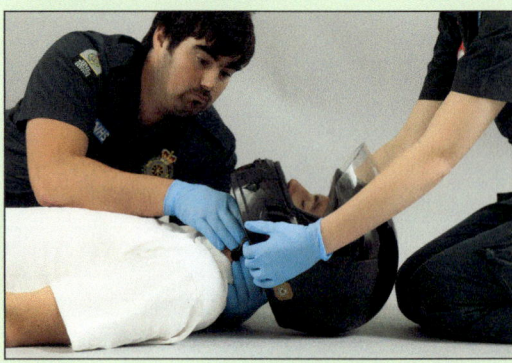

7. Rescuer one can now gently rock the helmet back and forth while pulling the sides of the helmet slightly apart and applying traction.
   Be careful when going past the nose that the helmet does not jam against it.

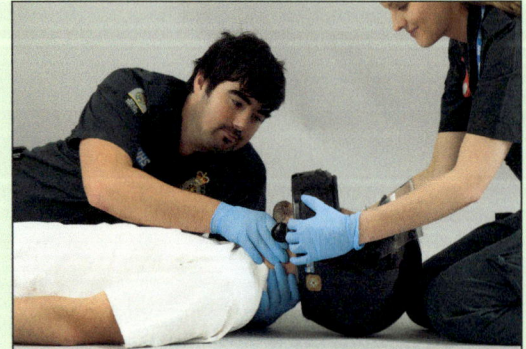

8. Once the helmet is approximately halfway off, rescuer one should stop moving the helmet and adjust their hands, so they can take over control of the head and neck through the helmet. Once they have control, they should say 'I'm on'.

Skeletal immobilisation

Procedure – *cont*

9. Rescuer two should adjust their hands to ensure they have a good grip. The hand against the back of the head should be moved up to take control of the occiput. It may be helpful to brace the elbow of the lower hand against the floor at this point. Once in position, with a firm grip controlling the head and neck, rescuer two should declare 'I'm on'.

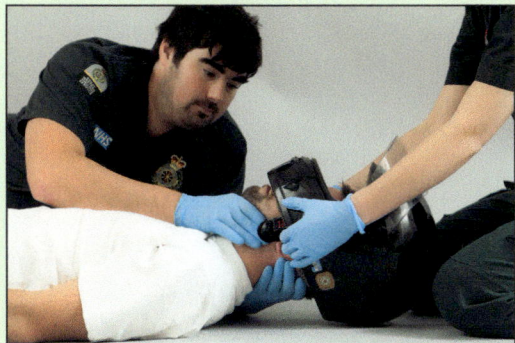

10. Rescuer one should continue to rock the helmet while applying traction until the head is released. Once this happens, set the helmet to one side ready to be conveyed to hospital with the patient.

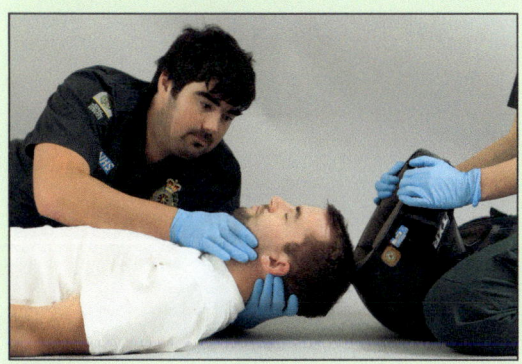

Procedure – *cont*

11. Rescuer one should now apply MILS and in a co-ordinated move (on 'Move' of 'Ready, Set, Move') lower the head to neutral alignment along with rescuer two. This may require a small amount of padding to be placed under the occiput.
If any resistance is felt while lowering to neutral alignment, cease immediately and pad in the current position.

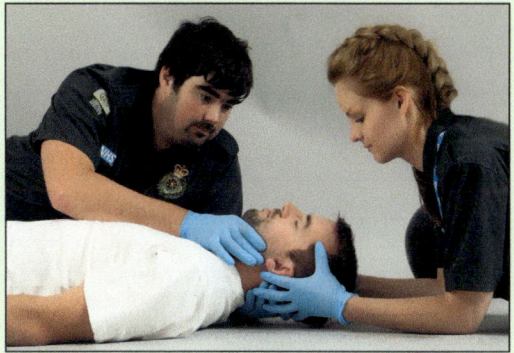

12. Document the procedure.

5.5.3 Cervical collars

The use of semi-rigid cervical collars to minimise the movement of the cervical spine when a traumatic injury of that area is suspected has been a mainstay of trauma management for many decades and remains a treatment intervention in modern trauma management guidelines [CoT, 2018; JRCALC, 2023]. Despite this, no high-quality studies have demonstrated an outcome benefit for patients when collars are utilised as part of pre-hospital immobilisation; moreover, in recent years an increasing number of concerns have been raised over the safety and consequences of their use [Sundstrøm, 2014].

National guidelines are beginning to acknowledge the limitations of cervical collars [Connor, 2013]. However, in the absence of high-quality evidence, their use by some ambulance services in the UK is likely to remain a part of pre-hospital spinal care treatment guidelines for some time, so knowing how to utilise them correctly to minimise potentially harmful situations caused by mis-sizing or poor application is important.

Chapter 16 – Trauma

Their use in paediatric patients is no longer recommended due to a lack of evidence for benefit and concerns that, among other issues, their application may lead to distress, causing a child to move their cervical spine more, rather than less [RCEM, 2019].

Indications
- To minimise movement of the cervical spine of an adult as part of spinal immobilisation.

Contra-indications
- Do not attempt to apply a collar when the patient has abnormal spinal anatomy (such as severe kyphosis).
- Where applying a collar is likely to cause distress that could result in increased cervical movement.

Advantages
- Helps to reduce rotational movement of the cervical spine.
- Provides a clear visual indicator that there is a concern for a potential cervical spine injury.

Disadvantages
- Raises intracranial pressure in head-injured patients.
- Can complicate airway management.
- Can cause pressure sores.
- Does not fully immobilise the cervical spine.

Procedure
Take the following steps to apply an Ambu Perfit ACE cervical collar [Pilbery & Lethbridge, 2022]:

Note that other types of collars may have different fitting instructions.
1. Explain the procedure to the patient and obtain consent unless the patient is unable to do so, for example due to being unconscious.
2. Don appropriate PPE, and undertake appropriate hand hygiene.
3. Ensure you have the correct equipment and, where possible, three people available to apply the collar.

Procedure – cont
4. Ensure the head is in a neutral position. This can only be accurately assessed by looking from the side of, and at the level of, the patient. Assign a rescuer to maintain MILS while the collar is applied.
5. Size the collar by measuring the distance with your fingers between an imaginary line drawn horizontally and immediately below the patient's chin, and another immediately on top of the patient's shoulder.
To help illustrate this, the patient here is shown sitting.

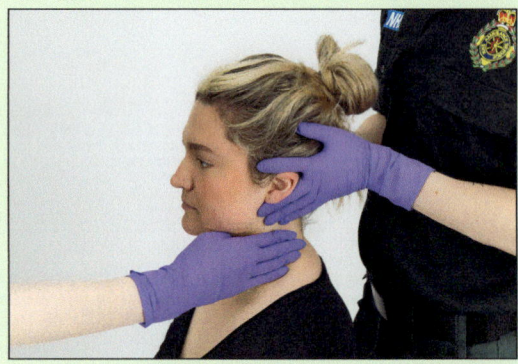

6. Compare the distance measured in step 5 with the space on the collar between the sizing line and the lower aspect of the plastic part of the collar body (not the foam).

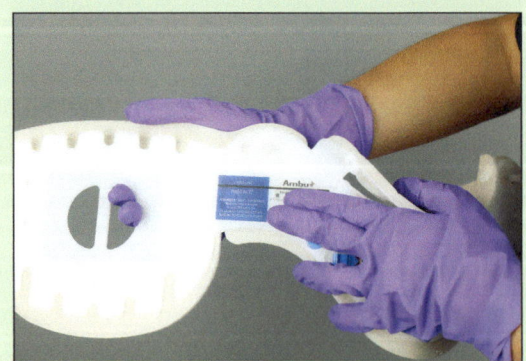

7. To initially increase the size of the collar:
    1. Disengage the locking pins by pulling them up.
    2. Adjust the collar to the appropriate size by pulling it apart until the distance between the sizing line and the collar body equals your finger measurements.

Skeletal immobilisation

Procedure – *cont*

3. Engage the locking pins by pushing them down.

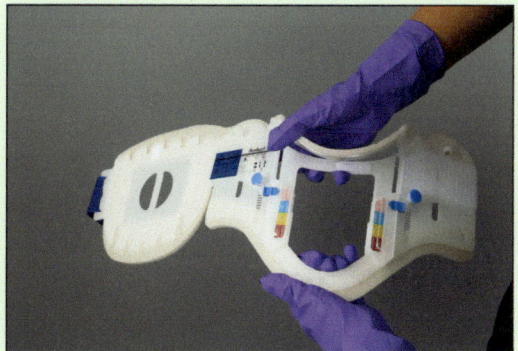

8. Ensure the chin piece has been flipped over from its storage position and is pointing towards the front of the device.

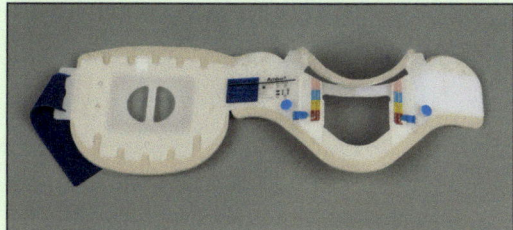

9. Offer the front of the collar up to the patient's chin and chest in order to see if the size is correct.
10. If you need to adjust from the original size:
    1. Disengage the locking tabs by pulling them up.
    2. Pull the ratchet tabs out.
    3. Adjust the collar to the correct size by sliding the ratchet tabs up or down.
11. Once the size is correct, ensure all ratchet tabs and the locking tabs are secured.

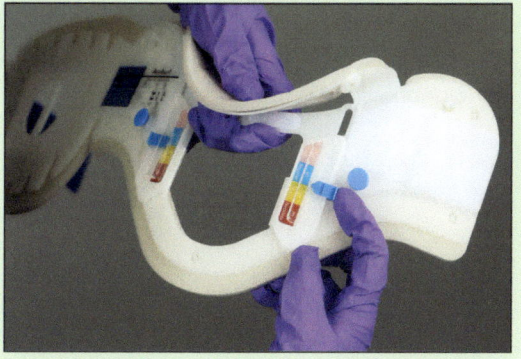

Procedure – *cont*

12. Roll the collar up to pre-form it prior to application.

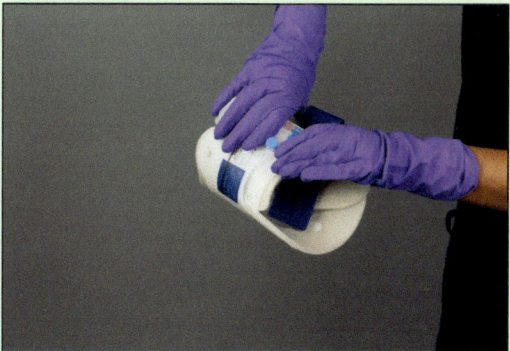

13. Slide the back part of the collar under the patient's neck until the Velcro can be seen appearing on the other side.

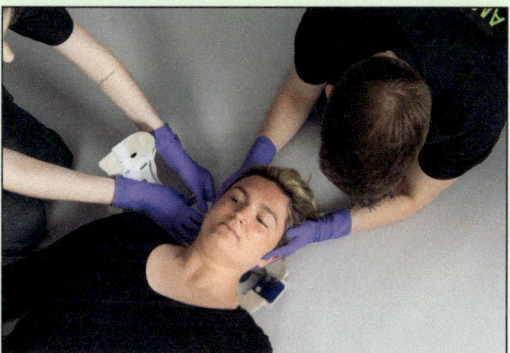

14. Position the chin piece under the chin.

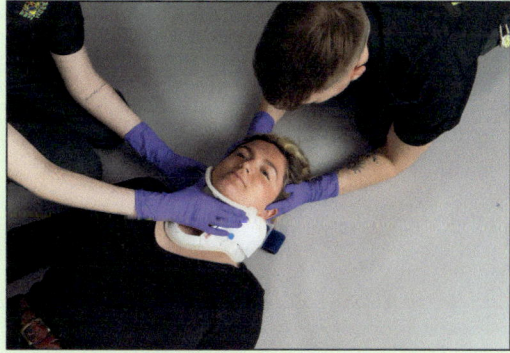

15. While keeping the front of the collar in the correct position with one hand, attach the Velcro with your other hand to achieve a secure fit.

Chapter 16 – *Trauma*

> **Procedure –** *cont*
>
> Maintain MILS until the patient's neck is fully immobilised in a vacuum mattress or similar appropriate device.
>
>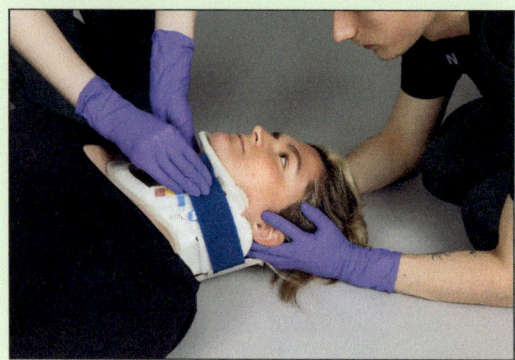
>
> 16. Document the procedure and the time it was completed.

5.5.4 Scoop stretcher

Orthopaedic stretchers (Figure 16.14) are the preferred tool to immobilise and transport patients who require spinal immobilisation [JRCALC, 2023]. This results in less movement of the spine while placing the patient on to the device, compared to the extrication board, and is also more comfortable [Krell, 2006].

Indications
- To provide immobilisation and to transport a patient.

Contra-indications
- Patient too heavy for the device (weighs more than 227 kg (36 st)).
- Any missing or defective components.
- Device regular inspection interval expired (check local policy).

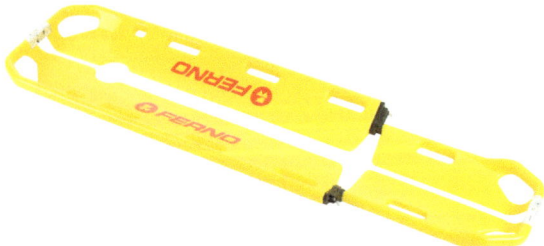

Figure 16.14 Scoop stretcher

Advantages
- Lightweight.
- Adjustable to suit most patients.
- Requires minimal casualty manoeuvring to position them on the stretcher.

Disadvantages
- Morbidly obese patients may not fit.
- Less comfortable and more likely to cause pressure injury than a vacuum mattress.

> **Procedure**
>
> Take the following steps to place a patient on a scoop stretcher [Pilbery & Lethbridge, 2022]:
>
> **Note:** This device is also sometimes referred to as an orthopaedic stretcher.
> 1. If the patient is conscious, explain the procedure and obtain consent if appropriate to do so.
> 2. Don appropriate PPE, and undertake appropriate hand hygiene.
> 3. If indicated, ensure MILS is being applied and a cervical collar has been fitted.
>
>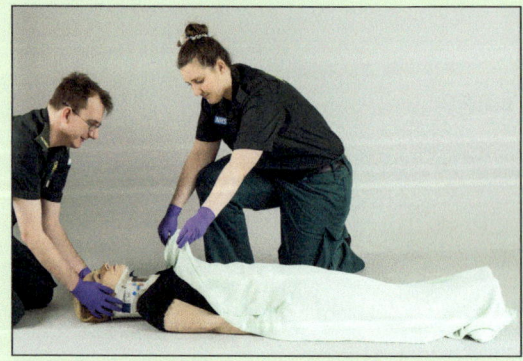
>
> 4. Ensure that the patient is exposed appropriately (being mindful of maintaining dignity) and any other equipment required has been gathered.

Skeletal immobilisation

Procedure – *cont*

5. Place the scoop on the ground next to the patient so that the head is in line with the area that is designed to accommodate the head on the scoop stretcher.

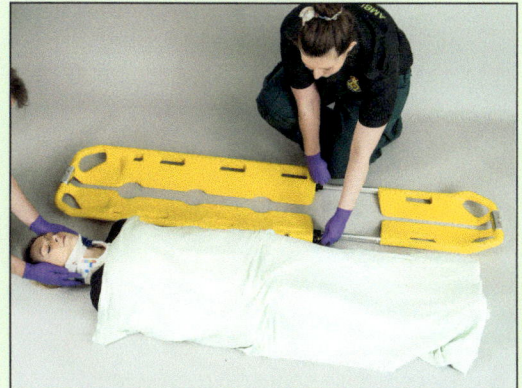

6. Move the locking pins on either side of the stretcher to the upright position. Adjust the length of the stretcher by pulling on the foot section until the scoop stretcher is the desired length.

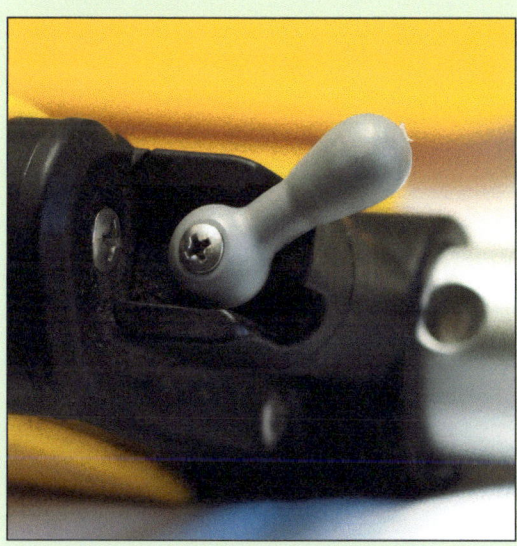

Procedure – *cont*

7. Move the locking pins to the downward position. Gently move the foot section up and down until it locks into place.

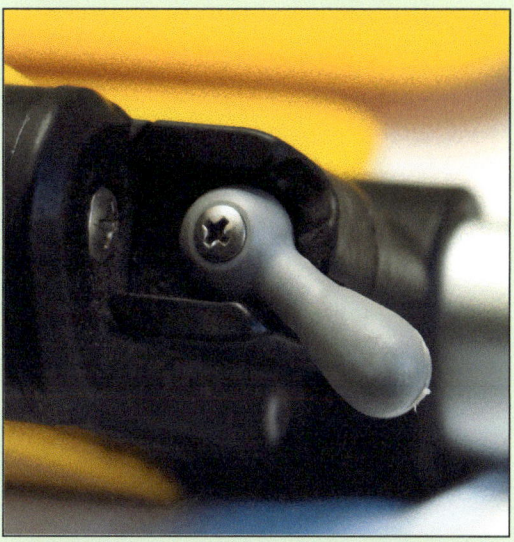

8. Separate the scoop stretcher by pressing the tabs on the Twin Safety Lock system at both the head and foot ends. Pull the two halves away from each other.

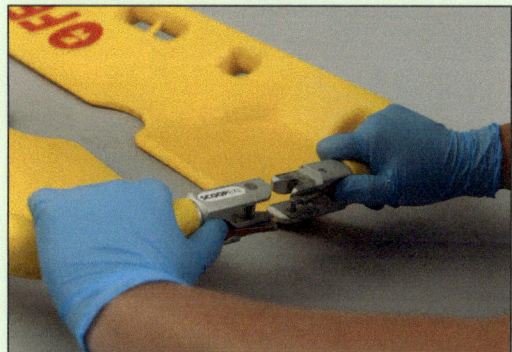

9. Ensure you have enough people to undertake the procedure. You will require people for each of the following:
    - MILS (if indicated)
    - two people to undertake the roll
    - one person to insert the scoop stretcher.

    The team leader should brief everyone as to their role and the steps involved.

Chapter 16 – Trauma

Procedure – *cont*

10. Position the rescuers:
    - One clinician should be positioned at the head of the patient to maintain MILS.
    - Two clinicians should kneel on the side the patient is being rolled towards, one level with the patient's chest, the other by the hips and legs.
    - Another person with the scoop stretcher should position themselves on the other side of the patient, ready to insert the first half of the board.

    All rescuers should consider the principles of safe moving and roll in a straight line with their back as straight as possible.
11. When all rescuers are ready, the clinician at the head end of the patient should issue the command 'Ready, Set, Move.' On 'move', the clinicians should conduct a co-ordinated roll. Once completed, the scoop stretcher should be inserted under the patient.

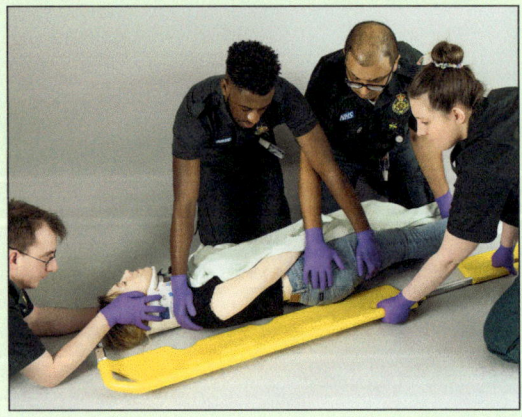

Procedure – *cont*

12. Once the scoop stretcher has been inserted, the patient should be lowered using the same 'Ready, Set, Move' command issued by the clinician at the head end of the patient.

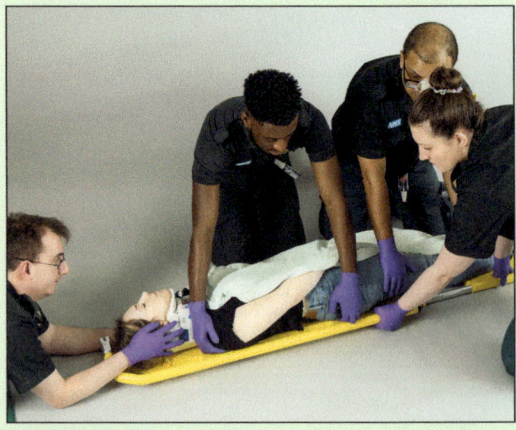

13. Repeat the procedure on the other side. Once both sections are in place, push the brackets of the Twin Safety Lock together until clicked into position. Start with the bracket at the head end.
14. Secure the patient to the stretcher by attaching the chest straps first. If possible, ask the patient to take a deep breath and to hold it before tightening the chest straps.

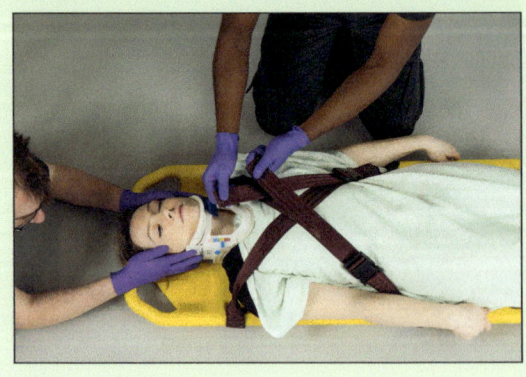

Procedure – *cont*

15. Apply the hip strap and secure.

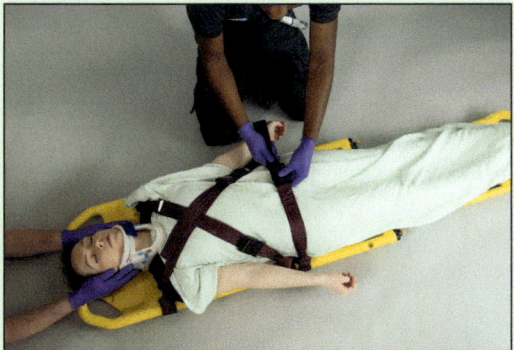

16. Apply the foot strap in a figure-of-eight configuration.

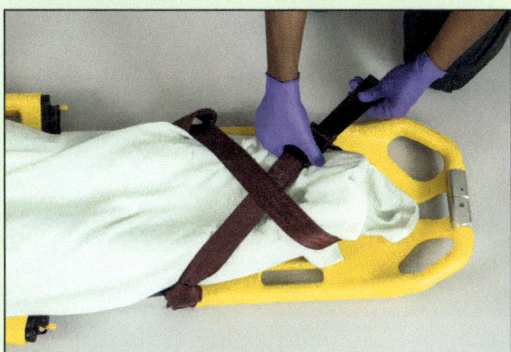

17. Secure the head using a system designed for use with a scoop stretcher. Here a disposable system is used.

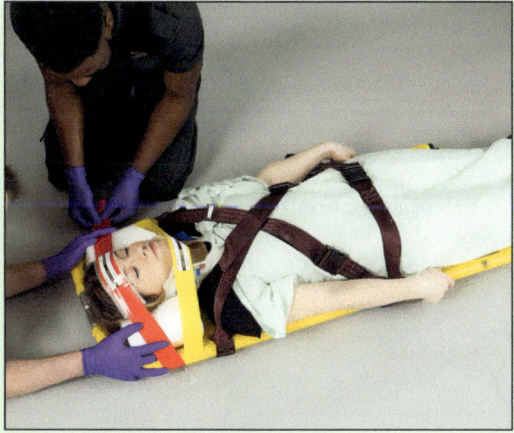

18. Document the procedure.

6   Burns

6.1   *Learning objectives*

By the end of this section you will be able to:
- explain what is meant by the term 'burn'
- describe the types of burn and their causes
- explain the safety considerations when dealing with burns
- state the rules associated with estimating the size of burns
- explain time-critical factors that affect the management of burns
- explain the complications associated with burns
- explain the treatment of burns
- explain why burns patients are transported to definitive care.

6.2   *Introduction*

A burn is an injury caused by energy transfer to the body's tissues, causing necrosis and an associated inflammatory reaction [Greaves, 2008].

Burns are commonly split into a number of types [JRCALC, 2023]:
- chemical
- cold
- electrical
- friction
- radiation
- thermal.

Note: Cold injury was discussed in Chapter 14, 'Exposure/Environment'.

6.3   *Assessment of burns*

6.3.1 History

It is important to identify the mechanism, including the cause of the burn, how it came into contact with the patient, and any first aid undertaken. Note when the injury occurred, how long the patient was exposed to the source and the duration of any cooling. Don't forget to be alert for signs of non-accidental injury.

Chapter 16 – Trauma

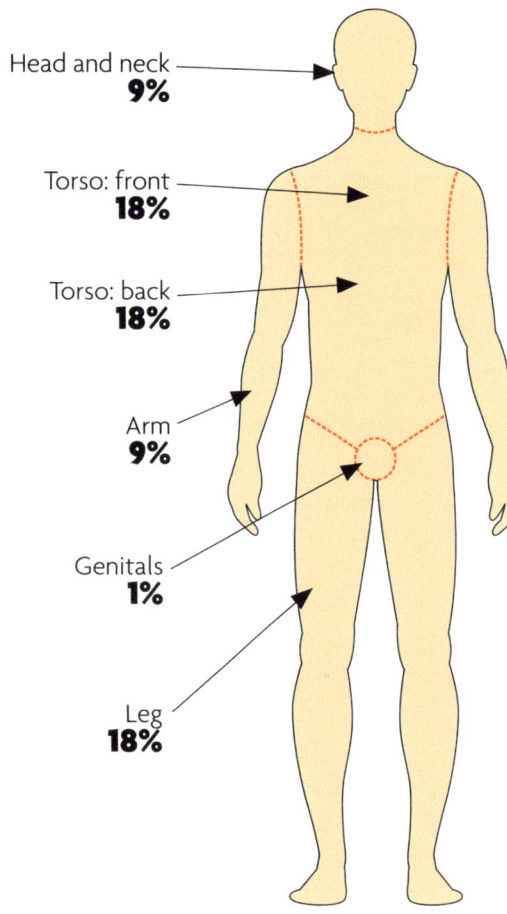

Figure 16.15 The 'rule of nines'

6.3.2 Assessment

Pre-hospital estimation of total body surface area (TBSA) of burn injury is poor, with the 'rule of nines' (Figure 16.15) underestimating burns of less than 20% and overestimating burns over 40%; also, it is not suitable for children under 14 years of age [Hettiaratchy, 2004].

The whole hand (palm and fingers) represents about 0.82% TBSA in adults and 0.77% in children, making accurate calculations tricky. However, the palm alone is 0.5% TBSA [Muehlberger, 2010] making it suitable for estimating burns less than 15% or greater than 85% TBSA. Note that these methods will generally underestimate %TBSA in obese patients [Butz, 2015].

Lund and Browder charts are more accurate, but these are cumbersome to complete in the back of an ambulance. An alternative that has been advocated is serial halving [Allison, 2004]. This involves determining whether greater than or less than 50%, 25% and finally 12.5% of the TBSA is burnt. This approximation is sufficient to determine whether the patient requires referral to a burns unit (if direct access is an option) and the need for intravenous fluids. Erythema (reddening) should not be included when calculating TBSA of burn injury [Enoch, 2009]. There are also mobile phone applications (such as the Mersey Burns App) which may help improve the accuracy of TBSA, although you should follow local guidance on the use of such tools [Chong, 2020].

6.3.3 Classification

Although important for subsequent burns management, the depth of a burn does not affect pre-hospital treatment, but may provide some indication as to the cause (Table 16.2) [NHS, 2022c].

6.4 Thermal burns

The most common type of thermal burns (sometimes referred to as thermal injuries) are flame, scald and contact. Flame burns are more common in adults and are often associated with smoke inhalation and other traumatic injuries. These are more likely to result in deep dermal or full-thickness burns.

Scalds are the most common cause of burn in children, usually due to spillages of hot drinks [Greaves, 2018]. They generally cause epidermal or superficial dermal burn injury [Hettiaratchy, 2004].

Direct contact burns are caused by brief contact with a very hot object, or (more commonly) prolonged contact with a cooler object. Typical patient groups include epileptics and those who misuse alcohol or drugs.

Irreversible damage to the epidermis can be caused by exposure to 44°C heat for 6 hours, or 65°C for 1 second [Moritz, 1947]. Burns injuries are characterised by a local response and, if the TBSA burnt is greater than 20%, a systemic response [Greaves, 2008].

Table 16.2 Burns classification

Classification	Other names	Example causes	Appearance	Sensation
Epidermal	Superficial, 1st degree	UV light, scalds	Dry and red, blanches with pressure, no blisters	May be painful
Superficial dermal	Superficial, partial thickness, 2nd degree	Scald (spill or splash)	Pale pink, fine blisters, blanches with pressure	Very painful
Mid-dermal	Superficial, partial thickness, 2nd degree	Scald (spill), flame	Dark pink with large blisters, delayed capillary refill	May be painful
Deep dermal	Deep partial thickness, 2nd degree	Scald (spill), flame	Blotchy red, may blister, no capillary refill	No sensation
Full thickness	3rd degree	Scald (immersion), flame, steam, high-voltage electricity	White, waxy or charred. No blisters or capillary refill. Children: dark lobster red with mottling	No sensation

6.4.1 Acute smoke inhalation injury

Smoke inhalation is a killer, with the majority of fire fatalities due to being 'overcome by gas or smoke' [HO, 2023]. Nasopharyngeal, oropharyngeal and mucosal burns are common [Toon, 2010], but thermal injury below the vocal cords is rare since heat is effectively exchanged in upper airway passages [Prien, 1988]. When air, steam and/or smoke are at sufficiently high temperatures to cause thermal injury to the lower airways, rapid oedema of the glottis develops, resulting in fatal airway obstruction.

Systemic toxins are the products of incomplete combustion and include CO and hydrogen cyanide. CO is an odourless, colourless gas that binds to haemoglobin with 250 times the affinity of oxygen. This results in a decrease in the oxygen-carrying capacity of the blood. Hydrogen cyanide adversely affects internal respiration by preventing aerobic production of adenosine triphosphate (ATP, the energy source for cells) [Toon, 2010].

6.4.2 Friction burns

Although friction burns are strictly speaking a thermal burn, they are the result of heat production caused by friction between the skin and another object. This can result in not just a burn, but abrasions too (see the section on 'Wounds and bleeding' earlier in the chapter).

6.4.3 Management

Safety first! The patient needs to be removed from the source of the burn if it is safe to do so, but don't get burnt yourself. Clothing should be removed unless it is sticking to the patient, as should jewellery, which may become constrictive as tissues swell.

Follow the <C>ABCDE approach for burns as you would any traumatic injury. However, inhalation injury is a particular concern and occurs in around 22% of all burns, 60% if facial burns are present [Toon, 2010].

Signs of inhalation injury include [Singer, 2010]:
- full-thickness or deep dermal burns to face, neck or upper torso
- singed nasal hair
- soot in sputum or oropharynx
- dyspnoea, hoarseness, cough or stridor
- cyanosis
- altered LOC.

Administer high-flow oxygen via a non-rebreathe mask. CO poisoning may make pulse oximetry readings unreliable [JRCALC, 2023].

Cooling
Thermal burns should be cooled for 20 minutes preferably with running water around 12°C [Battaloglu, 2020]. There is little evidence that ice causes damage to underlying tissues, but it runs the risk of making the patient hypothermic so is not recommended [Cuttle, 2008, 2009]. Cooling should commence immediately after the burn has occurred, but there is limited evidence to suggest that cooling up to 3 hours after the burn has occurred is still beneficial [Battaloglu, 2020].

Covering/dressing
Patients with burns lose heat from non-epithelialised areas of skin due to evaporation. With the thermoregulatory function of the skin disrupted, patients are at risk of hypothermia, even on a warm day. Hypothermia is part of the lethal triad in trauma, and for each 1°C reduction in body temperature the mortality rate increases significantly, although there is no evidence currently to suggest that pre-hospital cooling causes hypothermia [Lonnecker, 2001; Singer, 2010]. Once cooling has been completed, cover the burn with a clean sheet or Clingfilm, but take care not to apply it circumferentially as it can become constrictive as oedema develops [Battaloglu, 2020].

6.5 Chemical burns

Chemical burns generally result from exposure to acids, alkalis and other corrosive materials. This can be accidental, but increasingly commonly it is an intentional form of violence [JESIP, 2023b]. Alkali burns are generally more serious as they penetrate more deeply than other chemicals [NAEMT, 2020]. Their severity depends on the concentration of the chemical, the duration of exposure and the speed in applying first-aid measures [Greaves, 2008].

6.5.1 Management

Safety first! It is important that you do not become exposed to the chemical. If in doubt, do not approach the scene but wait for the HART or the fire and rescue service to attend. Wear appropriate PPE.

The following first-aid measures apply to chemical burns [FPHC, 2018]:
- Evacuate the casualty to a clean area away from the hazard.
- Remove contaminated clothing (cut it off and avoid removing it over the head).
- Remove excess contamination:
  - brush off solid material
  - gently blot (do not rub) excess and thickened liquids with absorbent material and discard.
- Rinse with copious amounts of water, with the patient leaning forward so that contamination does not run over themselves any more.
- Irrigate for at least 20 minutes, and ideally for up to an hour.

Be aware of local policy. Some hospitals have specialist treatments available for chemical burns patients.

6.6 Radiation burns

Radiation burns are most commonly caused by UV radiation from the sun or sunlamps (sunburn). However, in rare cases, it can be caused by exposure to radioactive materials.

Approximately 80% of skin cancer is preventable, and avoiding sunburn is key [NHS, 2022b]:
- Spend time in the shade between 11am and 3pm.
- Never burn.
- Cover up with suitable clothing and sunglasses.
- Take extra care with children.
- Use at least factor 30 sunscreen.

6.6.1 Management

Safety first! If the burns are due to exposure to radioactivity, do not approach but wait for the HART.

Sunburn

Basic first-aid measures are usually sufficient [SJA, 2021]:

- Cover the patient's skin with light clothing or a towel. Move them out of the sun, preferably indoors.
- Encourage them to drink frequent sips of cold water while cooling the affected area with cold water. If the area of sunburn is large, it may be more practical for the patient to soak the area in a cold bath for up to 20 minutes.
- If burns are mild, calamine or an after-sun lotion may help. Patients should be advised to stay inside or in the shade.

6.7 Electrical injuries

Electrical injuries are thankfully uncommon, but they cause significant damage and even death when they occur. The majority of electrical injuries in adults occur in the workplace and involve high voltages, whereas in children most injuries occur in the home with domestic voltage. Electrocution from lightning strikes is very rare, leading to around five deaths in the UK each year [JRCALC, 2023].

Electrical burns arise when a source of electrical power makes contact with the patient's body. They are frequently more serious than they appear, since rapid heat loss from the surface of the skin may leave it relatively undamaged, whereas the underlying tissues may have sustained serious injury, particularly between the entry and exit points (don't forget to look for both) [NAEMT, 2020].

6.7.1 Management

Safety first! Do not approach the patient until you are certain that the source of electricity has been cut off.

When dealing with electrical injuries, the thermal burns sustained may not be your highest priority. The patient may be in cardiac arrest, have airway or facial burns and be traumatically injured (fractures, serious internal injuries); this will need addressing first. Associated thermal burns can be managed as previously described.

17 Children and Infants

1 Why paediatric patients are different

1.1 Learning objective

By the end of this section you will be able to:
- explain how paediatric patients are anatomically, physiologically and developmentally different from adults.

1.2 Introduction

Paediatrics is a speciality of medicine that looks after people from birth to age 18 years. Children are generally divided into five main groups [Lissauer, 2007]:
- Infants: From birth to 12 months of age. In the first 4 weeks after birth, infants may also be called neonates.
- Toddler: Approximately 1–2 years of age.
- Pre-school: This is a young child aged 2–5 years.
- School-age: Generally 5–12 years (or the onset of puberty).
- Teenager: Also called adolescents. Generally from onset of puberty to 18 years, when, in the UK, they become an adult. Some guidance (such as the administration of certain drugs) treats this group the same as adults.

Note: For the purposes of resuscitation, an infant is a patient under 12 months of age and a child is a patient who is between 1 year and 18 years of age [Voorde, 2021].

1.3 Anatomy and physiology

As children get older, their bodies change anatomically and physiologically. This is important to remember when undertaking your assessment as you may need to modify your plan for their management.

1.3.1 Airway

Most of the changes in the infant and child airways have been covered in Chapter 10, 'Airway'. However, some extra points to consider are provided here.

Face and mouth

Infants' faces are small. This makes sizing of a face mask for resuscitation important if a good seal is to be achieved. It is important that pressure on the eyes is avoided as this can result in damage and reflex bradycardia. The floor of the mouth is also easy to compress, so care must be taken not to apply pressure to the soft tissues under the mandible during airway opening and positive-pressure ventilations (Figure 17.1) [Voorde, 2021].

Nose and pharynx

In the first 6 months, infants breathe through their nose, meaning that any nasal obstruction can result in increased work of breathing and respiratory compromise [AAP, 2018].

1.3.2 Breathing

Infants and small children have relatively small resting lung volumes, which means they have less oxygen capacity in reserve than adults. Therefore, early oxygenation is important when there are clinical signs of circulatory or respiratory failure [Voorde, 2021].

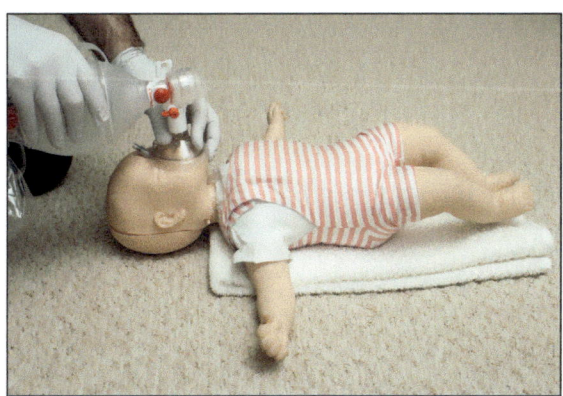

Figure 17.1 Infant positive-pressure ventilation

Chapter 17 – Children and Infants

The ribs of infants are cartilaginous and so are very pliable. In addition, they have weak intercostal muscles, which means that the diaphragm is their main muscle of respiration. If the diaphragm is impeded in any way, such as by gastric distension, for example, their ventilation may become ineffective [AAP, 2018].

As children get older, their intercostal muscles become more developed, contributing more to the mechanics of ventilation. Their ribs ossify, hardening and acting as an anchor for the developing intercostal muscles, making them less likely to collapse during periods of respiratory distress. As a result, intercostal recession in any child over the age of 5 years should be seen as an ominous sign of severe respiratory distress [RCUK, 2021b].

Infants have a relatively high metabolic rate, oxygen consumption and carbon dioxide production, requiring a higher respiratory rate than older children. This can be further increased by pain, fever and anxiety, resulting in changing 'normal' respiratory rates for infants and children (Table 17.1) [JRCALC, 2023].

Table 17.1 Respiratory rate ranges in infants and children

Age	Respiratory rate (breaths/min)
Birth–1 month	40–60
3–9 months	30–40
12–18 months	25–35
2–4 years	25–30
5–11 years	20–25
12 years and over	12–20

1.3.3 Circulation

The circulating blood volume in an infant is about 80 ml/kg, which means that in a newborn baby weighing 3 kg their blood volume is only 240 ml, making small blood losses significant.

Another important point to note is that oxygen delivery to the tissues is dependent on both arterial blood oxygen concentration and the cardiac output. In respiratory failure, a reduction in arterial blood oxygen can be compensated by increasing cardiac output. However, in circulatory failure, it is not possible to increase arterial blood oxygen content so tissue oxygen delivery falls immediately.

The stroke volume at birth is small, only 1.5 ml/kg, so increasing cardiac output is mainly achieved by increasing heart rate. Thus heart rates in infants and small children are higher than in older children (Table 17.2). In addition, systemic vascular resistance increases as children get older, a change reflected by increased 'normal' blood pressures (Table 17.3) [JRCALC, 2023; RCUK, 2021b].

Table 17.2 Paediatric heart rate ranges

Age	Heart rate (beats/min)
Birth–9 months	110–160
12–18 months	110–150
2–4 years	95–140
5–11 years	80–120
12 years and over	60–100

Table 17.3 Paediatric systolic blood pressure ranges

Age	Systolic blood pressure (mmHg)
Birth–9 months	70–90
12–18 months	80–95
2–4 years	80–100
5 years	90–100
6–11 years	90–110
12 years and over	100–120

1.4 Cognitive development

Children are also challenging because their brain develops as they age. This means that during your assessment of a child you will expect different levels of interaction and abilities in a 1-year-old compared to a 12-year-old child [AAP, 2018].

1.4.1 Infants

Under 2 months
Infants in this age group will spend the majority of their time feeding and sleeping. They are unable to tell the difference between their parents/carers and others, so do not display stranger anxiety. They will exhibit primitive reflexes, such as grasping objects placed in the palm of their hand, or turning their head towards a gentle stimulation on the side of their mouth (rooting).

2–6 months
Infants become more active during this period, making assessment a little easier. They begin to make eye contact, will smile and follow the light of your pen torch or a toy with their eyes. They will also turn their head in response to a loud noise or the voice of their parent/carer. Their motor skills develop and they will start to roll over and reach for objects. They will vocalise with coos and laughs when spoken to.

6–12 months
Infants are much more socially interactive at this age. They may be able to say single words such as 'mama' or 'dada', but will also develop stranger anxiety in the latter stages (typically after 9 months), so keep the infant with their parent/carer if possible. They will be able to feed themselves, sit unsupported, reach for objects and pass them between hands.

1.4.2 Toddlers

There is a rapid change in growth and cognitive development at this age. By 18 months, children will have a vocabulary of around 6–10 words, and will know the name of, and be able to point to, several parts of their body. They should be able to walk steadily and feed themselves with a spoon.

As they reach 2 years of age, children may be able to combine several words together to make a simple phrase. They will start to engage in symbolic play, feeding their teddy, for example. Stranger anxiety may be extreme and they are typically illogical thinkers, learning by trial and error, but have no sense of danger. They are self-centred and will be able to label objects as 'mine'. Toilet training may lead to children being dry during the day.

1.4.3 Pre-school

These children are creative and illogical thinkers, often confusing fantasy and reality. They are likely to have misconceptions about illness, injury and bodily functions. In addition, they may fear the dark, being left alone and the presence of monsters under the bed. They have good language skills and can participate in parallel play, taking it in turns with others, but their attention span is short.

1.4.4 School-age

Children at this age understand cause and effect and are capable of abstract thought. They can tell you about the progress of their current illness or injury but their ability to understand the seriousness of the situation is limited. They can be involved with their care if explanations are kept simple and clear. Peer-group support becomes important at this age, but they will still have separation anxiety from their parents/carers when ill, and fear pain and loss of control.

1.4.5 Teenagers

Teenagers (adolescents) are sometimes compared to toddlers: highly mobile but lacking common sense! However, they are able to rationalise and express themselves and their feelings in words. This is also a period of experimentation and risk-taking. Children at this age will typically transition from relying on their parents/carers for psychological support and development to their friends and peers. This typically leads to feelings of anxiety if they are 'different' from their peers. In addition, they may struggle with anxiety of independence, body image, sexuality and peer pressure.

2 Initial assessment and management of the paediatric patient

2.1 Learning objectives
By the end of this section you will be able to:
- conduct an initial assessment of the paediatric patient
- identify problems with a paediatric patient's airway, breathing, circulation and neurological status
- describe the principles that underpin the support of a seriously ill paediatric patient.

2.2 Introduction
The assessment of the paediatric patient is much the same as for adults, and you will follow the standard procedure you learnt about in Chapter 9, 'Patient Assessment'. As before, the primary survey is a chance to identify and correct life-threatening problems. In infants and children, prompt recognition and intervention when there are signs of respiratory and/or circulatory failure can prevent the majority of paediatric cardiorespiratory arrests [RCUK, 2021b].

2.3 Developmental approach to the paediatric patient
A child's cognitive development changes as they age, which requires modification in your method of assessment. In this section, you will be provided with some suggestions about how to conduct an assessment of the paediatric patient. Don't forget that you will also need to manage and reassure an often anxious and distressed parent/carer.

2.3.1 Infants
Conduct your assessment by taking account of the following principles [AAP, 2018]:
- Keep the environment comfortable, in terms of temperature and security for the infant. Familiar toys and blankets can help.
- Use the name of the patient while conducting your assessment.
- Where possible, assess an infant in the arms of a parent/carer.
- Approach the infant slowly and calmly. Loud voices and fast movements may scare them.
- Do not stand over an infant, but sit or kneel at their eye level.
- Look, listen and feel, in that order, to minimise infant distress.
- Warm your hands and tools such as stethoscopes.
- Be flexible in your assessment. If the infant is calm, count the respiratory rate and listen to the chest first. This is not possible to do accurately when the infant is crying.
- Observe the interaction between parent/carer and the infant. Consider if child abuse is a possibility.
- Toys can be used to distract the infant.
- Older infants may display stranger anxiety, so if you need to expose the infant, ask the parent/carer to do this. Don't let the infant get cold, though.
- Save painful procedures (such as blood sugar measurement) until last.

2.3.2 Toddlers
Conduct your assessment by taking account of the following principles [AAP, 2018]:
- Use the name of the patient while conducting your assessment.
- Approach slowly and don't touch them until they are familiar with you.
- Communicate using a firm, but friendly, tone of voice.
- Do not stand over a toddler, but sit or kneel at their eye level.
- Where possible, place the toddler on the lap of a parent/carer.
- Use play and distraction to help you conduct your assessment.
- If you need to use equipment, such as a stethoscope, let them hold it and become familiar and comfortable with it.
- Communicate directly with the toddler. Admire their clothes or ask about pets. Remember they are self-centred at this age.
- Provide limited choices. For example, 'Do you want me to listen to your belly or chest first?'
- Avoid questions that can be answered with a 'No'.

- Examine a toddler from toe to head.
- Involve the parent/carer. For example, place the pulse oximeter probe on their finger first, and ask them to remove the toddler's clothes or hold an oxygen mask near the toddler.
- Do not expect toddlers to sit still and co-operate. Be patient and opportunistic.

2.3.3 Pre-school

Conduct your assessment by taking account of the following principles [AAP, 2018]:
- Use the name of the patient while conducting your assessment.
- Use simple terms to explain what you are going to do.
- Choose your words carefully. Use age-appropriate language and avoid scaring the child.
- Teddies or dolls can be helpful to explain what you are going to do.
- Set limits on behaviour, if required. For example, 'You can cry or scream, but not kick or bite'.
- Praise good behaviour.
- Use games and toys to provide distraction. Ambulance bandages can be useful for this.
- Focus on one thing at a time and minimise the time between explaining a procedure, especially a painful one, and carrying it out.

2.3.4 School-age

Conduct your assessment by taking account of the following principles [AAP, 2018]:
- Use the name of the patient while conducting your assessment.
- Privacy becomes important in this age group. Make sure the environment is appropriate, and if you need to expose the child to examine them, cover them up afterwards.
- Speak directly to the child first, then include the parent/carer. Ask older children if they would like their parent/carer present.
- Involve the child in their care if they want this. Feeling out of control can distress children in this age group. However, do not negotiate unless the child really does have a choice.
- Anticipate the fears that the child has and address them straight away. Assure them that becoming ill or injured is not a punishment.
- Explain in simple terms what is wrong and what is going to be done.
- Explain procedures just prior to undertaking them. Don't lie to the child, for example by telling them a procedure won't hurt when it will.
- Praise the child for being co-operative, but do not chastise them if they are not.
- Physical assessments in this age group can usually be conducted head to toe.

2.3.5 Teenagers

Conduct your assessment by taking account of the following principles [AAP, 2018]:
- Use the name of the patient while conducting your assessment.
- Speak directly to the teenager and ask them first for information. If they do not know the answer, for example the name of their GP, check with them if it is okay to ask their parent/carer.
- Respect their modesty and privacy. Be confidential unless you have a duty to report or pass on their disclosures.
- Be honest and non-judgemental. Provide accurate information and allay fears, particularly concerns over body image or being 'different' as a result of their current illness or injury.
- Do not mistake the size of the teenager as a measure of their maturity.
- Avoid becoming frustrated or angry if the teenager does not want to communicate or is unco-operative.
- Enlist the help of their friends to assist when the teenager is being unco-operative, although keep in mind the teenager's right to confidentiality.

2.4 Recognising the sick infant and child

Unlike adults, infants and children generally have a cardiac arrest secondary to respiratory and/or circulatory failure. Outcome from cardiac arrest in infants and children is significantly worse than in adults, and intervening early on can prevent this from occurring.

2.4.1 Respiratory failure

Respiratory failure can be either compensated or decompensated. Compensated respiratory failure (sometimes known as respiratory distress) is characterised by increased work of breathing to overcome a respiratory problem, e.g. bronchiolitis. Respiratory failure is termed decompensated when the respiratory system can no longer maintain appropriate blood levels of oxygen and carbon dioxide. Since blood gases are not available out-of-hospital, a rough equivalent is a pulse oximetry (SpO_2) reading of less than 90% when breathing room air [RCUK, 2021b].

Occasionally, respiratory failure can be present in the absence of increased work of breathing, e.g. due to a decreased LOC or a morphine overdose.

2.4.2 Cardiac failure

As with respiratory failure, cardiac failure can also be compensated or decompensated. In compensated failure, vital organ (heart and brain) perfusion is maintained and blood pressure remains within normal limits. This is mostly achieved by peripheral vasoconstriction. Once there is insufficient circulation to deliver oxygen to the tissues (i.e. in shock), the infant or child will become hypotensive and their LOC will reduce.

2.5 *Primary survey*

The primary survey in the infant and child is the same as for adults, except for the general impression component, which should include use of the paediatric assessment triangle (PAT). The PAT is advantageous in children because it can be undertaken without actually touching the child and can be performed 'across the room' to avoid increasing a child's anxiety, by getting too close initially [AAP, 2018].

2.5.1 General impression

It is important to gain a general impression of the health of an infant or child from 'across the room', before your presence has an adverse effect on their level of anxiety or distress. To help you achieve this, use the PAT [Dieckmann, 2010].

As the name suggests, it consists of three key components:
- appearance
- work of breathing
- circulation to skin.

Appearance

The child's general appearance is probably the most significant aspect of the PAT, as it provides information about the perfusion of the brain. The parts of this component can be remembered using the mnemonic TICLS [AAP, 2018]:
- **Tone:** Is the infant/child moving spontaneously or are they floppy and listless?
- **Interactiveness:** Does the infant/child respond to people, objects and sounds or are they uninterested in their surroundings?
- **Consolability:** Can the infant/child be consoled by their parent/carer?
- **Look/Gaze:** Does the infant/child look at you or do they have a 'glass-eyed' stare into the distance?
- **Speech/Cry:** Is their speech or cry strong or weak, muffled or hoarse?

Work of breathing

In children, it is their work of breathing that provides a better indication as to the adequacy of oxygenation and ventilation, rather than the more traditional respiratory rate and/or auscultation in adults [AAP, 2018]. Look for signs of increased work of breathing as well as listening for abnormal airway sounds:
- **Abnormal airway sounds:** These include snoring, muffled or hoarse speech, stridor, grunting and wheezing.
- **Abnormal positioning:** Children who can sit up may adopt a 'sniffing the morning air' position, tripod position and/or refuse to lie down.
- **Recession:** Recession of the chest muscles provides an indication of increased work of breathing, as does head-bobbing in infants. Beware the child over 5 years who has signs of recession, as this is a sign of serious respiratory compromise [RCUK, 2021b].
- **Flaring:** Look for nasal flaring, an exaggerated opening of the nostrils during laboured inspiration.

Circulation to skin

When cardiac output is not sufficient to meet the body's metabolic demands, the circulation to non-essential organs, such as the skin, reduces. This can manifest in children as [AAP, 2018]:

- **Pallor:** White or pale skin indicating a reflex shunting of blood away from the skin. This may be the only sign of compensated shock.
- **Cyanosis:** This is blue discolouration of the skin caused by inadequate oxygenation. Note that blue hands and feet in newborns and infants under the age of 2 months (acrocyanosis) is a normal finding.
- **Mottling:** This is caused by abnormal blood vessel tone in the capillary beds of the skin. There are patchy areas of pallor and cyanosis. This can be normal when the child is exposed to a cold environment.

2.5.2 Airway

Obstruction of the airway is common in seriously ill children, causing hypoxia, which can lead to unconsciousness and cardiorespiratory arrest (such as in cases of choking) [RCUK, 2021b]. It is important to remember that chest movement does not imply a clear airway: you need to listen and feel for air movement.

Look for apparent difficulty in breathing or increased work of breathing. In conscious children, they may be in visible distress. Listen for additional noises, such as stridor, a high-pitched (usually) inspiratory sound [RCUK, 2021b].

Management

Children who are conscious should be allowed to adopt a position of comfort, ideally one that they themselves adopt to maximise the efficiency of their airway, and supplemental high-flow oxygen via a non-rebreathe mask should be administered.

For unconscious children, their head needs positioning appropriately to open the airway and prevent the tongue from falling backwards and occluding the airway. This can be achieved in children using a head tilt–chin lift, or jaw thrust manoeuvre as described in Chapter 10, 'Airway'. Remember that in infants, their head should be

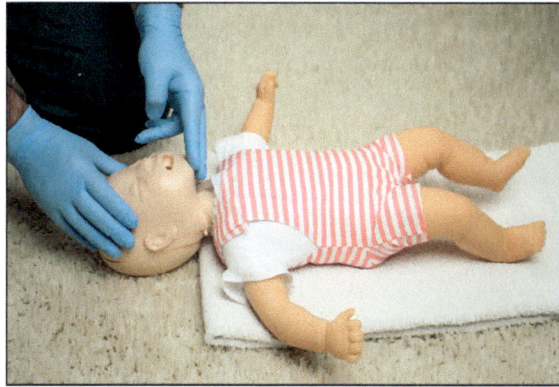

Figure 17.2 An infant, with their airway in neutral alignment

placed in the neutral position, with padding under the shoulders to account for their proportionally larger head (Figure 17.2).

Care must be taken not to compress the soft tissues under a child's jaw as this can also occlude the airway [RCUK, 2021b].

OPAs can be used in children as in adults. For small children and infants, it is generally recommended that the OPA is introduced the 'right way round' and not rotated 180°, although this is likely to require a tongue depressor, which you may not be equipped with.

2.5.3 Breathing

Assessment

The most effective way of determining whether the airway is obstructed is to look, listen and feel [Voorde, 2021]:

- Look for chest (and abdominal) movements.
- Listen at the child's mouth and nose for breath (plus added) sounds.
- Feel for air movement on your cheek.

Note: The chest may move in children, even with an obstruction, making it important to listen and feel.

As part of gaining a general impression, you will already have considered the patient's work of breathing, which includes [AAP, 2018]:

- abnormal airway sounds
- abnormal positioning

- recession
- flaring.

Other signs of increased work of breathing include an elevated respiratory rate and use of the accessory muscles.

Abnormal airway sounds

Stridor is a high-pitched inspiratory sound which indicates an upper airway obstruction. This may be an object or swelling due to infection. In severe cases, it can also occur on expiration. A wheeze, on the other hand, is usually an expiratory sound and is a sign of lower airway obstruction. You may be able to hear it with just your ears, but often it will only be heard on auscultation [AAP, 2018].

Grunting is usually heard in neonates and small infants, although it can occur in small children too. It occurs when the infant exhales against a partially closed glottis. This generates a small amount of end-expiratory pressure, keeping the small airways from collapsing at the end of expiration. It is an indication of severe respiratory compromise [RCUK, 2021b].

Abnormal positioning

Children in respiratory distress typically adopt a position that maximises their respiratory efficiency. In upper airway obstruction, this will be a 'sniffing the morning air' position. In lower respiratory problems they may adopt a 'tripod' position, sitting forward with their arms outstretched and resting on their knees [RCUK, 2021b].

Recession

Recession can be sternal, subcostal and/or intercostal. Note that significant recession can be seen in infants and young children, even in mild respiratory distress, due to their compliant chest wall (Figure 17.3). However, as previously mentioned, it is a serious sign in children over 5 years of age [AAP, 2018].

Flaring

Nostril flaring in infants and young children is a sign of increased respiratory effort.

Respiratory rate

An increased respiratory rate (tachypnoea) is often the first sign of respiratory problems, although it

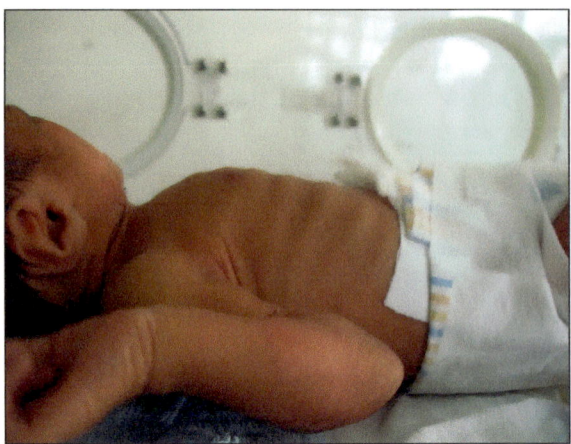

Figure 17.3 A newborn with intercostal recession
Source: Bobjgalindo (Own work) [CC-BY-SA-3.0-2.5-2.0-1.0], via Wikimedia Commons.

can be difficult to assess in the crying infant/child (see Table 17.1).

Use of accessory muscles

Additional muscles are often recruited when the work of breathing increases. One group is the sternocleidomastoid muscles in the neck. These cause 'head bobbing' in infants, who will nod their head up and down with each breath. However, this is not an efficient method of breathing [RCUK, 2021b].

Pulse oximetry

This can be unreliable when a child has poor peripheral circulation, but, if obtainable, a reading of less than 90% on air, or less than 95% on high-flow oxygen, is a sign of decompensated respiratory failure and urgent intervention is required [Voorde, 2021].

Management

All seriously ill children should receive high-flow oxygen via a non-rebreathe mask, unless their ventilation is insufficient. In this case, assistance should be provided with BVM ventilation. For children who are conscious, placing a mask over the child's face may be distressing. In this case, attempt administration using the least threatening method, for example by asking the parent/carer to hold an oxygen mask close to the patient's mouth and nose [JRCALC, 2023].

Watch for signs of decompensation, which include:
- changes to respiratory rate: increasing or sudden decrease
- reducing LOC/interaction with ambulance staff and parents/guardians
- exhaustion.

Unconscious children and infants whose airway is clear, and who are breathing normally, should be turned on to their side into the recovery position [Voorde, 2021]. While the adult recovery position can be used in children, modification is required for infants. Adopt the following principles when placing an infant in the recovery position:
- Place the child in as near true lateral position as possible, with their mouth suitably positioned to assist in the free drainage of fluid.
- The position needs to be stable. This may require a small pillow or a rolled-up blanket to be placed along the infant's back to maintain the position, to prevent the infant from rolling on to their back or front.
- Avoid any pressure on the infant's chest that might impair breathing.
- Whatever the position, it should be possible to turn the infant from their side on to their back (and vice versa) easily and safely.

2.5.4 Circulation

Assessment
When assessing circulation, look for signs of blood and other fluid losses, which are causing shock. Children can compensate very well, maintaining their blood pressure until they have significant fluid losses. However, you can spot the child in compensated circulatory failure by examining the following [RCUK, 2021b]:
- heart rate
- pulse volume
- capillary refill time.

Heart rate
Tachycardia is common in children and has a number of causes including pain, anxiety and fever. It is also often the first sign of circulatory failure. Bradycardia, defined as a heart rate of less than 60 beats/min in a child, is a serious sign and is normally an indication to start chest compressions [RCUK, 2021b].

Pulse volume
When a child develops shock, peripheral pulses will become weak and thready. If central pulses (such as a carotid pulse) become weak and thready, the child is in cardiorespiratory failure and arrest is imminent, so always ensure you compare central and peripheral pulses [RCUK, 2021b].

As children become peripherally vasoconstricted in response to shock, their extremities will become cool. Sometimes there is a clear demarcation line between cool skin and warm skin, that will either move towards the torso if shock progresses, or move distally if perfusion and circulation improve [JRCALC, 2023].

Capillary refill time
Capillary refill time can be a useful indicator of circulatory status, as was covered in Chapter 12, 'Circulation'.

Skin
Skin perfusion can provide valuable clues as to the infant's or child's circulatory status. Note the temperature of the skin, particularly the level of warm/cold demarcation lines on the limbs. Monitor this level frequently to see whether things are improving or heading to circulatory failure. The colour of the skin should also be assessed if it wasn't covered in the PAT.

End-organ perfusion
Although you will conduct a formal assessment of the LOC in 'Disability' (see section 2.5.5 of this chapter), consider whether there are any signs of poor cerebral perfusion. Early signs of compromise include a loss of interaction with the infant's or child's surroundings and irritability and agitation. Late signs include a loss of consciousness and loss of tone (e.g. a 'floppy' baby).

The kidneys are an essential organ and one clue that they are not being adequately perfused is a reduction in urine output. A simple way of assessing this is to ask about the number of wet nappies or the number of times the child has passed urine.

Management

The principal method of maintaining circulation is to ensure that airway and breathing are adequately addressed. As with breathing, watch for signs of decompensation:
- changes in heart rate: increasing or sudden fall
- increasing peripheral vasoconstriction:
  - capillary refill time increasing
  - warm/cold demarcation line moving up the limb towards the body
  - loss/reduction of peripheral pulses
- reduced LOC
- hypotension (late sign).

2.5.5 Disability

Assessment

Often you will already have an idea about the patient's LOC from the general impression. Use the AVPU mnemonic to quickly gauge the child's LOC:
- **A:** Alert
- **V:** Responds to voice
- **P:** Responds to pain
- **U:** Unresponsive.

Pupils should be checked for dilation, equality and reactivity. Seriously ill children are typically hypotonic and floppy, but in cases of serious brain dysfunction, posturing (particularly in response to pain), such as abnormal flexion and extension, may be seen [RCUK, 2021b].

Management

Ensure that airway, breathing and circulation are managed adequately. Don't forget to check blood glucose if you are authorised, and during the history determine whether there is a risk of poisoning or meningococcal septicaemia [JRCALC, 2023].

2.5.6 Exposure

In order to complete the primary survey it may be necessary to remove some of the child's clothing, but be mindful that children lose heat rapidly, particularly infants. Use this time to thoroughly examine infants and children who are ill for rashes. Keep in mind the possibility of an NAI, and check for bruises and other signs of injury.

18 Learning Disabilities

1 Supporting the care of people with learning disabilities

1.1 Learning objectives

By the end of this section you will be able to:
- define the term 'learning disability'
- explain the needs of a person with a learning disability in emergency care situations.

1.2 Introduction

A learning disability is a reduced intellectual ability and difficulty with everyday activities – for example household tasks, socialising or managing money – that affects someone for their whole life [Mencap, 2023a].

Learning disability includes the presence of a significantly reduced ability to understand new or complex information and to learn new skills (impaired intelligence), coupled with a reduced ability to cope independently (impaired social functioning) that started before adulthood, with a lasting effect on development [DoH, 2001].

There are estimated to be 1.3 million people with a learning disability in England, including 950,000 adults aged 18 or over [PHE, 2023].

A profound and multiple learning disability (PMLD) is when a person has a severe learning disability and other disabilities that significantly affect their ability to communicate or be independent [NHS, 2023c].

Learning disabilities are distinct from learning difficulties. Learning disability is characterised by the presence of reduced intellectual ability, whereas people with learning difficulties have a normal intellectual ability and ability to deal with everyday activities. Some of the most common learning difficulties include dyslexia, dyspraxia and attention deficit hyperactivity disorder.

1.3 Learning disabilities legislation and rights

Several pieces of legislation have already been reviewed in the 'Legal and Ethical Issues' chapter; however, you should be aware how a number of pieces of legislation apply to people with learning disabilities.

1.3.1 Legislation

Equality Act 2010
According to the Equality Act 2010, a person is disabled if a physical or mental impairment has a substantial and long-term negative effect on their ability to carry out normal daily activities [HMG, 2023]. This definition will apply to nearly all of those having a learning disability.

The Equality Act extends certain rights to those recognised as having a disability [HMG, 2023b], including:
- **Employment rights:** It is against the law for employers to discriminate against a person because of a disability. All employers must make reasonable adjustments so those with disabilities are not disadvantaged.
- **Education:** It is unlawful for education providers to treat students with disabilities unfavourably. This may be due to direct, or indirect, discrimination or forms of harassment or victimisation. As with employers, education providers must make reasonable adjustments to ensure students with disabilities are not discriminated against.
- **Police:** A person with learning disabilities should only be interviewed when a responsible person is present. The responsible person, or 'appropriate adult', should not work for the police and should have experience of working with people with learning disabilities.

Chapter 18 – Learning Disabilities

Consent and capacity

Having a learning disability does not automatically mean a person lacks mental capacity; in fact, the majority will have full capacity. As always, you must assess your patient as the individual they are and have no pre-conceived ideas as to their potential mental ability until you have completed a formal and structured assessment. The legislation for consent and capacity and the tests used to judge a person's capacity are the same for those with or without learning disabilities. Remember it is your responsibility to make reasonable adjustments, appropriate to the context in which you are working, to support someone to make their own decision where possible.

Down Syndrome Bill

The Down Syndrome Bill was introduced in 2022 and places a statutory duty on relevant authorities (which include the NHS, social care authorities, housing authorities, and education and youth offending authorities) to ensure they take account of the specific needs of people with Down's syndrome when exercising their relevant functions [Parliament, 2021]. This may include making changes to the way people access services or the services they provide to meet the specific challenges that people with Down's syndrome face.

Care Act

The 2014 Care Act helps to improve people's independence and well-being. It makes clear what services local authorities must provide and also the rights for both a person with care needs and also a carer to request a care needs assessment. Both persons requiring care and those providing care are extended a number of new rights under the act [DoH, 2023].

1.3.2 Rights

As we have outlined above, people with learning disabilities have the same rights as all other people; these rights are detailed within the Human Rights Act 1998.

People with learning disabilities have the same right to access healthcare as all other people; however, due to a number of factors, patients with learning disabilities find it far harder to access healthcare and therefore suffer the consequences, including earlier death and poor long-term condition management, as identified by Sir Jonathan Michael (2008) in his public inquiry into accessing healthcare for those with learning disabilities.

When responding, remember that patients with learning disabilities have the same rights and expectations of receiving healthcare as any other patient, and try to practise in such a way as to promote these rights and to assist with overcoming any barriers that stand in the way.

1.4 Causes of learning disabilities

There are four main causes that are responsible for learning disabilities [Holland, 2011]:
- genetics
- events before birth
- events during birth
- events after birth.

1.4.1 Genetics

Chromosomal conditions, such as Down's syndrome or fragile X syndrome, are not in themselves learning disabilities, but they do frequently cause learning disabilities.

1.4.2 Events before birth

Infections during pregnancy can be transmitted from the mother to the fetus, leading to developmental problems and learning disabilities. Other maternal factors, including dietary deficiencies, excessive alcohol consumption during the pregnancy, and endocrine disorders such as phenylketonuria, can also cause learning disabilities.

1.4.3 Events during birth

If during a traumatic or difficult delivery a baby's oxygen supply is interrupted for a significant period of time, brain damage may occur, which will cause a learning disability.

1.4.4 Events after birth

In the early years of life, a child is susceptible to many factors that may cause long-term impairment and learning disabilities as a result. Examples of this include infections, particularly meningitis or encephalitis, and traumatic injuries of the brain, sustained by falls, road traffic accidents or non-accidental injuries.

1.5 Categories of learning disabilities

Learning disabilities are categorised as mild, moderate, severe or profound [Holland, 2011]. As with all conditions, the way in which any individual is challenged by their disability will be unique to them. Many people diagnosed with learning disability will be able to lead largely independent lives, whereas others may need more significant help and support.

For people with mild learning disabilities, some occasional support for complex issues may be all that is required, whereas many people with profound and multiple learning disabilities will require more intense help, potentially through to round-the-clock care.

You must always assess any patient with learning disabilities as an individual. Understand how they would normally manage, and what level of support they require on a day-to-day basis. Do not assume, just because a person has a diagnosis of a learning disability that they are incapable of making decisions about their own care needs.

2 Disabilities and healthcare

2.1 Introduction

By the end of this section, you will be able to:
- describe how learning disabilities lead to inequality in healthcare
- describe how you may need to adapt your methods of communication when assisting a person with a learning disability
- give examples of sources of information, advice and guidance to support the well-being of people with learning disabilities
- describe how learning disabilities influence a person's vulnerability
- define 'hate crime' and what to do if you think your patient is a victim of disability hate crime.

2.2 Inequality in healthcare

People with learning disabilities tend to have poorer health than people without a learning disability, as they are more likely to have additional health problems. This includes a higher incidence of weight-related problems, mental health issues and respiratory diseases.

People with learning disabilities are also more likely to have poor health outcomes as a result of not receiving equal healthcare. This means that people with learning disabilities die younger than those in the general population and a recent study found as many as 42% of deaths in patients with learning disabilities could have been avoided if they had received better healthcare [White, 2023].

Mencap identifies the main barriers for people with a learning disability from accessing healthcare as being [Mencap, 2023b]:
- a lack of *accessible* transport links
- patients not being identified as having a learning disability
- staff having little understanding about learning disability
- failure to recognise that a person with a learning disability is unwell
- failure to make a correct diagnosis
- anxiety or a lack of confidence for people with a learning disability
- lack of joint working from different care providers
- not enough involvement allowed from carers
- inadequate aftercare or follow-up care.

2.2.1 Tackling inequality

All providers of healthcare have a legal and ethical duty to make reasonable adjustments when providing care to patients with learning disabilities [PHE, 2020]. Many of these relate to longer-term care, but as a responder you should also consider what adjustments you may need to make to your practice when caring for a patient with learning disabilities in an emergency situation. You should make all reasonable adjustments necessary to ensure that patients with learning disabilities receive the same standard of care as any other patients. Modifications required will be unique based on the situation, but very importantly you will very likely need to adjust your communication techniques.

2.3 Communication

As discussed previously, every individual will be affected by their own disability in a unique way, so in order to be able to communicate effectively you need to first understand what is normal for your patient.

For a patient with a mild or moderate learning disability you may be able to communicate in a near to normal manner, maybe just ensuring you use language that is not overly complex or challenging to understand and avoiding the use of jargon. For patients with more severe or profound learning disabilities it is likely you will need to make more significant adjustments.

Patients with profound, multiple or severe learning disabilities frequently may rely on non-verbal communication, including facial expressions, vocal sounds, body language and behaviour.

Some may have a small range of formal communication, including words, drawings, gestures or symbols. Others may not have reached any form of intentional communication and you may be relying on feedback from carers as to how changes in behaviour may be indicating pain or distress. In these situations you should seek out the advice of those who know the patient best, as they may be able to better interpret signs the patient is displaying.

You should also consider the use of specialist assessment tools, such as the Abbey pain scale, which is used to assess pain in patients who cannot verbalise, and be mindful that many people with profound learning disabilities also have some degree of visual and/or hearing disability [FPLD, 2023].

Some further guidelines for communicating with people who have learning disabilities include [Mencap, 2023c]:
- Find a good place to communicate in, somewhere quiet without distractions. If you are talking to a large group, be aware that some people may find this difficult.
- Ask open questions.
- Check with the person that you understand what they are saying, e.g. 'The TV isn't working? Have I got that right?'
- If the person wants to take you to show you something, go with them.
- Watch the person. They may tell you things by their body language and facial expressions.
- Learn from experience. You will need to be more observant and don't feel awkward about asking parents/carers for their help.
- Try drawing. Even if your drawing is not great, it might still be helpful.
- Take your time, do not rush your communication.
- Use gestures and facial expressions. If you are asking if someone is unhappy, make your facial expression unhappy to reinforce what you are saying.
- Be aware that some people find it easier to use real objects to communicate, but photos and pictures can really help too.

2.4 Learning disabilities and vulnerability

People with learning disabilities are more vulnerable to harm due to their disability. As with other types of abuse, this harm could take the form of physical abuse, mental abuse, financial abuse or sexual abuse.

People with learning disabilities are also often victims of hate crimes. Disability hate crime is any incident/crime which is perceived by the victim or any other person to be motivated by a hostility or prejudice based on a person's disability or perceived disability [CPS, 2022].

It is thought that the vast majority of hate crimes go unreported at present, with as little as 1% leading to a prosecution [Leonard Cheshire, 2022]. As with all vulnerable people, you should do all you can to tackle a person's vulnerability and ensure their safety. Any activity that may be described as a hate crime should be reported to the police.

Refer to Chapter 4, 'Legal and Ethical Issues', and Chapter 5, 'Safeguarding Adults and Children', for more information on safeguarding and how to make a safeguarding referral when appropriate. If you believe a person is in imminent danger, then you should contact the police for immediate assistance.

2.5 Further support

In the management of an individual incident, you should look to friends, family and carers to help support your patient where possible. You may also be able to get further advice and support from:

- social workers
- support agencies.

Also consider what local expertise may be available through specialist learning disability nurses or charities, such as Mencap (www.mencap.org.uk).

Chapter 19 Older People

1 Ageing

1.1 Learning objective

By the end of this section you will be able to:
- describe the anatomical and physiological changes that occur as a person ages.

1.2 Introduction

Older people are generally defined as those aged over 65 years; however, ageing is a highly unique process and there may be patients at a lower age who have the same conditions and vulnerabilities as those aged 65 and over. So, although being aged over 65 is still the most accepted definition of older people, you should consider that those aged 50–64 may also have the same issues, depending on the unique progression of their own disease, vulnerabilities or risk factors [NICE, 2013].

The percentage of the population classed as older is growing rapidly, with over 18% of the UK population aged over 65 years in the 2021 Census [ONS, 2022] and predictions indicating that by 2037 this will reach nearly 25% [ONS, 2018b].

Although there are no national statistics relating to the number of older people who call the ambulance service, around 45% of the 4,374,611 people who attended an emergency department in 2012/13, and arrived by ambulance, were over the age of 65 [HSCIC, 2014].

1.3 Anatomy and physiology of ageing

There is no single mechanism of ageing. Instead, there are a range of mechanisms that over time result in the worsening of cell function, causing cellular damage and impairing the body's ability to repair itself. This results in a range of anatomical and physiological changes (Figure 19.1).

1.3.1 Musculoskeletal system

Bones, joints and muscles are all affected by ageing.

Bones

Bone formation is greatest in the period from birth to adolescence, but equalises with bone absorption in a person's twenties, before bone absorption becomes more dominant. This leads to a reduction in body calcium, impairing the body's ability to create bone matrix and increasing the risk of fractures. Cancellous bones, such as those found in the vertebral bodies, wrists and hips, are especially vulnerable. Calcium supplements are often prescribed, as absorption of calcium from the digestive system also declines with age [Farley, 2011].

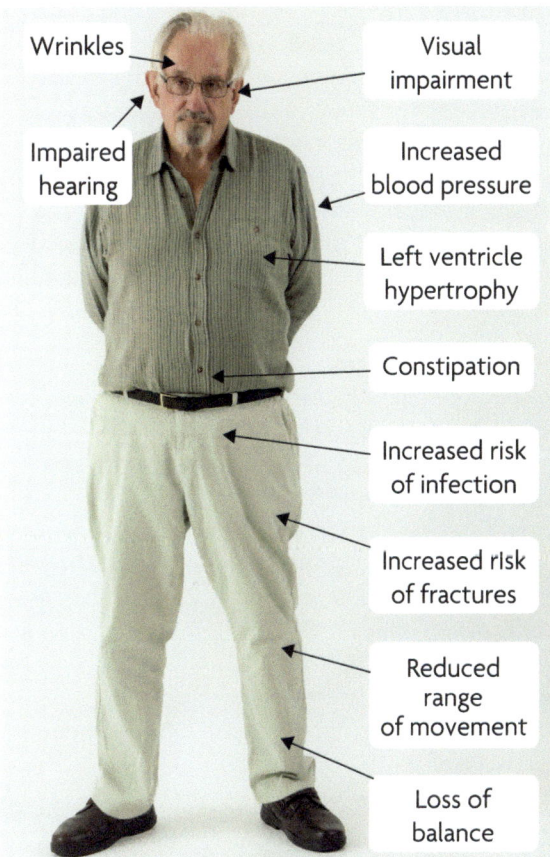

Figure 19.1 Changes related to ageing

Joints

The loss of fluid within the intervertebral discs results in kyphosis, the familiar stooped posture of older age, which also reduces the height of the person. With stooping comes a change in the person's centre of gravity and changes to their gait, which becomes slower, shorter and more cautious [Knight, 2008d].

Muscles

Muscles degrade (atrophy), leading to a reduction in muscle strength and mass. The rate of decline is variable, with some muscles, such as the diaphragm, remaining unchanged, whereas the lower limbs can experience noticeable wasting. Coupled with the decline in nervous system function, movement speed is reduced, and increased muscle rigidity results in limited movement in the neck, shoulders, hips and knees [Farley, 2011].

1.3.2 Respiratory system

The respiratory system is in steady decline from around the age of 25, following a functional peak at 20 years of age. There are a variety of external factors which adversely affect the respiratory system, including poor nutrition, lack of physical exercise and smoking [Farley, 2011]. Changes due to ageing are fairly insignificant compared to the external factors, as there is usually sufficient spare capacity in lung function to offset any decline due to older age.

Ventilatory changes

Respiratory function does deteriorate with age, in tandem with the decline of the musculoskeletal system. The strength of the respiratory system declines from around 55 years of age, with intercostal muscle wasting, increasing the work of breathing and making the respiratory system more reliant on the diaphragm [Knight, 2008a]. Shortness of breath on exertion (SOBOE) is more common in older people due to [Farley, 2011]:
- decreasing muscle strength
- muscles being more prone to fatigue when work of breathing increases
- muscle wasting
- decreased blood supply to the muscles of respiration.

Most measurements of lung function decline with age, but in healthy patients this is mostly offset by a large reserve capacity of the respiratory system [Farley, 2011].

1.3.3 Cardiovascular system

Blood vessels

As the body ages, blood vessels (particularly the arteries) lose their elasticity and become less compliant. The arteries thicken, which makes them more rigid, and the normally smooth inner layer (tunica interna) becomes roughened, which increases the resistance to blood flow [Knight, 2008b]. This contributes to a rise in systolic blood pressure.

Heart

In order to overcome the increase in systemic vascular resistance, the heart needs to pump with greater force; like all muscles that are exercised, it thickens (hypertrophies) over time, particularly in the left ventricle.

There are also changes in the electrical conduction system, with the loss of around 50–75% of pacemaker cells by the age of 50 leading to an increased chance that the heart will go into an abnormal rhythm.

1.3.4 Nervous system

Brain and senses

In healthy people the ageing brain functions normally, and learning, for example, is still able to occur. However, brain weight does decline by approximately 5–10% over a lifetime with little change up to the age of 50 years. Indeed, it is not until 60 years of age and older that there is a significant reduction in weight [Farley, 2011].

About 10% of neurons are lost by the age of 75, but this does not result in significant loss of mental function. However, the loss of sensory neurons leads to impaired hearing, vision, smell, temperature regulation and appreciation of pain. In addition, older people become increasingly reliant on visual, tactile and auditory cues to stay on their feet since their brain becomes less able to sense balance, which increases the risk of falling, particularly if any/all of these senses are impaired [Knight, 2008c].

1.3.5 Immune system

From a functional peak around puberty, there is a gradual reduction in immune system capacity over a person's lifetime of between 5% and 30%, but the immune system does continue to function even in very old adults. However, older people are more likely to die of infectious diseases, such as pneumonia, influenza and gastroenteritis, for example. In addition, older adults respond to infection differently from younger adults, including the following responses [Farley, 2011]:

- Fewer micro-organisms are required to cause symptomatic infection.
- Confusion prior to a raised temperature is more common.
- Symptoms can be masked and/or mistaken for other diseases.
- There is an increased risk from chronic diseases such as diabetes and COPD.

1.3.6 Integumentary system

The skin is probably the most visible sign of older age and all layers are affected [Farley, 2011]:

- **Epidermis:** Loss of skin cells leads to decreased surface contact between the dermis and epidermis, which reduces the exchange of nutrients and other products of metabolism. In addition, the epidermis degrades, causing roughened skin that takes longer to heal and provides less of a barrier.
- **Dermis:** This layer also degrades, becoming thinner. The dramatic reduction in dermal blood vessels leads to pallor, decreased temperature and impaired thermoregulation compounded by a loss of sensory nerve endings, increasing the risk of injury.
- **Hypodermis:** A reduction in subcutaneous fat leads to increased conductive heat loss, and the redistribution of the fat leads to bony prominences, which are vulnerable to pressure ulcers and fractures following trauma. Clinically, the skin looks dry, lax and wrinkly. The wrinkles are due to a combination of gravity, decreasing subcutaneous fat and, in the face, repeated traction by facial muscles. In addition, photo-ageing caused by UV radiation from the sun increases the number of skin lesions, which are usually benign, although they can become cancerous later in life.

1.3.7 Digestive system

Food intake declines with age, with about a 10% reduction in calorific intake each decade after 50 years of age. Older people may experience altered taste, linked mainly to a decrease in the sense of smell and smell discrimination. In addition, they are more likely to have missing teeth and poorly fitting dentures, all of which contribute to weight loss and malnutrition becoming more common. Increased intake of sugar and salt can contribute to the development of diabetes and high blood pressure [Nigam, 2008].

Muscular contractions that initiate the swallowing reflex also decline with age, leading to an increased risk of choking. Lower down the GI tract, there is impaired absorption of essential fats and other nutrients, while in the large intestine the process of moving the contents through (peristalsis) slows, increasing the transit time of bowel contents, which can cause constipation. This in turn can lead to the formation of haemorrhoids due to the increased straining required to defecate [Nigam, 2008].

2 Caring for older patients

2.1 *Learning objectives*

By the end of this section you will be able to:
- Identify a range of common conditions associated with ageing
- describe the impact co-morbidities (the presence of other diseases) will have on your treatment plans
- discuss attitudes towards ageing.

2.2 *Age-related conditions*

The following are a range of conditions commonly associated with older patients; however, these conditions are not necessarily unique to older

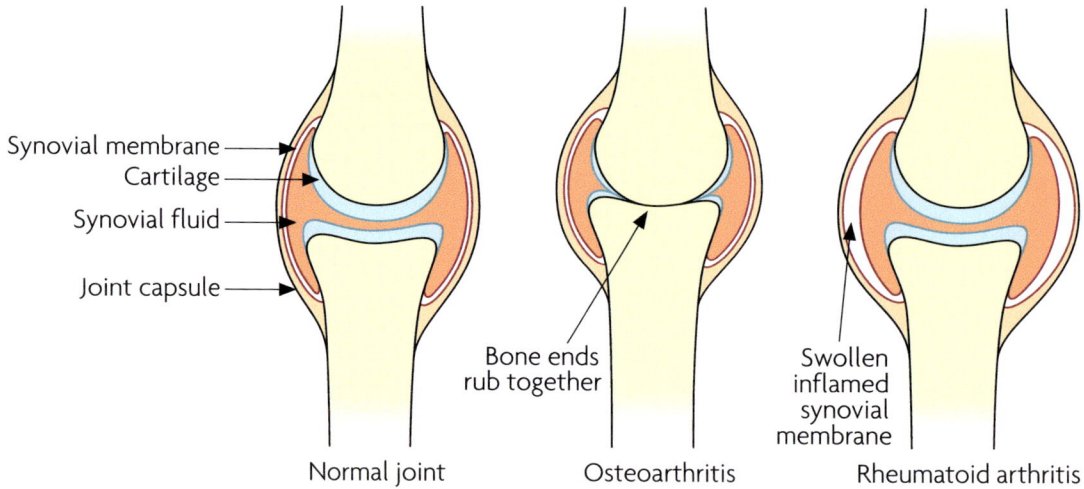

Figure 19.2 Normal and arthritic joints

patients and can be seen in younger people as well in certain circumstances.

2.2.1 Parkinson's

Due to the death of cells in the brain, patients with Parkinson's disease don't have enough of the neurotransmitter dopamine. One in 500 people in the UK suffers from the disease for which there is no cure and no known cause [Parkinson's UK, 2015]. The main symptoms of Parkinson's are tremor, rigidity and slowness of movement but may also include:

- tiredness
- pain
- depression
- constipation.

Parkinson's is treated with a combination of medication, therapy and occasionally surgery to help alleviate symptoms and slow the progression of the disease.

2.2.2 Arthritis

Arthritis is defined as inflammation within a joint. There are many different forms of the condition, but the two main ones are osteoarthritis and rheumatoid arthritis [NHS, 2022d].

Osteoarthritis

A normal joint is covered at the ends of the bone in smooth cartilage, to allow bone ends to glide across each other. In degenerative forms of arthritis, these smooth cartilage ends have been worn away. The underlying bone tries to repair this but often overgrows, altering the shape of the joint, known as osteoarthritis.

Osteoarthritis is particularly common in joints that see heavy use, including the hips and knees, base of the thumb and big toe (Figure 19.2).

Rheumatoid arthritis

Inflammation is a normal response as part of the body's healing process, but in patients with this form of arthritis the inflammation happens for no obvious reason. This is an autoimmune condition (the body's own immune system is attacking the joints) and instead of helping to repair the body it causes damage to the joint, pain and stiffness. This type of arthritis often affects several joints at once. As well as joint pain, other symptoms of rheumatoid arthritis include:

- tiredness
- depression
- irritability
- flu-like symptoms.

2.2.3 Osteoporosis

Bones are constantly going through a process of regenerating themselves by breaking down old matter and replacing it with new. Up to around the late twenties bone density increases slowly, and from around 35 years onwards it starts (very gradually at first) to decrease as part of the natural ageing process. However, in certain people this can be accelerated and lead to weaker bones, which are more likely to fracture as a result.

Osteoporosis occurs when the mesh-like structure within bones becomes thin, causing bones to become fragile and break easily [ROS, 2021]. Women are more susceptible to osteoporosis due to increased bone loss in the years following the menopause.

The main risk of osteoporosis is the increased risk of fractures from just minor forces, rather than the significant force we would normally expect to cause a fracture. Broken hips and wrists are common injuries, as is a broken neck or back in a fall from just standing height.

2.2.4 Elderly mental illness

It is thought by some that mental health problems are a normal part of ageing, but this is not necessarily the case, with most older people developing no mental health problems, and many of those that do can be helped or treated, or the onset even prevented with the right action early on [MHF, 2015].

Dementia

Dementia is one of the most common causes of mental illness in older patients, and we will look at this in some detail in the next section of this chapter.

Depression

Depression is another common mental illness in later life that makes people feel sad and lack motivation [Age UK, 2022]. We all have these feelings at times, but depression occurs when these feelings are more intense and persist for weeks, months or longer. Depression is often linked to loss, which is common as people grow older. These losses can influence people's self-esteem and feeling of value and include:
- loss of job
- loss of good health
- loss of independence
- loss of spouse or friends
- loss of social network.

As with depression at any age, a number of treatment options, including medication and talking therapies, are available. It is also possible that certain things can be done to prevent the development of depression to begin with.

Many elderly people are isolated and spend prolonged periods of time on their own. Arranging for appropriate social interactions can help to alleviate these feelings of isolation and prevent the development of depression in the first place.

When treating elderly patients, make sure you consider the risk of depression as part of your holistic assessments. Mental and physical health are closely intertwined and you should be looking to always promote an individual's mental well-being as well as their physical.

2.3 *Attitudes to ageing*

Attitudes towards ageing are fundamental for ageing well and current attitudes towards ageing in society and the media may be negatively impacting on the older population [AAA, 2015]. As has already been discussed, ageing is unique to every individual and age itself is no marker for a person's independence, or ability to contribute to society. Some people will have a range of age-related illnesses in their sixties whereas others will live long into their nineties with limited if any illness or disability.

Everyone, regardless of age, should be encouraged to live the best-quality life that they can and you must not judge anyone's ability on purely their age, as doing so would not just lead to an inaccurate assessment, but would also be considered discrimination under the Equality Act.

2.4 *Patients with co-morbidities*

When treating elderly patients, it is often the case that they have a number of simultaneous co-morbidities, for example a patient with cardiovascular disease and type 2 diabetes; both of these are serious long-term conditions that can be life limiting, especially if not managed correctly.

Chapter 19 – Older People

They also interact with each other and can make the other disease worse. This makes caring for patients very challenging as a number of conditions may be interacting with each other and causing varied presentations.

Many of these patients will have specialist medical or nursing support and might be under the care of a chronic condition management team, or community matron.

When dealing with patients with a range of co-morbidities, be sure to consider all of the conditions that may be influencing the current presentation: do not become fixated on just one element of the patient's illness. These cases are complex and in elderly patients, who may already have compromised immune systems or compensatory mechanisms, can represent significant dangers. Be prepared to seek additional help and support early on in such situations and recognise the limitations of your own scope of practice and knowledge where necessary.

3 Dementia

3.1 Learning objectives

By the end of this section you will be able to:
- define dementia
- explain the differences between dementia and delirium
- describe a number of strategies that can assist when communicating with a patient with dementia
- identify a number of causes of challenging behaviour
- explain how to manage challenging behaviour.

3.2 Introduction

Dementia is not a disease in its own right. Instead, it is an umbrella term to cover a range of conditions and diseases that result in the gradual death of cells within the brain, leading to progressive cognitive decline. The most common symptoms include: memory loss, confusion, mood and personality changes, and problems with planning and performing tasks in the right order [Alzheimers Society, 2024].

Dementia is an 'organic' disorder, meaning there is an associated physical deterioration of the brain tissue, which can be seen via a brain scan or, after death, at autopsy, though depending on the exact type of dementia, different physical changes will be seen. Dementia is progressive – the damage and symptoms get worse over time and are irreversible. It is therefore not a normal result of ageing, but rather is the result of a disease.

3.2.1 Dementia in context

As of early 2024, there are around 900,000 people in the UK living with dementia [Alzheimer's Society, 2024]. One in 11 people aged over 65 have dementia in the UK and the prevalence is more common in women than men. Dementia is an increasing challenge as people are living longer, and by 2030 it is estimated that the number of people in the UK living with dementia will have reached over 1 million [NHS, 2023d].

3.3 Dementia

Dementia tends to affect people in three different ways:
- **Cognitive:** As the areas of the brain responsible for cognition are damaged and the number of cells are reduced, patients are less able to deal with complex thought processes or store memories so easily.
- **Behavioural:** As different areas of the brain are affected, a person's behaviour may change. This is particularly seen in frontotemporal dementia where the person may lose a sense of inhibition.
- **Neurological:** Physical changes to the structure of the brain mean that the brain of those with dementia is not able to function appropriately. A loss of brain cells and a change to the types and quantity of chemicals in the brain lead to a vast alteration in neurological function. In some forms, including dementia with Lewy bodies, physical signs such as shaking may develop, showing changes to the neurological system.

3.3.1 Different types of dementia

There are many different types of dementia, with Alzheimer's disease being the most common single cause in the UK, making up around two-thirds of cases, and vascular dementia coming in second. However, multiple-disease processes are even more common than single-disease processes, with Alzheimer's disease and vascular dementia, and Alzheimer's disease and Lewy bodies dementia, being common combinations.

3.3.2 Causes of dementia

Different forms of dementia have different underlying causes; here we will consider some of the most common types [Alzheimer's Society, 2015c; NHS Choices, 2015]. Dementia is normally caused by gradual changes in the brain, often associated with brain cells dying quicker than they should as part of the normal ageing process. It is thought that an abnormal protein present within the brain is responsible for a lot of this premature degeneration.

Some causes include:
- Lewy bodies
- frontotemporal dementia
- infections, including encephalitis
- some brain tumours
- lack of thyroid hormone
- head injury
- long-term alcohol abuse.

Alzheimer's disease
In Alzheimer's disease loss of brain cells leads to the brain shrinking. The cerebral cortex, the area of the brain responsible for processing thought and other complex functions including memory, calculation and some communication skills, is most affected.

Clumps of protein gather in the brain and it is thought that they are responsible for the increased rate of brain cell death. Connections between brain cells are also lost and the chemicals that normally carry signals, known as neurotransmitters, are greatly reduced, all of which leads to the cognitive impairment seen.

Vascular dementia
Vascular dementia occurs when cells are damaged due to a lack of blood and therefore oxygen reaching brain tissue. As people age, their vessels tend to become narrower and harden where fatty deposits develop. This process, called atherosclerosis, means that less blood can get through the vessels and surrounding brain tissue is starved of oxygen. Patients who have been diagnosed with small vessel disease or have previously had a stroke or a TIA are at increased risk of developing vascular dementia.

3.3.3 Disease progression

Every patient will have a unique disease progression; however, the main forms of dementia are all progressive, i.e. they will all get worse with time. The speed at which any individual's disease progresses will vary widely and is based on many factors, including their age at time of onset, genetics, and other physical and mental health [Alzheimer's Society, 2015b]. Patients with a history of poorly controlled heart disease or diabetes are likely to experience a faster deterioration.

The Alzheimer's Society (2015b) divides the progression of the disease in three broad stages:

Early (mild) stage
Dementia normally begins with mild, subtle changes in a person's abilities or behaviour. The changes are often incorrectly thought to just be part of the normal ageing process, and include:
- loss of memory of recent events
- mislaying items around the house
- becoming confused easily
- losing track of the day or date.

Middle (moderate) stage
As the disease progresses changes become more obvious and a greater degree of help is required in day-to-day life. Changes may include:
- needing frequent reminders or help to eat, wash, dress and use the toilet
- increasingly forgetful – especially of names
- becoming confused about where they are, and may try to walk off to find somewhere else

- experiencing difficulty with perception, and may start to have delusions.

Changes in behaviour are more commonly seen in this stage and patients can become easily upset, angry or even aggressive – perhaps because they are misinterpreting events or do not understand what is happening.

Late (severe) stage

At this stage individuals will need increasing levels of help with daily activities and may gradually become totally dependent on others for nursing care. Loss of memory can become severe and they may not recognise people and their surroundings, though they may have occasional moments of clarity or recognition.

Behaviour changes can become very severe with restlessness, agitation and angry outbursts, occurring particularly during close personal care, usually because the person does not understand what is happening.

This stage of the disease can be very distressing for both the patient and their family and carers and needs to be managed gently and tactfully.

3.3.4 Dementia and other diseases

When assessing a patient with dementia, be careful not to attribute changes in their status to the on-going deterioration of the condition without good evidence to do so. Dementia normally progresses slowly and any sudden changes should trigger a search for a different cause. Many patients with dementia will have other co-morbidities and a detailed assessment will be required to identify any underlying illness.

Asking people who are familiar with the patient for detailed information on their condition is a good way to find out what is normal for them.

3.3.5 Treating patients with dementia

Responding for the ambulance service, it is likely that you will frequently meet patients with dementia, at various stages of the disease progression. Managing these patients may require some significant modifications to your usual approach, and although every encounter will be unique, you should consider the following guidance:

- Approach all situations in a calm manner: Your patient may be confused, scared or not understand what is happening. A calm manner on your part can help to relax your patient and make them feel safe.
- Communicate clearly and be patient: more details for communicating with a patient with dementia is included in the next section.
- Use relatives, friends and carers wherever possible to aid communication and to help the patient feel more relaxed by having a friendly familiar face present.

Be compassionate: Remember that every person is different and will need different management – there is no one way to manage 'patients with dementia'.

3.3.6 Dementia and pain management

Pain management is a difficult issue, especially for those who are not able to communicate effectively. It is well recognised that patients with dementia frequently receive inadequate pain relief [Chandler, 2014], and that is especially true of emergency care patients.

One of the key challenges is that patients are unable to express their pain, so healthcare staff tend to underestimate the amount of pain a patient is suffering and therefore not provide adequate pain management techniques.

It is likely that the ambulance crews that back you up will use specialist tools, to help determine whether or not a patient with dementia is in pain. One such tool designed for use with patients with late-stage dementia is the Abbey pain scale (Figure 19.3) [Abbey, 2004].

3.3.7 Dementia and discrimination

The Equality Act 2010 defines a disability as any physical or mental impairment that has a 'substantial' and 'long-term' negative effect on a person's ability to carry out normal daily activities. Clearly, dementia meets these criteria, so those that have dementia are protected by the Equality

The Abbey Pain Scale

For measurement of pain in people with dementia who cannot verbalise.

How to use scale: While observing the resident, score questions 1 to 6.

Name of resident:..

Name and designation of person completing the scale:..

Date: .... Time: ....

Latest pain relief given was.. at ....hrs.

Q1. Vocalisation
eg whimpering, groaning, crying
Absent 0   Mild 1   Moderate 2   Severe 3

Q1 [ ]

Q2. Facial expression
eg looking tense, frowning, grimacing, looking frightened
Absent 0   Mild 1   Moderate 2   Severe 3

Q2 [ ]

Q3. Change in body language
eg fidgeting, rocking, guarding part of body, withdrawn
Absent 0   Mild 1   Moderate 2   Severe 3

Q3 [ ]

Q4. Behavioural change
eg increased confusion, refusing to eat, alteration in usual patterns
Absent 0   Mild 1   Moderate 2   Severe 3

Q4 [ ]

Q5. Physiological change
eg temperature, pulse or blood pressure outside normal limits, perspiring, flushing of pallor
Absent 0   Mild 1   Moderate 2   Severe 3

Q5 [ ]

Q6. Physical changes
eg skin tears, pressure areas, arthritis, contractures, previous injuries
Absent 0   Mild 1   Moderate 2   Severe 3

Q6 [ ]

Add scores for Q1 to Q6 and record here ➔ Total pain score [ ]

Now tick the box that matches the Total Pain Score ➔

0–2	3–7	8–13	14+
No pain	Mild	Moderate	Severe

Finally, tick the box which matches the type of pain ➔

Chronic	Acute	Acute on chronic

Abbey J, De Bellis A, Piller N, Esterman A, Gilles L, Parker D, Lowcay B. The Abbey Pain Scale. Funded by the JH & JD Gunn Medical Research Foundation 1998–2002.
(This document may be reproduced with this reference retained.)

Figure 19.3 The Abbey pain scale

Source: Abbey, Piller, De Bellis, et al. (2004). 'The Abbey pain scale: a 1-minute numerical indicator for people with end-stage dementia', *International Journal of Palliative Nursing.* 10:1, 6–13. Copyright © 2004 MA Healthcare Ltd. Reproduced courtesy of MA Healthcare Ltd.

Act, which makes it illegal to discriminate against them on the basis of their disability. Nonetheless, the Alzheimer's Society (2015a) identifies that patients with dementia are frequently discriminated against for a broad range of reasons, including:

- **Stigma:** Dementia is still highly stigmatised and a failure to understand the broad nature of the disease is common.
- **Impaired mental capacity:** It is often assumed that patients are unable to make even simple

decisions for themselves so others decide for them, without having taken all reasonable steps to support the person in making the decision themselves.
- **Ageism:** Dementia is generally an illness of older persons, meaning that many symptoms are put down to 'getting old' rather than being tackled and treated appropriately.

When caring for patients with dementia, remember that every patient is an individual, with a unique illness and unique needs. Therefore, you must tailor your treatment so it is uniquely appropriate for each patient you come into contact with.

3.3.8 Dementia vs delirium

If dementia can be thought of as chronic brain failure, then delirium is acute brain failure [Barrett, 2014]. Unlike dementia, it is usually temporary and there is an underlying cause which can normally be corrected, for example an acute infection. It is a common and serious condition that is characterised by disruptions in thinking, consciousness, attention, cognition and perception. Unlike dementia, its onset is over a short period of time (typically hours to days). To complicate matters, patients with dementia can also develop delirium and this has been associated with serious complications and a poor outcome, including death [Fick, 2002].

Delirium is often divided into three subtypes [Hosker, 2017]:
- **Hyperactive:** Characterised by anxiety, restlessness, irritability, anger and frustration. Patients may be easily startled and distracted, and unable to sit still. Speech can be loud, but incoherent with frequent topic-hopping.
- **Hypoactive:** Patients with hypoactive delirium are typically lethargic, apathetic, slow in movement, withdrawn, drowsy and difficult to wake.
- **Mixed:** A combination of the two other variants, with patients fluctuating between hyperactive and hypoactive delirium throughout the day.

Differentiating between delirium and dementia can be difficult, especially in the pre-hospital setting where you do not know the patient and it can be hard to clearly establish a baseline. If in doubt, it is safer to assume delirium, as this is more commonly associated with acute illness, and ensure patients receive prompt medical attention [SAS, 2014].

3.4 Communication

Although the principles of communication have already been covered in Chapter 3, 'Communication', there are some additional points to consider when you are caring for a patient with dementia:
- **Get their attention:** Approach the patient from the front so they can see you coming. Try to make eye contact and ensure they can see your face and body movements.
- **Use their name:** Using their name can help them understand that you are not a stranger (although this may not be true), which can be reassuring.
- **Frequently remind them who you are:** This can reduce anxiety and avoid the patient becoming alarmed at being treated by a stranger.
- **Keep ambient noise and activity to a minimum:** Reducing distractions, activity and noise will help a patient with dementia (indeed most patients) to concentrate on what you are saying.
- **Do not rush:** Take your time. Slowing your rate of speech can help, but increase the time spent speaking AND listening. It may help if you silently count to seven between short sentences, and then give the patient the same time to answer.
- **Keep calm:** Adopt a calm tone and manner to reduce distress and make the patient feel more comfortable with you. Patients with dementia maintain the ability to determine your body language even after their ability to understand speech has been lost.
- **Keep things simple:** Avoid jargon and speak in short and simple to understand sentences. When giving instruction, break down the task into simple stages. Give clear instructions; for example, rather than saying 'sit there' you could try saying 'sit in this blue chair, please'.
- **Use the patient's preferred method of communication:** Establish this early on from

the patient and others who know them. This includes speaking to the patient in their first language or using communication aids such as pictures or talking mats.

3.5 *Challenging behaviour*

Many patients with dementia are placid and sweet-tempered, but over 90% will exhibit some form of challenging behaviour. This includes [Barrett, 2014]:
- sleeplessness
- wandering
- agitation
- pacing
- aggression (including spitting)
- disinhibition
- jealousy (especially sexual jealousy).

Challenging behaviour needs to be seen as a manifestation of unmet need, which the patient may not be able to express, such as boredom, frustration and/or annoyance.

3.5.1 Managing challenging behaviour

It is important to appreciate that each patient will be slightly different, so the best way of managing challenging behaviour will need to be tailored to them. Advice from carers and/or relatives may help, but general principles include [SAS, 2014]:
- Trying to find out what is the cause of the behaviour.
- Reducing the stress and/or demands placed on the patient.
- Explaining what is happening using the patient's name and saying who you are. You are likely to have to repeat this process often.
- Giving patients time to respond to your requests or questions.
- Trying not to show criticism or irritation and avoiding confrontation with patients.
- Watching for warning signs that they are becoming more anxious or agitated. Get help if the situation does not calm down quickly.
- Referring to carers and/or relatives who know the patient and who will have experience in managing the patient's challenging behaviour.
- Avoiding making sudden movements or using a sharp tone; instead, remain calm and keep your voice low.

Chapter

20 Cardiac Arrest

1 Basic life support (BLS) and defibrillation

1.1 Learning objectives

By the end of this section you will be able to:
- explain the benefits of the chain of survival to BLS
- describe the types of cardiopulmonary arrest
- recognise when it is appropriate to use a defibrillator
- explain the safety considerations when using a defibrillator.

1.2 Introduction

Cardiac arrest is the ultimate medical emergency, but you will have the ability to undertake the two most effective treatments for this: CPR (more commonly called BLS in healthcare circles) and defibrillation. However, the role of the responder and ambulance service is just one link in a chain which maximises the patient's chance, not only of a return of spontaneous circulation (ROSC), but also of surviving to hospital discharge neurologically intact (i.e. with normal or near-normal brain function) [Olasveengen, 2021]. That chain is known as the chain of survival [RCUK, 2021a].

1.3 Chain of survival

The chain of survival encompasses four key principles that are required if a resuscitation is to be successful in adults (Figure 20.1) [Olasveengen, 2021]:
- early recognition and call for help
- early bystander CPR
- early defibrillation
- post-resuscitation care.

1.3.1 Early recognition and call for help

This relies on patients and the public calling for help early on and can be influenced by the ambulance service with public education and training sessions. Recognition of cardiac chest pain is particularly important as around 21–33% of patients with acute myocardial ischaemia will suffer a cardiac arrest in the first hour following onset [Müller, 2006].

1.3.2 Early CPR

Performing CPR immediately following cardiac arrest can double or triple the chance of the patient surviving [Semeraro, 2021]. When a member of the public calls 999, they will be given advice on how to perform chest compressions only, based on the thought that initiation of chest compressions is more important than a delay in starting ventilation.

1.3.3 Early defibrillation

Providing good-quality CPR and defibrillating in the first 3–5 minutes of a cardiac arrest can produce survival rates of 50–70%, but, conversely, the chance of surviving to hospital discharge falls by 10–12% for every minute of delay [RCUK, 2021a].

1.3.4 Post-resuscitation care

Restarting your patient's heart and palpating a pulse (ROSC) is a great feeling, but the patient is not out of the woods yet. The true measure of success is returning the patient to their pre-cardiac arrest state, with brain function intact so that they can leave hospital. Providing post-resuscitation care on

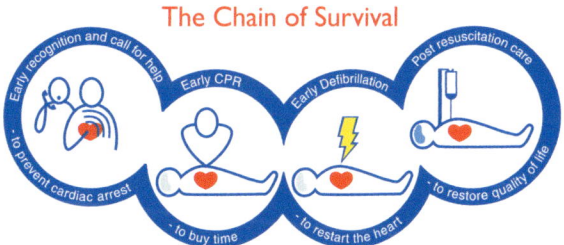

Figure 20.1 The chain of survival
Source: Image reproduced courtesy of Laerdal Medical

Chapter 20 – Cardiac Arrest

scene, en route and in hospital is crucial if this is to happen [RCUK, 2021a].

1.3.5 Children

In stark contrast to adults, children usually suffer a cardiac arrest secondary to hypoxia. The outcomes from these secondary cardiac arrests are very poor and the emphasis with children is to intervene before their heart arrests [RCUK, 2021b].

1.4 Defibrillation

Heart rhythms associated with cardiac arrest are divided into shockable and non-shockable rhythms, depending on whether they should receive an electric current across the myocardium (heart muscle) to depolarise a sufficient amount of the heart muscle simultaneously and allow the normal heart pacemaker (the sinoatrial node) to resume control of the electrical conduction system. Delivering electricity to the heart in this way is known as defibrillation [RCUK, 2021a].

In patients who have a shockable rhythm, the sooner they receive defibrillation, the greater the chance it will be successful and the patient will survive. However, it is equally important to ensure that defibrillation minimises the interruption of CPR. For each 5-second delay in CPR prior to delivering a shock, the chance of the shock being successful is halved [RCUK, 2021a].

1.4.1 Shockable rhythms

There are two shockable rhythms: ventricular fibrillation (VF) and pulseless ventricular tachycardia.

Ventricular fibrillation (VF)
VF is a rapid and disorganised ventricular rhythm and is never associated with a palpable pulse. On an ECG, you will not see any discernible P, QRS or T waves and complexes, and the rate of the undulations is typically between 150 and 500 [Garcia, 2004]. The height (amplitude) of the electrical activity you can see is often referred to as its coarseness (Figure 20.2). As a rule of thumb, if you find it difficult to decide whether the rhythm is VF or asystole (more on this shortly), you should not shock the patient [Soar, 2021].

Ventricular tachycardia (VT)
VT is known as a broad- or wide-complex tachycardia because the QRS complexes are >0.12 seconds in duration (typically 0.16–0.20 seconds). It usually originates from the ventricles, is monomorphic (has one shape), and has a regular rhythm at a rate of 100–300/minute (Figure 20.3) [Garcia, 2004; RCUK, 2021a]. Unlike patients with VF, patients with VT may have a pulse and/or signs of life, so always check before defibrillating.

1.4.2 Non-shockable rhythms

As with shockable rhythms, there are two non-shockable rhythms: asystole and pulseless electrical activity (PEA). As the name implies, these are patients who will not benefit from defibrillation.

Asystole
Asystole is the term given to the absence of electrical activity from the heart. On an ECG, you will see a flat (isoelectric) or almost flat line (Figure 20.4) [Garcia, 2004]. A variant of asystole is

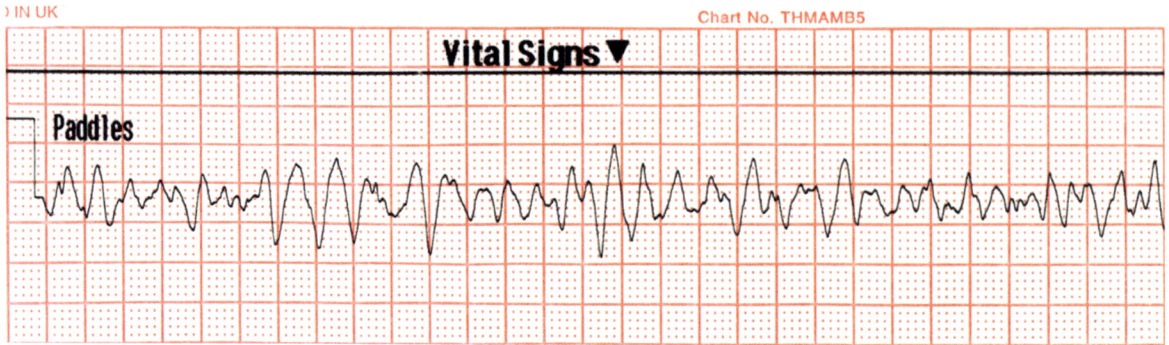

Figure 20.2 Ventricular fibrillation

Basic life support (BLS) and defibrillation

an agonal rhythm, which is characterised by a slow (rate of <20/minute), irregular and wide ventricular complexes, often varying in shape (morphology).

Pulseless electrical activity (PEA)

PEA is organised electrical activity in the absence of a palpable pulse (Figure 20.5). Typically, patients in PEA will have some mechanical myocardial activity, but it is not sufficiently strong to produce an adequate cardiac output to lead to a detectable pulse or blood pressure [RCUK, 2021a]. PEA is associated with a number of reversible causes that are a key component of advanced life support. As with VT, it is important to feel for a pulse and/or look for signs of life prior to determining the need for CPR.

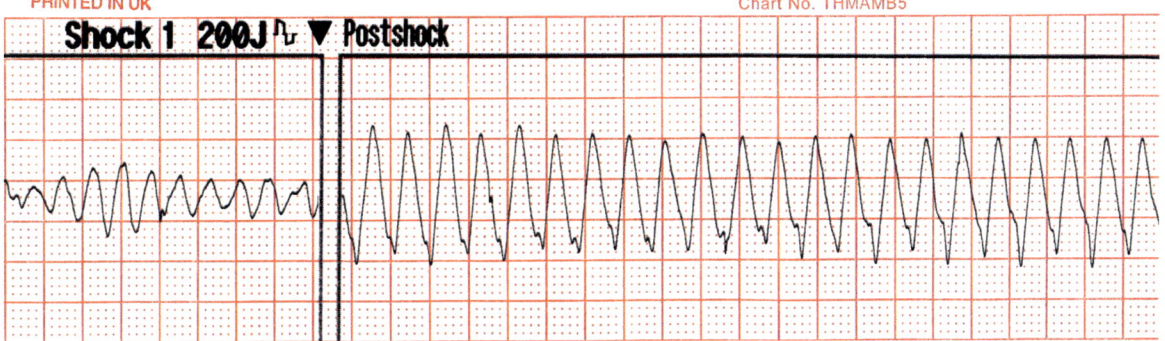

Figure 20.3 VT following a 200 J shock. The patient was in VF prior to the shock

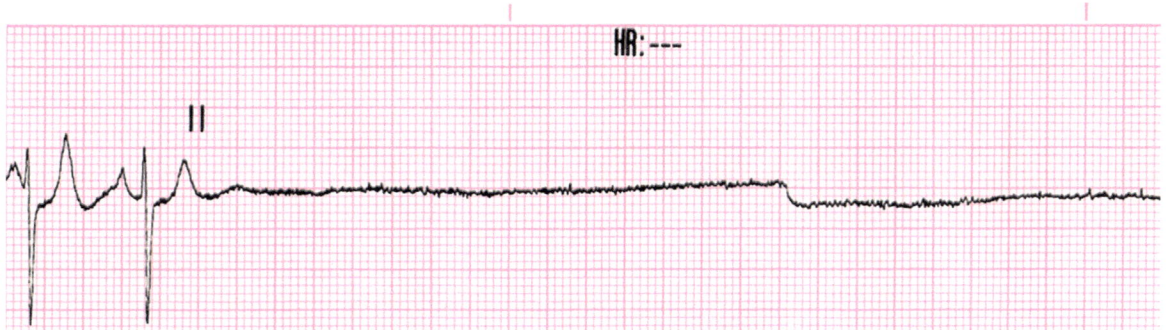

Figure 20.4 Asystole. Note the two complexes on the left-hand side of the ECG before the start of asystole. The baseline is not always completely straight in asystole

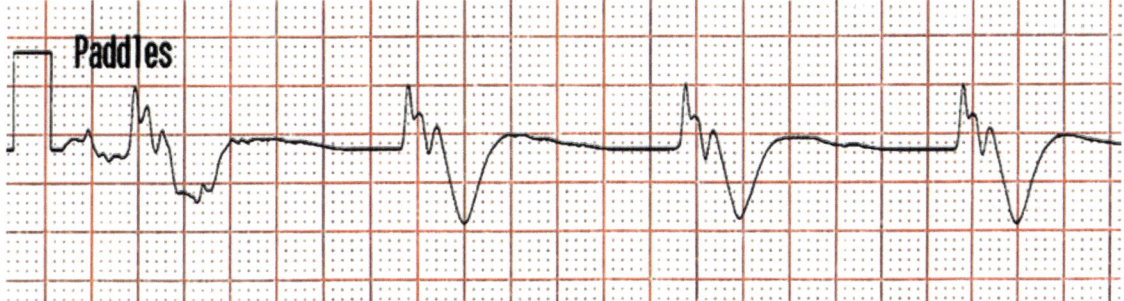

Figure 20.5 An example of an ECG showing PEA

1.4.3 Defibrillators

There are many brands and types of defibrillator on the market and it is important that you are familiar with the equipment you have in your workplace/ ambulance. Broadly, they fall into two types: automated external defibrillators (AEDs) and manual defibrillators. You will be issued with an AED.

AEDs

These 'shock boxes' are devices that provide voice and visual prompts to guide the public and healthcare professionals to defibrillate safely. AEDs are now widely available in public places such as shopping centres, sports centres, airports and railway stations [BHF, 2017]. Despite their name, some AEDs can be manually overridden by healthcare providers proficient in rhythm interpretation, but they are capable of recognising shockable and non-shockable rhythms [RCUK, 2021a].

Difficult environments and defibrillation

You will frequently encounter challenging environments that make resuscitation difficult. In terms of defibrillation, some of these can increase the risk of injury due to inadvertent electrocution. However, prompt defibrillation is life-saving and so it is important that you make a DRA and do not delay a shock unnecessarily.

Specific defibrillation scenarios include [RCUK, 2021a]:
- **Wet surfaces:** This is safe as long as you are not in contact with the patient and the patient's skin (if wet) is dried to ensure good contact is made by the self-adhesive pads to the patient's chest.
- **Metal surfaces:** As before, this is safe as long as you are not in contact with the patient. Metal surfaces actually conduct any current that leaks from the pads through the metal and away from the crew and bystanders.
- **In-flight:** Defibrillation in aircraft and helicopters is safe, particularly if the patient is in contact with metal surfaces for the reason given above. Oxygen use in a confined cabin could potentially increase the risk of fire, although there are no reports of these occurring. Consider restricting oxygen use in aircraft cabins or confined spaces.

Safety

The only person who should receive a shock when a defibrillator is used is the patient. This can be achieved as long as members of the resuscitation team communicate well, so that everyone is well clear of the patient at the time of defibrillation.

Other ways of maximising safety include [Kerber, 2012; RCUK, 2021a]:
- Do not defibrillate patients while they are in water or near an explosive or combustible environment.
- Ensure that the rescuers do not hold intravenous infusion equipment or the ambulance trolley during defibrillation.
- Wear gloves.
- Shave the patient's chest, if required, to obtain a good skin-to-electrode contact.
- Avoid placing the pads over jewellery, piercings, medication patches, wounds and tumours.
- Ensure that the pads are well away from pacemaker sites (>8 cm in adults and 12 cm in children).
- Remove oxygen from the patient unless the ventilation bag is directly connected to an endotracheal tube or supraglottic airway device. It should be at least 1 m away from the patient's chest.

2 Paediatric BLS

2.1 Learning objectives

By the end of this section you will be able to:
- explain how the causes of cardiac arrest in children are usually different from adults
- explain the procedure for providing BLS with an AED to paediatric patients.

2.2 Introduction

You will recall from the 'Children and Infants' chapter that paediatric patients are not small adults. This is true of cardiac arrest where, unlike adults, who experience a primary cardiac arrest typically due to a cardiac arrhythmia, infants and children usually suffer a secondary cardiac arrest [RCUK, 2021b]. This is not the sudden event experienced by adults, but a progressive worsening of the patient's condition until they cannot continue to compensate. Outcome from secondary cardiac arrest is poor.

Paediatric BLS is different from that of adults, and there are also some differences between infants (paediatric patients under 1 year of age) and children (between 1 and 18 years of age) and so they are presented separately in this section.

2.3 Infant BLS with AED

Indications
- Infant (0–12 months) patient with no apparent signs of life.

Contra-indications
- Newborn who requires resuscitation. (Follow local guidelines.)
- Patient whose condition is unequivocally associated with death.
- Patient has a Recommended Summary Plan for Emergency Care and Treatment (ReSPECT), relevant to their current clinical presentation, indicating that CPR attempts are not recommended.
- Patient has a valid 'do not attempt cardiopulmonary resuscitation' (DNACPR) form.

Advantages
- Provides blood flow to the brain and other vital organs.
- Good chance of a ROSC if the primary cause is cardiac (although less common in infants).

Disadvantages
- Unlikely to lead to ROSC without other interventions, particularly effective ventilation and oxygenation, and treatment for reversible causes.

Procedure

Take the following steps to perform BLS on an infant with an AED [Voorde, 2021]:
1. Ensure the scene is safe for you, the patient and bystanders.
2. Don appropriate PPE, and undertake appropriate hand hygiene.

Procedure – cont
3. Check for responsiveness by placing a hand on the infant's forehead to stabilise it and tug their hair while calling their name. If they have no hair, apply another method of tactile stimulation.

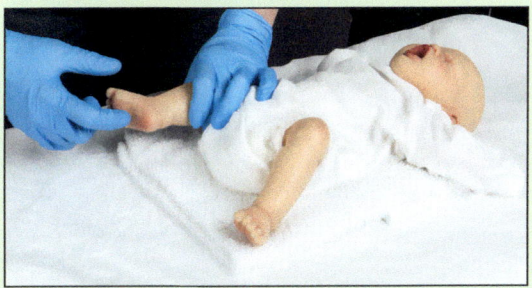

4. If the patient responds, assess the infant's ABCDE, call for assistance and reassess regularly. If they do not respond, summon additional assistance and remove outer clothing.
5. Open the infant's airway by placing one hand on their forehead and gently tilt it back until it is in a neutral position. Perform a chin lift by placing the fingertips of your other hand on the bony part of the lower jaw and lift upwards. Do not compress the soft tissues under the jaw as this will occlude the airway.

Placing a towel under the infant's shoulders and upper body can help keep their head in a neutral position.

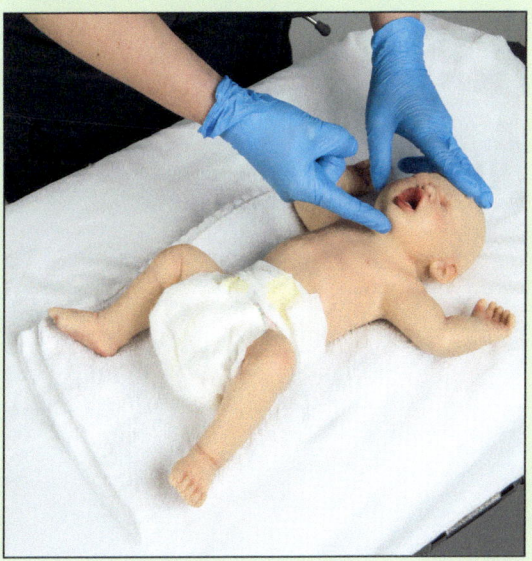

Chapter 20 – *Cardiac Arrest*

Procedure – *cont*

6. If a head tilt–chin lift does not effectively open the airway or you suspect a cervical spinal injury, you can use a jaw thrust to open the airway:
    1. Position yourself behind the infant.
    2. Place one or two fingers under both angles of the jaw.
    3. Rest your thumbs on the infant's cheeks.
    4. Lift the jaw upwards.

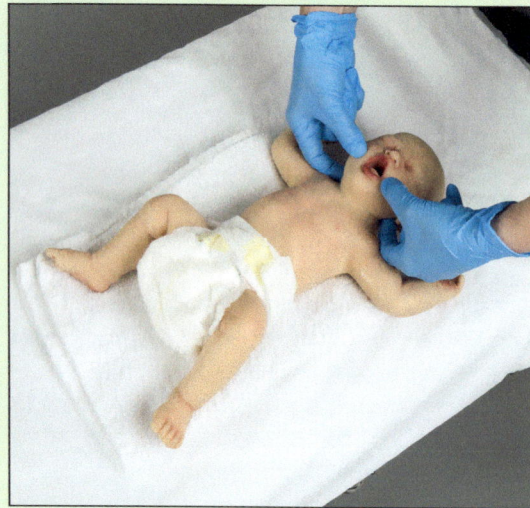

7. Look, listen and feel for normal breathing and check for signs of life (swallowing, vocalising, coughing or normal breathing) for no longer than 10 seconds, by placing your face close to the infant's face:
    - look for chest and abdominal movements
    - listen for airflow at the mouth and nose
    - feel for airflow at the mouth and nose.
8. If the infant is breathing normally, place them into the recovery position.
9. If the infant is not breathing or there are no signs of life (no swallowing, vocalising, coughing or normal breathing), check for and carefully remove any airway obstruction, and provide five rescue breaths:
    1. Where possible, use a two-handed BVM technique and ensure the bag is connected to high-flow oxygen.

Procedure – *cont*

2. Ventilate the chest steadily for 1 second, just enough to make the chest rise.
3. Maintain head tilt–chin lift and watch the chest fall.

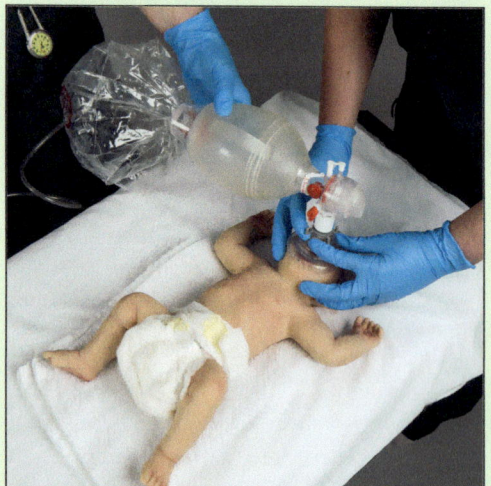

10. If the infant's chest is not rising and falling in a similar fashion to normal breathing, open their mouth and check for any visible obstruction. Do not blindly sweep in the infant's mouth. Reposition the head, using a jaw thrust if the head tilt–chin lift manoeuvre is not effective. The use of an airway adjunct, such as an OPA, may help too.

Make no more than five attempts to achieve effective ventilation before moving on to chest compressions.

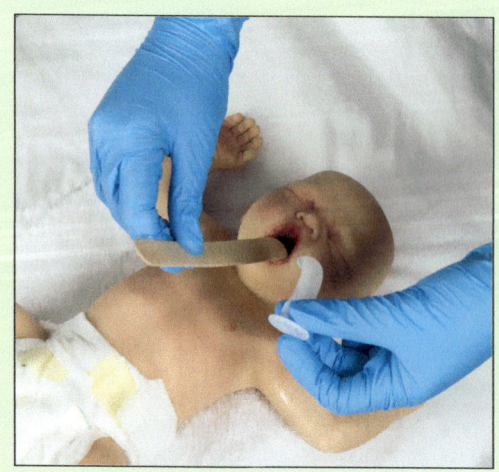

Paediatric BLS

Procedure – *cont*

11. Check for signs of life (swallowing, vocalising, coughing or normal breathing) and if they are absent (or you are not sure), start chest compressions. If there are signs of life, continue ventilation until the infant starts breathing effectively on their own.
12. If there are no signs of life (or you are unsure), start chest compressions:
    1. If you are on your own, use the tips of two fingers; otherwise, adopt the encircling technique by placing both thumbs side by side on the lower sternum and spreading the remaining fingers around to the infant's back.
    2. Avoid compressing the abdomen by placing your fingers one finger's width above the xiphisternum.
    3. Compress the sternum at least one-third of the depth of the chest (or by 4 cm) and then fully release the pressure while maintaining contact with the sternum. If this is difficult, use the two-handed technique as you would for adults.
    4. Repeat the compressions at a rate of 100–120 per minute for 15 compressions and then give 2 ventilations.
    5. Continue compressions and ventilations at a ratio of 15:2.

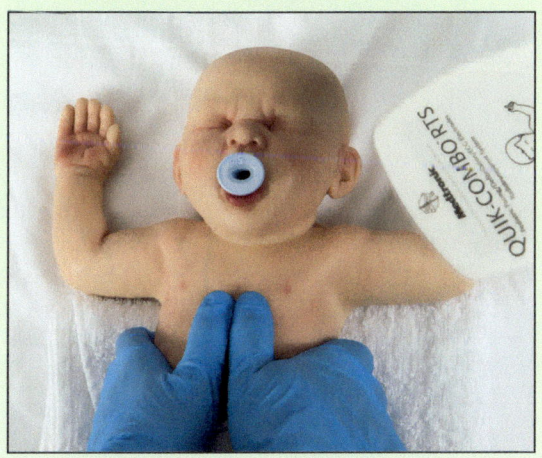

Procedure – *cont*

13. If possible, recruit another person on scene to provide BLS and coach them to provide high-quality chest compression while you expose the infant's chest and prepare for defibrillation by ensuring that the pad sites are free from jewellery, piercings, medication patches, pacemakers, wounds and tumours.

    If you are on your own and cannot get anyone on scene to help, you will have to decide whether to continue BLS or, if you suspect that the likelihood of a primary cardiac arrest is very high because the infant suddenly collapsed or has a known heart problem, for example, stop BLS and apply defibrillator pads. Follow local guidance.
14. Switch on the AED and attach the pads to the patient, ensuring they make good contact. Use paediatric pads if available.

    In infants, it may be more practical to place the pads in the anterior–posterior position in order to provide enough gap between the pads.

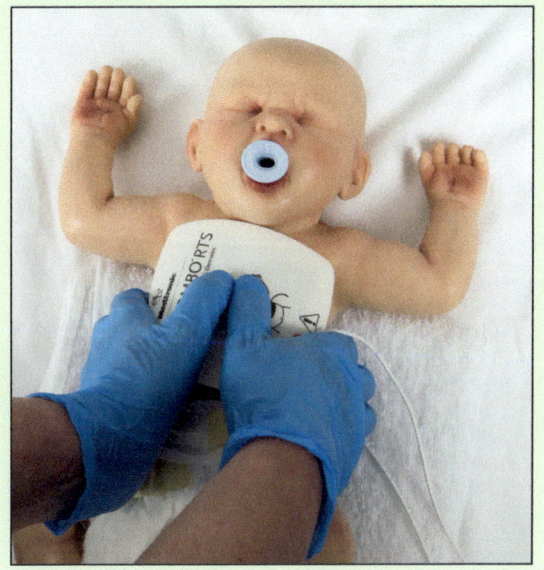

Chapter 20 – Cardiac Arrest

Procedure – *cont*

15. Follow visual and voice prompts, ensuring that no one touches the patient while the AED is analysing the rhythm.

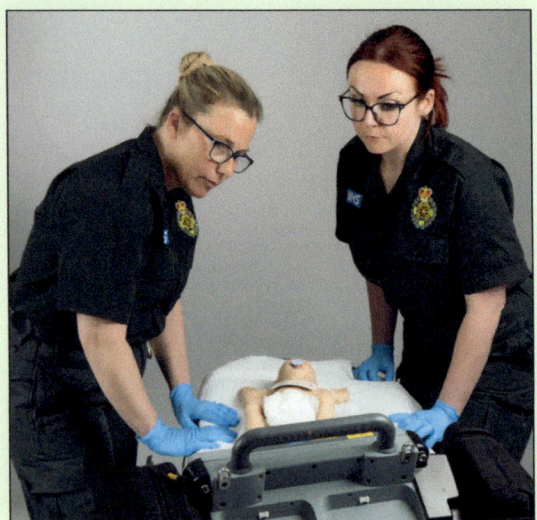

16. If a shock is advised, make sure everyone is clear of the patient, oxygen is kept at least 1 m away from the patient and push the shock button.
    If a shock is not advised, skip to step 17.

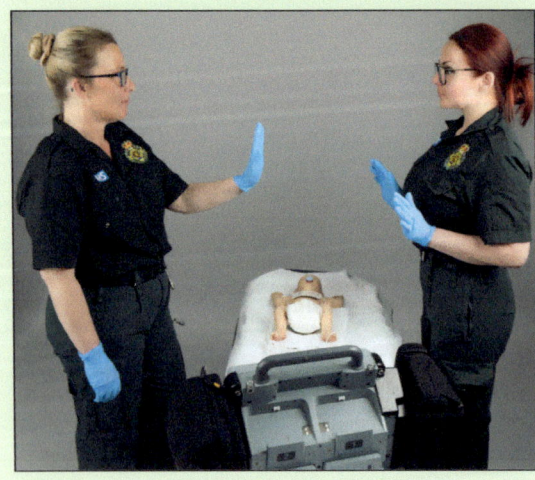

Procedure – *cont*

17. Immediately restart CPR at a ratio of 15:2. If possible, you should alternate chest compressions with another person every 2 minutes, but keep the changeover time to a minimum.

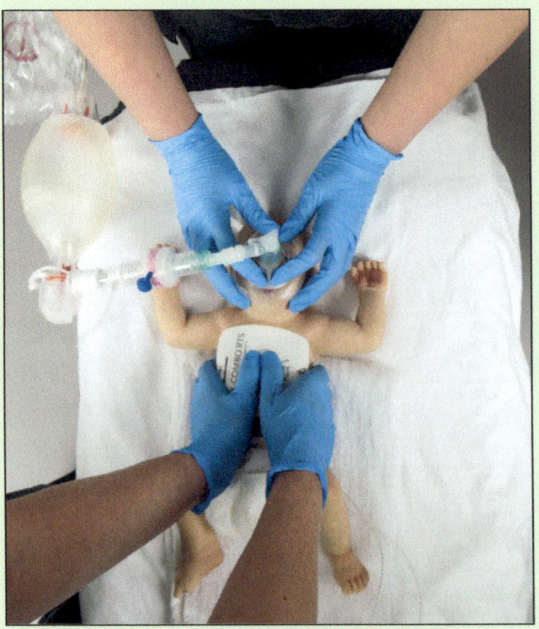

18. Continue to follow visual and voice prompts from the AED, ensuring that no one touches the patient while the AED is analysing the rhythm, and that oxygen is kept at least 1 m away from the patient if defibrillation is required.
19. Document the procedure.

2.4 Child BLS with AED

Indications
- Child over 1 year with no apparent signs of life.

Contra-indications
- Patient whose condition is unequivocally associated with death.
- Patient has a ReSPECT, relevant to their current clinical presentation, indicating that CPR attempts are not recommended.
- Patient has a valid DNACPR form.

Advantages
- Provides blood flow to the brain and other vital organs.
- Good chance of a ROSC if the primary cause is cardiac (although less common in children).

Disadvantages
- Unlikely to lead to ROSC without other interventions, particularly effective ventilation and oxygenation, and treatment for reversible causes.

Procedure

Take the following steps to perform BLS on a child with an AED [Voorde, 2021]:
1. Ensure the scene is safe for you, the patient and bystanders.
2. Don appropriate PPE, and undertake appropriate hand hygiene.
3. Check for responsiveness by placing a hand on the child's forehead to stabilise it and tug their hair while calling their name.

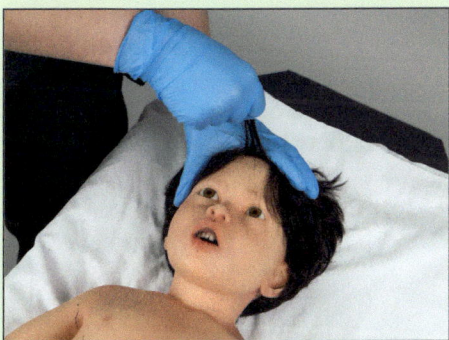

4. If the patient responds, assess the child's ABCDE, call for assistance and reassess regularly. If they do not respond, summon additional assistance and remove outer clothing.
5. Open the child's airway by placing one hand on their forehead and gently tilt it back until it is in a 'sniffing' position. Perform a chin lift by placing the fingertips of your other hand on the bony part of the lower jaw and lift upwards. Do not compress the soft tissues under the jaw, as this will occlude the airway. Younger children typically do not require any padding of

Procedure – cont

the shoulders or head, but older children may benefit from a towel or pillow under the occiput (as with adults) to obtain good airway alignment.

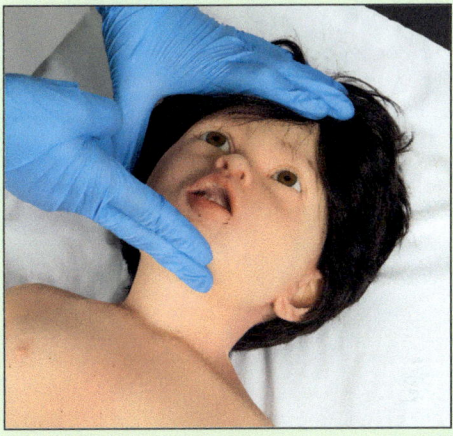

6. If a head tilt–chin lift does not effectively open the airway or you suspect a cervical spinal injury, you can use a jaw thrust to open the airway:
   1. Position yourself behind the child.
   2. Place two fingers under both angles of the jaw.
   3. Rest your thumbs on the child's cheeks.
   4. Lift the jaw upwards.

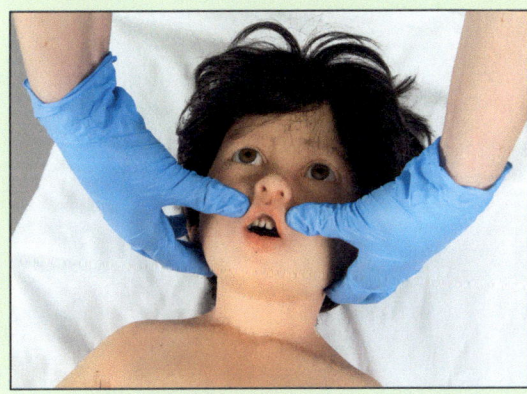

7. Look, listen and feel for normal breathing and check for signs of life (swallowing, vocalising, coughing or normal breathing) for no longer than 10 seconds, by placing your face close to the child's face:
   - look for chest and abdominal movements

Chapter 20 – *Cardiac Arrest*

Procedure – *cont*

- listen for airflow at the mouth and nose
- feel for airflow at the mouth and nose.

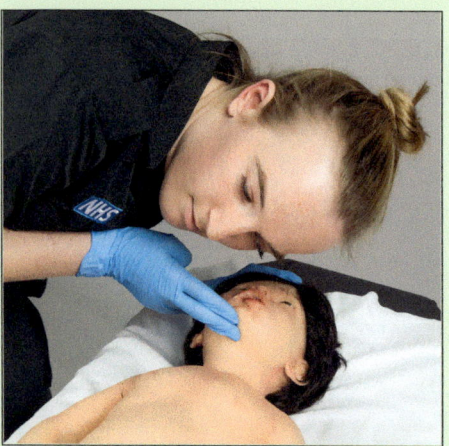

8. If the child is breathing normally, place them into the recovery position.
9. If the child is not breathing or there are no signs of life (no swallowing, vocalising, coughing or normal breathing), check for and carefully remove any airway obstruction, and provide five rescue breaths:
   1. Ensure the head is in a 'sniffing' position and apply a chin lift.
   2. Where possible, use a two-handed BVM technique and ensure the bag is connected to high-flow oxygen.
   3. Ventilate the chest steadily for 1 second, just enough to make the chest rise.
   4. Maintain head tilt–chin lift and watch the chest fall.

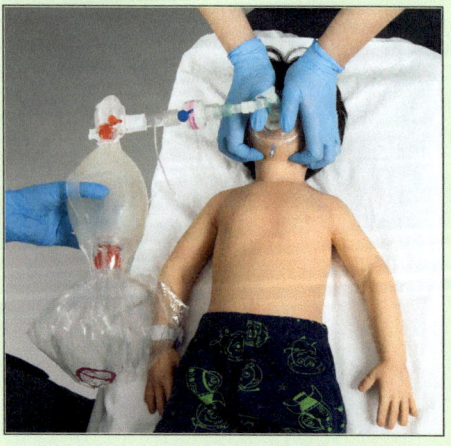

Procedure – *cont*

10. If the child's chest is not rising and falling in a similar fashion to normal breathing, open their mouth and check for any visible obstruction. Do not blindly sweep in the child's mouth. Reposition the head, using a jaw thrust if the head tilt–chin lift manoeuvre is not effective. The use of an airway adjunct, such as an OPA, may help too.

    Make no more than five attempts to achieve effective ventilation before moving on to chest compressions.
11. Check for signs of life (swallowing, vocalising, coughing or normal breathing) and if they are absent (or you are not sure), start chest compressions. If there are signs of life, continue ventilation until the child starts breathing effectively on their own.
12. If there are no signs of life (or you are unsure), start chest compressions:
    1. Position yourself by the side of the child.
    2. Avoid compressing the abdomen by placing your hand a finger's width above the xiphisternum.
    3. Lock your elbow and position your body so that your shoulder is directly over the child's chest.
    4. Compress the sternum by at least one-third of the depth of the chest (or by 5 cm) and then fully release the pressure while maintaining contact with the sternum. If this is difficult, use the two-handed technique as you would for adults.
    5. Repeat the compressions at a rate of 100–120 per minute for 15 compressions and then give 2 ventilations.

Procedure – cont

6. Continue compressions and ventilations at a ratio of 15:2.

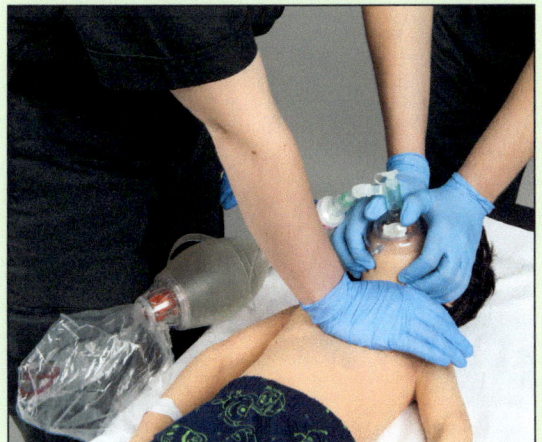

13. If possible, recruit another person on scene to provide BLS and coach them to provide high-quality chest compression while you expose the child's chest and prepare for defibrillation by ensuring that the pad sites are free from jewellery, piercings, medication patches, pacemakers, wounds and tumours.

    If you are on your own and cannot get anyone on scene to help, you will have to decide whether to continue BLS or, if you suspect that the likelihood of a primary cardiac arrest is very high because the child suddenly collapsed or has a known heart problem, for example, stop BLS and apply defibrillator pads. Follow local guidance.
14. Switch on the AED and attach the pads to the patient, ensuring they make good contact. Use paediatric pads if available.

Procedure – cont

In smaller children, it may be more practical to place the pads in the anterior–posterior position in order to provide enough gap between the pads.

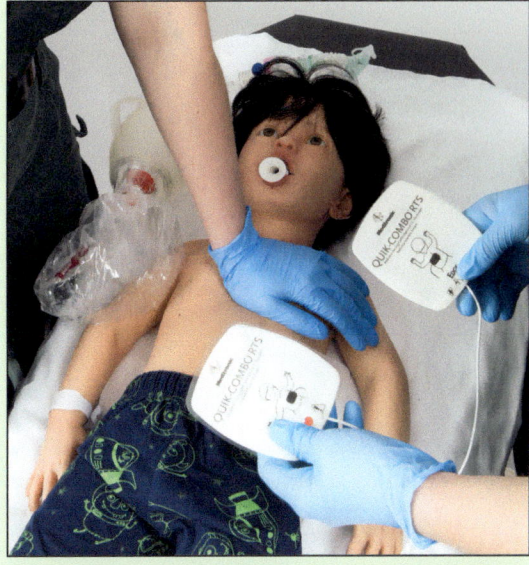

15. Follow visual and voice prompts, ensuring that no one touches the patient while the AED is analysing the rhythm.

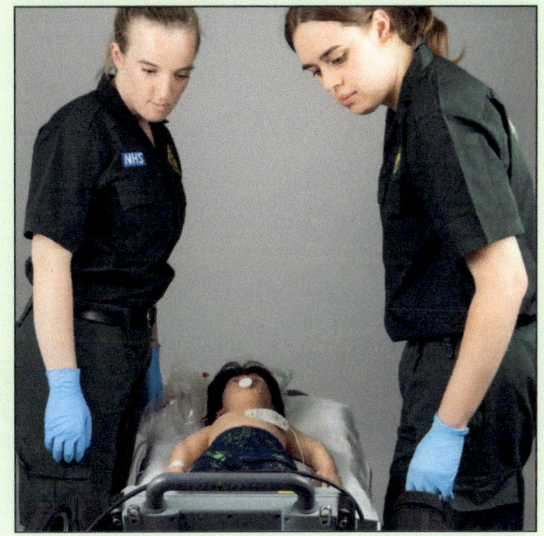

Chapter 20 – Cardiac Arrest

Procedure – *cont*

16. If a shock is advised, make sure everyone is clear of the patient, oxygen is kept at least 1 m away from the patient and push the shock button.

    If a shock is not advised, skip to step 17.

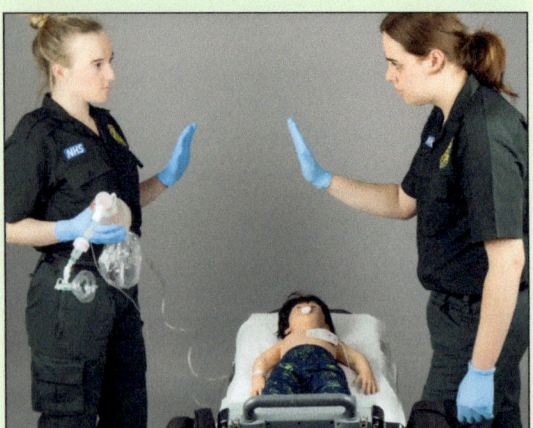

17. Immediately restart CPR at a ratio of 15:2. If possible, you should alternate chest compressions with another person every 2 minutes, but keep the changeover time to a minimum.

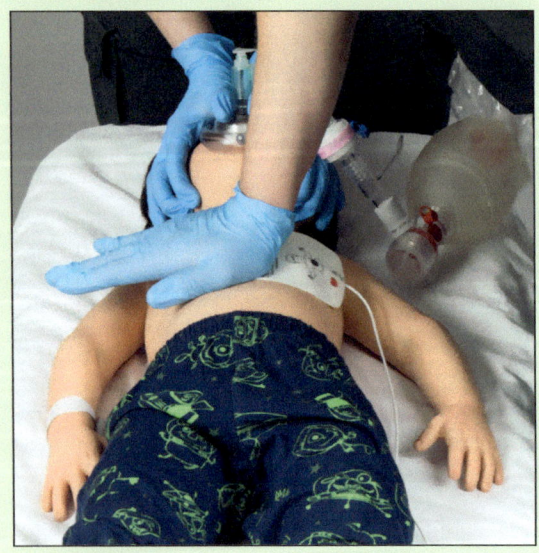

Procedure – *cont*

18. Continue to follow visual and voice prompts from the AED, ensuring that no one touches the patient while the AED is analysing the rhythm, and that oxygen is kept at least 1 m away from the patient if defibrillation is required.
19. Document the procedure.

3 Adult BLS

3.1 Learning objectives

By the end of this section you will be able to:
- explain how the causes of cardiac arrest in children are usually different from adults
- explain the procedure for providing BLS with an AED to adult patients.

3.2 Causes of cardiac arrest in adults

The commonest cause of cardiac arrest in adults is an irregular heart rhythm (arrhythmia) caused by myocardial ischaemia or infarction [RCUK, 2021a]. Most victims of sudden cardiac death (SCD) have a history of cardiac disease and commonly experience warning signs, such as chest pain in the hours prior to a cardiac arrest [Semeraro, 2021].

Other circulatory causes of cardiac arrest are most commonly due to hypovolaemia in patients who become suddenly ill. Of course, adults are also prone to cardiac arrests due to a primary airway or breathing problem, just like children. Ideally, you will intervene before an airway or breathing problem deteriorates into cardiac arrest [RCUK, 2021a].

3.3 Adult BLS with AED

Indications
- Adult patient with no apparent signs of life.

Adult BLS

Contra-indications
- Patient whose condition is unequivocally associated with death.
- Patient has an advance decision to refuse treatment (ADRT) or a ReSPECT that applies to their current clinical presentation.
- Patient has a valid DNACPR form.

Advantages
- Provides blood flow to the heart and brain.
- Increases the likelihood that the heart will resume an effective rhythm and cardiac output.
- Most likely combination to result in ROSC in patients with a shockable rhythm.

Disadvantages
- Unlikely to lead to ROSC in a non-shockable rhythm without advanced life support.

Procedure

Take the following steps to perform BLS with an AED [JRCALC, 2023; Olasveengen, 2021]:
1. Ensure the scene is safe for you, the patient and bystanders.
2. Don appropriate PPE, and undertake appropriate hand hygiene.
3. Check the patient to see if they are responsive by gently shaking their shoulders and asking if they are all right.

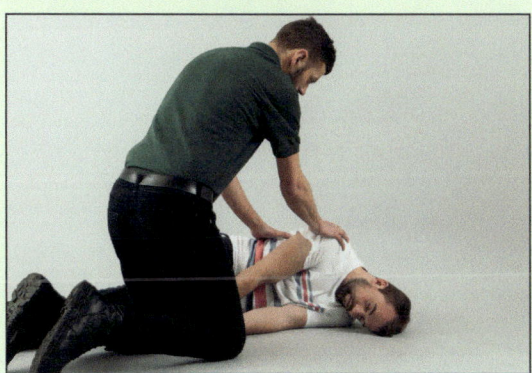

4. If the patient responds, obtain a history and undertake a further patient assessment. If the patient does not respond, request assistance and turn the patient on to their back.

Procedure – *cont*

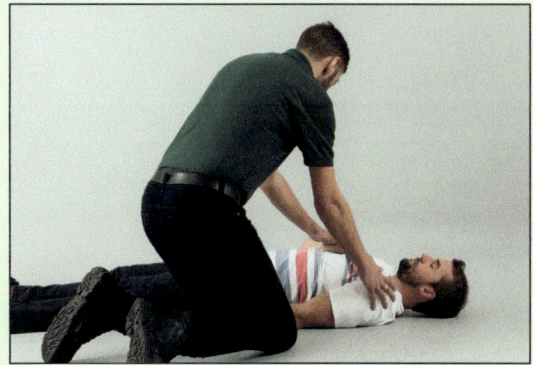

5. Open the patient's airway and look, listen and feel for breathing for no more than 10 seconds. Note that agonal breathing (occasional gasps) is common immediately following cardiac arrest, and should not be confused with normal breathing or taken as a sign of life.

If the patient is breathing normally, place them into the recovery position.

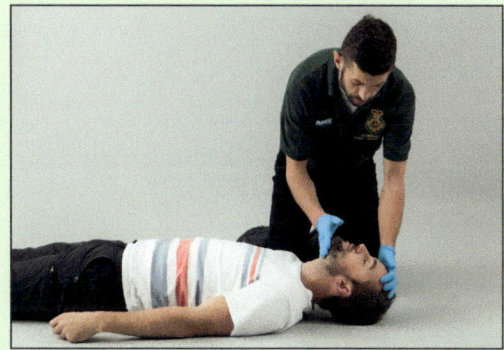

6. If the patient is not breathing normally or there are no signs of life (not moving, no normal breathing or coughing) and there is another person who can provide chest compressions, coach them to provide high-quality chest compressions:
   1. Kneel beside the patient.
   2. Place the heel of one hand in the centre of the chest (lower half of the sternum).
   3. Place the heel of your other hand on top of the first.

Chapter 20 – Cardiac Arrest

Procedure – *cont*

4. Interlock your fingers and ensure that pressure is not applied over the patient's ribs.
5. Position yourself directly over the patient's chest with your arms straight, and apply downward pressure to compress the chest to a depth of 5 cm but not more than 6 cm.
6. After each compression release the pressure on the chest, but maintain contact with the patient's skin.
7. Repeat at a rate of 100–120 compressions per minute.

If you are on your own, the priority is to apply the AED as soon as possible, so skip to step 7.

7. Expose the patient's chest and ensure that the pad sites are free from jewellery, piercings, medication patches, pacemakers, wounds and tumours. Shave the chest if required.

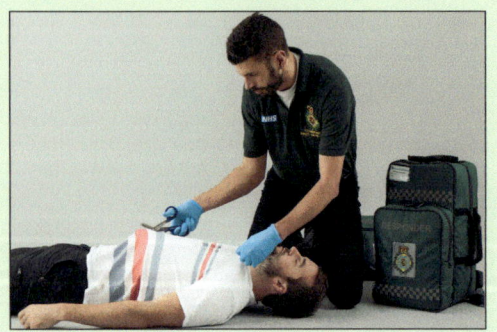

8. Switch on the AED and attach the pads to the patient, ensuring they make good contact. Do not interrupt chest compressions (if they are being performed) while applying the self-adhesive pads.

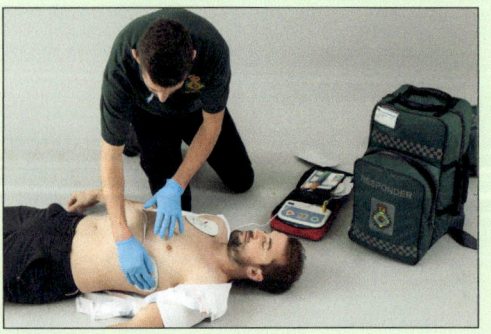

Procedure – *cont*

9. Follow visual and voice prompts, ensuring that no one touches the patient while the AED is analysing the rhythm.

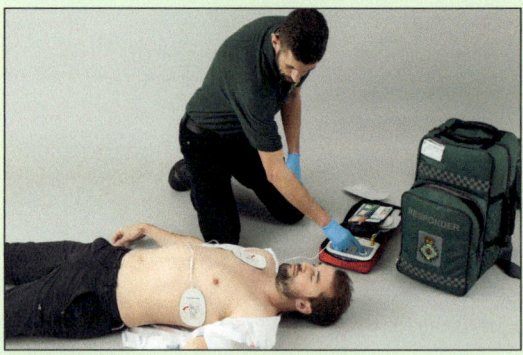

10. If a shock is advised, make sure everyone is clear of the patient and push the shock button.

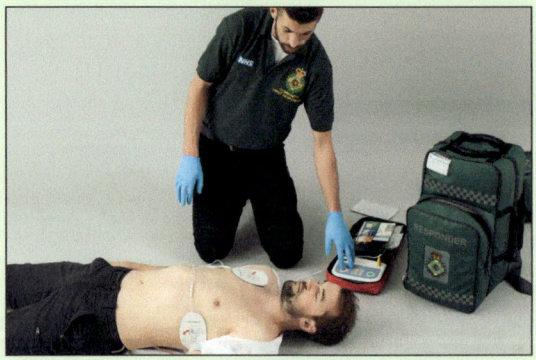

If a shock is not advised, skip to step 11.

11. Immediately restart chest compressions.
12. After 30 compressions, open the airway (you can insert an OPA if available) and provide two rescue breaths with a BVM.

    Each ventilation should cause the chest to rise and take about 1 second to deliver.
13. Continue with chest compressions and ventilations at a ratio of 30:2. If possible, you should alternate chest compressions with another person every 2 minutes, but keep the changeover time to a minimum.

Cardiac arrest in special circumstances

Procedure – *cont*

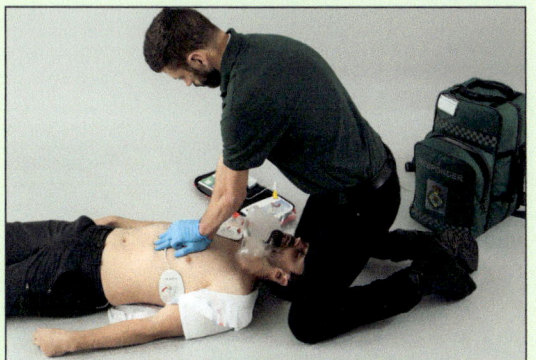

14. Follow visual and voice prompts from the AED, ensuring that no one touches the patient while the AED is analysing the rhythm and that oxygen is kept at least 1 m away from the patient if defibrillation is required.
15. Document the procedure.

4 Cardiac arrest in special circumstances

4.1 Learning objectives

By the end of this section you will be able to:
- explain the considerations for a pregnant patient in cardiac arrest
- explain the considerations for a hypothermic patient in cardiac arrest
- explain the management of a drowned patient in cardiac arrest.

4.2 Introduction

In this chapter, you have been introduced to the principles and techniques of resuscitation of a patient in cardiac arrest. However, in some circumstances the techniques need to be modified and/or alternative techniques used.

4.3 Cardiac arrest in pregnancy

The general procedure for resuscitating a pregnant patient is the same as for any other patient. However, for patients who are more than 20 weeks pregnant, there is a risk that their fetus-filled uterus can press down on the inferior vena cava and aorta, restricting venous return and leading to a reduction in cardiac output and uterine perfusion [RCUK, 2021a].

To prevent this from occurring, the pregnant patient must not lie supine. In the conscious patient, the left lateral position is often used, but this is not practicable in a cardiac arrest when chest compressions need to be provided. Instead, the uterus should be manually displaced to the left [JRCALC, 2023].

The hand position for patients in advanced pregnancy (over 28 weeks) may need to be 2–3 cm higher on the sternum. In addition, you may not be able to place the defibrillator pads in their usual positions, if the breasts are large. In these cases, use alternative pad placements, such as an anterior–posterior or bi-axillary placement [JRCALC, 2023].

During the latter stages of pregnancy, the patient is more likely to regurgitate their stomach contents and aspirate them into the lungs, particularly with over-enthusiastic BVM ventilation, so take care to provide just enough PPV to see the chest rise [Mansfield, 2018].

4.4 Cardiac arrest in hypothermic patients

In cases of moderate and severe hypothermia, signs of life can be difficult to identify. Unless there is a clear indication that the cardiac arrest has been caused by a lethal injury or fatal illness, patients should be resuscitated [JRCALC, 2023].

4.5 Cardiac arrest in drowned patients

Resuscitation is difficult while in the water and should consist of ventilations only. Chest compressions are futile in deep water, so wait until the patient is on a firm surface, such as the shore or the deck of a boat [Szpilman, 2012]. The incidence of spinal injuries is very low (around 0.5%) and immobilising the spine delays effective resuscitation, so only immobilise the spine when there is a clear MOI that could cause spinal injury (such as diving into shallow water or water-skiing) [Watson, 2001].

Get the victim out of the water as soon as possible and place them supine (on their back), with head and torso at the same level, and check for breathing. If your patient is not breathing, or is breathing abnormally, administer five rescue breaths via a BVM connected to high-flow oxygen. Note that this is different from the usual ABC approach that the current resuscitation guidelines advocate for adults but reflects that correction of hypoxia is the most important aspect in the management of the drowned patient. It can be difficult to differentiate post-arrest gasping from initial respiratory efforts of the drowning patient, so if you are unsure, administer ventilations and start CPR. Pulse checks are unreliable, so try to utilise other diagnostic tests if available, such as ECG and end-tidal carbon dioxide ($EtCO_2$) monitoring. If in doubt, commence chest compressions with ventilations at a ratio of 30:2 [Lott, 2021].

Large amounts of foam can be generated by the mixing of moving air with water and surfactant from the lungs. If this occurs, do not waste time trying to suction it, but continue to provide ventilations until an appropriate clinician can intubate the patient.

Resuscitation efforts should not be stopped unless it is clear that it would be futile to continue (e.g. due to the patient having sustained massive traumatic injuries). There are no completely accurate prognostic indicators in drowning, although duration of submersion is correlated with risk of death or severe neurological impairment [Szpilman, 2012].

5 Post-resuscitation care

5.1 Learning objectives
By the end of this section you will be able to:
- explain the management of the post-resuscitation patient.

5.2 Introduction
A ROSC in a patient who you have resuscitated is a great feeling, but it is just the first step on the path to complete recovery from a cardiac arrest. A complex pathophysiological process occurs as a result of whole-body ischaemia during a cardiac arrest and subsequent reperfusion when ROSC is achieved. This is known as post-cardiac arrest syndrome [Nolan, 2021].

5.3 Management
There is a bundle of care that ambulance clinicians will undertake following a ROSC. Some of them you can undertake if ROSC occurs prior to ambulance clinician arrival [JRCALC, 2023]:
- Reassess the patient's airway and breathing:
  - Provide ventilation, if required, at a rate of 10–12 breaths/minute.
  - Oxygen therapy should be titrated to maintain an SpO_2 of 94–98%.
- Reassess the patient's circulation:
  - Perform frequent pulse and blood pressure checks.
- Check blood glucose if able to do so.

6 Cardiac arrest decisions

6.1 Learning objective
By the end of this section you will be able to:
- explain when a resuscitation attempt may be stopped or not commenced.

6.2 When to start and stop resuscitation
Whenever there is a chance that a patient may survive from a cardiac arrest, resuscitation should be attempted unless a patient has stated, via an ADRT or ReSPECT, that this should not occur, or there is a valid DNACPR [JRCALC, 2023].

However, there are certain patients who have an injury or presenting condition that is unequivocally associated with death, irrespective of age [JRCALC, 2023]:
- Decapitation.
- Massive cranial and cerebral destruction.
- Hemicorporectomy (complete amputation of the body below the waist) or similar massive injury.
- Decomposition/putrefaction: tissue damage suggests that the patient has been dead for hours, days or even longer.

- Incineration: full-thickness burns and charring covering more than 95% of the TBSA.
- Hypostasis: the pooling of blood in the dependent part of the body (i.e. those parts affected by gravity) after death.
- Rigor mortis: stiffness of the body and limbs following death.
- Fetal maceration.

6.2.1 Conditions when resuscitation can be discontinued

Even if resuscitation has been commenced, this should be stopped if any of the following are present [JRCALC, 2023]:

- A DNACPR or ReSPECT form that advises resuscitation is not to be attempted.
- An ADRT clearly states that the patient is not to be resuscitated.
- The patient is in the final stages of a terminal illness and the senior clinician determines that CPR would not be successful even if no formal DNACPR decision has been documented.
- The patient has been submerged for more than 90 minutes (although submersion time is often difficult to accurately determine).
- There is no realistic chance that CPR would be successful because all of the following are present:
  - More than 15 minutes have elapsed since the onset of cardiac arrest.
  - No bystander CPR was provided in the 15 minutes prior to the arrival of the ambulance service.
  - There are no exclusion factors, such as drowning, hypothermia, poisoning or pregnancy, and the patient is an adult.
  - The ECG shows asystole for more than 30 seconds.

6.3 End of life decisions

6.3.1 Advance care planning

In terminal conditions, death can often be anticipated, which provides patients with the opportunity to consider their wishes and preferences about future care, particularly as they are likely to be unable to do so when close to death. Unfortunately, only 5% of people put these wishes and preferences in writing by means of an advance care plan (ACP, sometimes also called a preferred priorities for care document, or treatment escalation plan).

The contents of an ACP are not legally binding, but any best-interests decision about patients must take into account the patient's wishes and preferences. One example of an ACP is the ReSPECT [Blackmore, 2020]. This is a personalised plan specifying a person's recommended clinical care during an emergency when they do not have capacity to make decisions. This will include cardiac arrest and death (and takes the place of a DNACPR in this instance), but is not limited to only those events. Ask about the presence of such a plan as part of your patient assessment.

6.3.2 ADRT

ADRTs (also known as living wills) are documents that outline specific aspects of care that the patient does not wish to receive. This is then typically referred to when the patient is unable to make these wishes clear. Examples of the interventions that a patient may refuse include being ventilated, being tube fed, receiving antibiotics, and being admitted to hospital unless they are suffering from a complaint with a treatable cause.

Unlike the ACP, this is a legal document and, as long as the phrase 'even if life is at risk' is present, and the document is signed, dated and witnessed, the contents must be respected by healthcare staff. Note that treatment can only be declined and not requested, and the ADRT only comes into effect once the patient loses mental capacity [JRCALC, 2023].

6.3.3 DNACPR decision

DNACPR decisions are made by a senior clinician, usually with involvement from the patient's clinical team. There are four broad situations when a DNACPR decision will be made [JRCALC, 2023]:

- A mentally competent patient refuses resuscitative treatment.

Chapter 20 – Cardiac Arrest

- A valid advanced directive clearly states that the patient does not want CPR.
- CPR is unlikely to be successful.
- Successful CPR is possible, but the length and quality of life following resuscitation is not in the patient's best interests.

Ideally, this is written and agreed ahead of time and documentary evidence of the decision will be presented to you before you commence resuscitation. However, even if there is no formal DNACPR in place, the senior clinician can still elect not to start or continue resuscitation if the patient is in the final stages of a terminal illness and they think that CPR would not be successful. Ultimately, if you are unsure about the validity of previously made decisions, then commencing resuscitation is defendable if you believe it is in the patient's best interests [JRCALC, 2023].

References

A & Ors v East Sussex CC, 2003
A & Ors, R (on the application of) v East Sussex County Council & Anor [2003] EWHC 167 (Admin). Available at: https://www.bailii.org/ew/cases/EWHC/Admin/2003/167.html [Accessed 27 August 2014].

AAA, 2015
Age Action Alliance, 2015. Attitudes to Ageing. Available at: http://ageactionalliance.org/theme/attitudes-to-ageing/ [Accessed 6 December 2015].

AACE, 2016
Association of Ambulance Chief Executives, 2016. *UK Ambulance Services Clinical Practice Guidelines 2016*. Bridgwater: Class Professional Publishing.

AAOS, 2011
American Academy of Orthopaedic Surgeons and American College of Emergency Physicians, 2011. *Critical Care Transport*. Sudbury: Jones and Bartlett Publishers.

AAP, 2018
American Academy of Pediatrics, 2018. *Pediatric Education for Prehospital Professionals* (3rd edition). Burlington, MA: Jones & Bartlett Learning.

Aaronson, 2012
Aaronson PI, Ward JPT and Connolly MJ, 2012. *The Cardiovascular System at a Glance* (4th edition). Wiley-Blackwell.

Abbey, 2004
Abbey J, Piller N, DeBellis A, et al., 2004. The Abbey pain scale: a 1-minute numerical indicator for people with end-stage dementia. *International Journal of Palliative Nursing*, 10(1), 6–13.

Abrassart, 2013
Abrassart S, Stern R and Peter R, 2013. Unstable pelvic ring injury with hemodynamic instability: what seems the best procedure choice and sequence in the initial management? *Orthopaedics and Traumatology: Surgery & Research*, 99(2), 175–182. https://doi.org/10.1016/j.otsr.2012.12.014

Adults with Incapacity (Scotland) Act 2000
The Scottish Government, 2008. Adults with Incapacity (Scotland) Act 2000. Available at: http://www.gov.scot/publications/2008/06/13114117/0 [Accessed 5 January 2015].

Age UK, 2022
Age UK, 2022. Depression and Anxiety. Available at: https://www.ageuk.org.uk/information-advice/health-wellbeing/conditions-illnesses/depression-anxiety/ [Accessed 28 July 2024].

Age UK, 2023
Age UK, 2023. Safeguarding older people from abuse and neglect. Available at: https://www.ageuk.org.uk/globalassets/age-uk/documents/factsheets/fs78_safeguarding_older_people_from_abuse_fcs.pdf [Accessed: 8 May 2024].

Ali, 2017
Ali M, 2017. Communication skills 2: overcoming barriers to effective communication. *Nursing Times*, 114(1), 40–42.

ALK-Abello, 2023
ALK-Abello, 2013. Jext 150 and 300 micrograms solution for injection in pre-filled pen: patient information leaflet. Available at: https://www.medicines.org.uk/emc/files/pil.5747.pdf [Accessed 5 May 2024].

Allan, 2004
Allan MA and Marsh J, 2004. *History and Examination* (2nd edition). Mosby's crash course. Edinburgh: Mosby.

Allen, 2007
Allen LA and O'Connor CM, 2007. Management of acute decompensated heart failure. *Canadian Medical Association Journal*, 176(6), 797–805.

Allison, 2004
Allison K, Porter KJEM and Royal PC, 2004. Consensus on the prehospital approach to burns patient management. *Emergency Medicine Journal*, 21, 112–114.

Althaus, 1982
Althaus U, Aeberhard P, Schüpbach P, et al., 1982. Management of profound accidental hypothermia with cardiorespiratory arrest. *Annals of Surgery*, 195(4), 492.

Alzheimer's Society, 2015a
Alzheimer's Society, 2015. Equality, discrimination and human rights. Available at: https://www.alzheimers.org.uk/site/scripts/documents_info.php?documentID=1674 [Accessed 29 November 2015].

References

Alzheimer's Society, 2015b
Alzheimer's Society, 2015. The progression of Alzheimer's disease and other dementias. Available at: https://www.alzheimers.org.uk/site/scripts/documents_info.php?documentID=133 [Accessed 29 November 2015].

Alzheimer's Society, 2015c
Alzheimer's Society, 2015. Types of dementia. Available at: https://www.alzheimers.org.uk/Facts_about_dementia/What_is_dementia/ [Accessed 29 November 2015].

Alzheimer's Society, 2024
Alzheimer's Society, 2024. What is dementia? Available at: https://www.alzheimers.org.uk/about-dementia/types-dementia/what-is-dementia [Accessed 2 March 2024].

Amodio, 2014
Amodio D, 2014. The neuroscience of prejudice and stereotyping. *Nature Review Neurosciences*, 15, 670–682. https://doi.org/10.1038/nrn3800

Asbury, 2014
Asbury S and Jacobs E, 2014. *Dynamic Risk Assessment: The Practical Guide to Making Risk-Based Decisions with the 3-Level Risk Management Model* (1st edition). Abingdon, Oxon: Routledge.

Athanassiadi, 2010
Athanassiadi K, Theakos N, Kalantzi N, et al., 2010. Prognostic factors in flail-chest patients. *European Journal of Cardio-Thoracic Surgery: Official Journal of the European Association for Cardio-Thoracic Surgery*, 38(4), 466–471. https://doi.org/10.1016/j.ejcts.2010.02.034

Austin, 2010
Austin MA, Wills KE, Blizzard L, et al., 2010. Effect of high flow oxygen on mortality in chronic obstructive pulmonary disease patients in prehospital setting: randomised controlled trial. *British Medical Journal*, 341, c5462.

Balvers, 2016
Balvers K, Van der Horst M, Graumans M, et al., 2016. Hypothermia as a predictor for mortality in trauma patients at admittance to the Intensive Care Unit. *Journal of Emergencies, Trauma, and Shock*, 9(3), 97–102. https://doi.org/10.4103/0974-2700.185276

Barrett, 2014
Barrett E and Burns A, 2014. Dementia revealed: what Primary Care needs to know. Available at: https://www.england.nhs.uk/wp-content/uploads/2014/09/dementiarevealed-toolkit.pdf [Accessed 15 January 2015].

Battaloglu, 2020
Battaloglu E, Greasley L, Leon-Villapalos J, et al., 2020. *Expert Consensus Meeting: Management of Burns in Pre-Hospital Trauma Care*. Available at: https://fphc.rcsed.ac.uk/media/2957/2020-09-20-burns-consensus.pdf [Accessed 5 May 2024].

Benger, 2009
Benger J, Nolan J and Clancy M (eds), 2009. *Emergency Airway Management*. Cambridge; New York: Cambridge University Press.

Betsy, 2012
Betsy T and Keogh JE, 2012. *Microbiology Demystified* (2nd edition). New York: McGraw-Hill.

BHF, 2017
British Heart Foundation and Resuscitation Council (UK), 2017. A guide to automated external defibrillators (AED). Available at: https://www.resus.org.uk/publications/a-guide-to-aeds/ [Accessed 6 May 2024].

Blaber, 2008
Blaber A, 2008. *Foundations for Paramedic Practice: A Theoretical Perspective* (1st edition). Maidenhead: Open University Press.

Blackmore, 2020
Blackmore T, 2020. Palliative and End of Life Care for Paramedics. Bridgwater: Class Professional Publishing.

Bledsoe, 2014
Bledsoe BE, Porter RS and Cherry RA, 2014. *Paramedic Care: Principles and Practice. Vol. 3*. Harlow: Pearson.

BMA, 2019
British Medical Association, 2019. Consent and refusal by adults with decision-making capacity. Available at: https://www.bma.org.uk/media/2481/bma-consent-toolkit-september-2019.pdf [Accessed 22 January 2024].

BOC, 2013
BOC Healthcare, 2013. ENTONOX® (50%nitrous oxide/50%oxygen). Available at: https://www.boconline.co.uk/en/images/entonox-integral-valve-cylinder-instructions_tcm410-675418.pdf [Accessed 27 April 2024].

BOC, 2022
BOC, 2022. Medical oxygen. Available at: https://www.boconline.co.uk/en/images/Medical-Oxygen-Integral-Valve-Cylinders-leaflet_tcm410-671502.pdf [Accessed 27 April 2024].

References

Bose, 2006
Bose P, Regan F and Paterson-Brown S, 2006. Improving the accuracy of estimated blood loss at obstetric haemorrhage using clinical reconstructions. *BJOG: An International Journal of Obstetrics and Gynaecology*, 113(8), 919–924. https://doi.org/10.1111/j.1471-0528.2006.01018.x

Boulton, 2018
Boulton AJ, Lewis CT, Naumann DN, et al., 2018. Prehospital haemostatic dressings for trauma: a systematic review. *Emergency Medicine Journal: EMJ*, 35(7), 449–457. https://doi.org/10.1136/emermed-2018-207523

Bowers, 2007
Bowers B and Scase C, 2007. Tracheostomy: facilitating successful discharge from hospital to home. *British Journal of Nursing*, 16(8), 476–479.

Boyett, 2009
Boyett MR, 2009. 'And the beat goes on.' The cardiac conduction system: the wiring system of the heart. *Experimental Physiology*, 94(10), 1035–1049.

Boyle, 2009
Boyle JS, Bechtel LK and Holstege CP, 2009. Management of the critically poisoned patient. *Scandinavian Journal of Trauma, Resuscitation and Emergency Medicine*, 17(1), 29. https://doi.org/10.1186/1757-7241-17-29

Breakell, 2001
Breakell A, 2001. The clinical evaluation of the Respi-check mask: a new oxygen mask incorporating a breathing indicator. *Emergency Medicine Journal*, 18(5), 366–369. https://doi.org/10.1136/emj.18.5.366

Briar, 2003
Briar C and Lasserson D, 2003. *Nervous System* (2nd edition). London: Mosby.

Briscoe, 2006
Briscoe VJ and Davis SN, 2006. Hypoglycemia in type 1 and type 2 diabetes: physiology, pathophysiology, and management. *Clinical Diabetes*, 24(3), 115–121.

Bryan, 2022
Bryan Y, 2022. Assessment of coma. Available at: https://bestpractice.bmj.com/topics/en-gb/417.

BSI, 2011
British Standards Institution, 2011. *BS EN 1089-3:2011*. London: BSI.

Buss, 2010
Buss J and Thompson G (eds), 2010. *Auscultation Skills: Breath & Heart Sounds* (4th edition). Philadelphia: Wolters Kluwer/Lippincott Williams & Wilkins Health.

Butz, 2015
Butz DR, Collier Z, O'Connor A, et al., 2015. Is palmar surface area a reliable tool to estimate burn surface areas in obese patients? *Journal of Burn Care & Research*, 36(1), 87–91. https://doi.org/10.1097/BCR.0000000000000146

Byrne, 2023
Byrne RA, Rossello X, Coughlan JJ, et al., 2023. 2023 ESC Guidelines for the management of acute coronary syndromes: developed by the task force on the management of acute coronary syndromes of the European Society of Cardiology (ESC). *European Heart Journal*, 44(38), 3720–3826. https://doi.org/10.1093/eurheartj/ehad191

Canto, 2012
Canto AJ, Kiefe CI, Goldberg RJ, et al., 2012. Differences in symptom presentation and hospital mortality according to type of acute myocardial infarction. *American Heart Journal*, 163(4), 572–579.

Cardona, 2020
Cardona V, Ansotegui IJ, Ebisawa M, et al., 2020. World Allergy Organization Anaphylaxis Guidance 2020. *World Allergy Organization Journal*, 13(10), 100472. https://doi.org/10.1016/j.waojou.2020.100472

Chandler, 2014
Chandler R and Bruneau B, 2014. Barriers to the management of pain in dementia care. *Nursing Practice*, 110(28), 12–16.

Chapin, 2013
Chapin MM, Rochette LM, Annest JL, et al., 2013. Nonfatal choking on food among children 14 years or younger in the United States, 2001–2009. *Pediatrics*, 132(2), 275–281.

Chauhan, 2018
Chauhan R, Conti BM and Keene D, 2018. Marauding terrorist attack (MTA): Prehospital considerations. *Emergency Medicine Journal: EMJ*, 35(6), 389–395. https://doi.org/10.1136/emermed-2017-206959

Chin, 2004
Chin RFM, Neville BGR and Scott RC, 2004. A systematic review of the epidemiology of status epilepticus. *European Journal of Neurology*, 11(12), 800–810.

References

Chong, 2020
Chong HP, Quinn L, Jeeves A, et al., 2020. A comparison study of methods for estimation of a burn surface area: Lund and Browder, e-burn and Mersey Burns. *Burns*, 46(2), 483–489. https://doi.org/10.1016/j.burns.2019.08.014

CKS, 2023
Clinical Knowledge Summaries, 2023. Gastroenteritis. Available at: https://cks.nice.org.uk/topics/gastroenteritis/ [Accessed 21 January 2024].

Connor, 2013
Connor D, Greaves I, Porter K, et al., 2013. Pre-hospital spinal immobilisation: an initial consensus statement. *Emergency Medicine Journal*, 30(12), 1067–1069. https://doi.org/10.1136/emermed-2013-203207

CoP, 2023
College of Paramedics, 2023. Paramedic Career Framework. Available at: https://collegeofparamedics.co.uk/COP/ProfessionalDevelopment/post_reg_career_framework.aspx [Accessed 28 July 2024].

Corwell, 2014
Corwell B, Knight B, Olivieri L, et al., 2014. Current diagnosis and treatment of hyperglycemic emergencies. *Emergency Medicine Clinics of North America*, 32(2), 437–452.

CoT, 2018
Committee on Trauma, 2018. *ATLS Advanced Trauma Life Support Student Course Manual* (10th edition). Washington DC: American College of Surgeons.

CPS, 2022
Crown Prosecution Service, 2022. Disability hate crime and other crimes against disabled people – prosecution guidance. Available at: https://www.cps.gov.uk/legal-guidance/disability-hate-crime-and-other-crimes-against-disabled-people-prosecution-guidance [Accessed 23 December 2023].

CQC, 2022
Care Quality Commission, 2022. Regulation 20: Duty of candour. Available at: https://www.cqc.org.uk/guidance-providers/all-services/regulation-20-duty-candour [Accessed 22 January 2024].

Crook, 2013
Crook J and Taylor RM, 2013. The agreement of fingertip and sternum capillary refill time in children. *Archives of Disease in Childhood*, 98(4), 265–268.

CSCB, 2014
Coventry Safeguarding Children's Board, 2014. Serious case review: Daniel Pelka. Available at: http://www.coventry.gov.uk/lscb [Accessed 21 January 2015].

Cuttle, 2008
Cuttle L, Kempf M, Kravchuk O, et al., 2008. The optimal temperature of first aid treatment for partial thickness burn injuries. *Wound Repair and Regeneration: Official Publication of the Wound Healing Society [and] the European Tissue Repair Society*, 16(5), 626–634. https://doi.org/10.1111/j.1524-475X.2008.00413.x

Cuttle, 2009
Cuttle L, Pearn J, McMillan JR, et al., 2009. A review of first aid treatments for burn injuries. *Burns*, 35(6), 768–775. https://doi.org/10.1016/j.burns.2008.10.011

Czura, 2011
Czura CJ, 2011. 'Merinoff Symposium 2010: Sepsis' – Speaking with One Voice. *Molecular Medicine*, 17(1–2), 2–3. https://doi.org/10.2119/molmed.2010.00001.commentary

Data Protection Act 2018
UK Government, 2018. *Data Protection Act 2018*. London: HM Stationery Office.

Deary, 1993
Deary IJ, Hepburn DA, MacLeod KM, et al., 1993. Partitioning the symptoms of hypoglycaemia using multi-sample confirmatory factor analysis. *Diabetologia*, 36(8), 771–777.

DHG, 2023
DHG Healthcare, 2023. Raizer II User Manual. Available at: https://www.felgains.com/app/uploads/2020/10/LIT-00155-Raizer-II-User-Manual-Issue-1-Jan-2023-EN-1.pdf [Accessed 30 January 2024].

DHSC, 2023
Department of Health and Social Care, 2023. The NHS Constitution for England. Available at: https://www.gov.uk/government/publications/the-nhs-constitution-for-england/the-nhs-constitution-for-england [Accessed 22 January 2024].

Dieckmann, 2010
Dieckmann RA, Brownstein D and Gausche-Hill M, 2010. The pediatric assessment triangle: a novel approach for the rapid evaluation of children. *Pediatric Emergency Care*, 26(4), 312.

Dobson, 2009
Dobson T, Jensen J, Karim S, et al., 2009. Correlation of paramedic administration of furosemide with emergency

physician diagnosis of congestive heart failure. *Journal of Emergency Primary Health Care*, 7(3), 3.

DoH, 2000
Department of Health, 2000. No secrets: guidance on protecting vulnerable adults in care. Available at: https://www.gov.uk/government/publications/nosecrets-guidance-on-protecting-vulnerable-adults-in-care [Accessed 21 January 2015].

DoH, 2001
Department of Health, 2001. Valuing people. Available at: https://www.gov.uk/government/uploads/system/uploads/attachment_data/file/250877/5086.pdf [Accessed 14 June 2015].

DoH, 2006
Department of Health. (2006). Medical gases: health technical memorandum 02-01: medical gas pipeline systems. Available at: https://www.england.nhs.uk/wp-content/uploads/2021/05/HTM_02-01_Part_A.pdf [Accessed 27 April 2024]

DoH, 2013
Department of Health, 2013. Managing healthcare fire safety. Available at: https://www.gov.uk/government/publications/managing-healthcare-fire-safety [Accessed 28 July 2014].

DoH, 2013b
Department of Health, 2013. Winterbourne View Hospital: Department of Health review and response. Available at: https://www.gov.uk/government/publications/winterbourne-view-hospital-departmentof-health-review-and-response [Accessed 21 January 2015].

DoH, 2023
Department of Health, 2023, Factsheet 1: General responsibilities of local authorities: prevention, information and advice, and shaping the market of care and support services. Available at: https://www.gov.uk/government/publications/care-act-2014-part-1-factsheets/care-act-factsheets [Accessed 18 December 2023].

DoHSC, 2024
Department of Health and Social Care, 2024. Guide to donning (putting on) and doffing (removing) PPE (non-AGP) in adult social care settings. Available at: https://www.gov.uk/government/publications/ppe-guide-for-non-aerosol-generating-procedures/guide-to-donning-putting-on-and-doffing-removing-ppe-non-agp-in-adult-social-care-settings-text-only-version#:~:text=Put%20on%20eye%20protection.%20Put%20on%20gloves%20if

Dougherty, 2015
Dougherty L, Lister S and West-Oram A, 2015. *Royal Marsden Manual of Clinical Nursing Procedures* (9th edition). John Wiley & Sons Inc.

Douglas, 2005
Douglas G, Nicol EF, Robertson C, et al., 2005. *Macleod's Clinical Examination* (11th edition). Edinburgh: Elsevier Churchill Livingstone.

Drake, 2019
Drake R, Vogl AW and Mitchell AWM, 2019. *Gray's Anatomy for Students* (4th edition). Elsevier.

DSFRS, 2024
Devon & Somerset Fire & Rescue Service, 2024. Car and vehicle fires. Available at: https://www.dsfire.gov.uk/safety/on-the-road/car-and-vehicle-fires [Accessed 21 January 2024].

Dunn, 2005
Dunn L, 2005. Pneumonia: classification, diagnosis and nursing management. *Nursing Standard*, 19(42), 50–54.

Durrer, 2003
Durrer B, Brugger H, Syme D, et al., 2003. The medical on-site treatment of hypothermia: ICAR-MEDCOM recommendation. *High Altitude Medicine & Biology*, 4(1), 99–103.

Dykes, 2002
Dykes M, 2002. *Crash Course: Anatomy* (2nd edition). London: Mosby.

EC, 2013
European Commission, 2013. *Chemicals at Work – A New Labelling System*. Available at: http://ec.europa.eu/social/blobservlet?docid=10450&langid=en [Accessed 15 December 2014].

Elliott, 2011
Elliott J and Heller S, 2011. Hypoglycaemia unawareness. *Practical Diabetes International*, 28(5), 227–232.

Enoch, 2009
Enoch S, Roshan A and Shah M, 2009. Emergency and early management of burns and scalds. *British Medical Journal*, 338, b1037. https://doi.org/10.1136/bmj.b1037

Equality Act 2010
UK Government. Equality Act 2010. Available at: http://www.legislation.gov.uk/ukpga/2010/15/contents [Accessed 11 January 2015].

References

Evans, 2012
Evans JDW and Sutton P, 2012. *Cardiovascular System*. Edinburgh: Mosby/Elsevier.

Falk, 2003
Falk E and Thuesen L, 2003. Pathology of coronary microembolisation and no reflow. *Heart*, 89(9), 983–985.

Farley, 2011
Farley A and Hendry C, 2011. *The Physiological Effects of Ageing* (1st edition). Chichester: Wiley-Blackwell.

Feber, 2006
Feber T, 2006. Tracheostomy care for community nurses: basic principles. *British Journal of Community Nursing*, 11(5), 186.

Fick, 2002
Fick DM, Agostini JV and Inouye SK, 2002. Delirium superimposed on dementia: a systematic review. *Journal of the American Geriatrics Society*, 50(10), 1723–1732.

FPHC, 2017
Faculty of Pre-hospital Care, 2017. *Position statement on the application of tourniquets*. Available at: https://fphc.rcsed.ac.uk/media/2876/position-statement-on-the-application-of-tourniquets-july-2017.pdf [Accessed 5 May 2024].

FPHC, 2018
Faculty of Pre-hospital Care, 2018. *Corrosive Substance Attack*. Available at: https://fphc.rcsed.ac.uk/media/2490/corrosive-substance-attack_28032018.pdf [Accessed 5 May 2024].

FPLD, 2023
Foundation for People with Learning Disabilities, 2023. Hearing loss. Available at: https://www.learningdisabilities.org.uk/learning-disabilities/a-to-z/h/hearing-loss [Accessed 23 December 2023].

Francis, 2013
Francis R, 2013. Final report – Mid Staffordshire NHS Foundation Trust Public Inquiry. Available at: http://webarchive.nationalarchives.gov.uk/20150407084003/http://www.midstaffspublicinquiry.com/report [Accessed 31 December 2014].

Frank, 2010
Frank M, Schmucker U, Stengel D, et al., 2010. Proper estimation of blood loss on scene of trauma: tool or tale? *The Journal of Trauma: Injury, Infection, and Critical Care*, 69(5), 1191–1195. https://doi.org/10.1097/TA.0b013e3181c452e7

Gabbe, 2011
Gabbe BJ, de Steiger R, Esser M, et al., 2011. Predictors of mortality following severe pelvic ring fracture: results of a population-based study. *Injury*, 42(10), 985–991. https://doi.org/10.1016/j.injury.2011.06.003

Garcia, 2004
Garcia TB and Miller GT, 2004. *Arrhythmia Recognition: The Art of Interpretation*. Sudbury, MA: Jones and Bartlett Publishers.

Garcia, 2015
Garcia TB, 2015. *12-lead ECG: The Art of Interpretation* (2nd edition). Burlington, MA: Jones & Bartlett Learning.

Garlapati, 2012
Garlapati AK and Ashwood N, 2012. An overview of pelvic ring disruption. *Trauma*, 14(2), 169–178. https://doi.org/10.1177/1460408611434375

Ginsberg, 2004
Ginsberg L, 2004. *Lecture Notes: Neurology* (8th edition). Oxford: Wiley-Blackwell.

Gitelman, 2008
Gitelman A, Hishmeh S, Morelli BN, et al., 2008. Cauda equina syndrome: a comprehensive review. *American Journal of Orthopedics*, 37(11), 556–562.

GMC, 2024
General Medical Council, 2024. Disclosing patients' personal information: a framework. Available at: https://www.gmc-uk.org/professional-standards/professional-standards-for-doctors/confidentiality/disclosing-patients-personal-information-a-framework [Accessed 22 January 2024].

Goldberg, 2007
Goldberg A, Southern DA, Galbraith PD, et al., 2007. Coronary dominance and prognosis of patients with acute coronary syndrome. *American Heart Journal*, 154(6), 1116–1122.

Golden, 1997
Golden FSC, David GC and Tipton MJ, et al., 1997. *Review of Rescue and Immediate Post-Immersion Problems: A Medical/Ergonomic Viewpoint*. Sudbury: HSE Books.

Graveling, 2009
Graveling AJ and Frier BM, 2009. Hypoglycaemia: an overview. *Primary Care Diabetes*, 3(3), 131–139.

Greaves, 2008
Greaves I, Porter K, Ryan J, et al., 2008. *Trauma Care Manual* (2nd edition). London: Hodder Arnold.

References

Greaves, 2010
Greaves I, Porter K and Smith J, 2010. *Practical Prehospital Care: The Principles and Practice of Immediate Care* (1st edition). London: Churchill Livingstone.

Greaves, 2018
Greaves I, Porter K and Wright C (eds), 2018. *Trauma Care Pre-Hospital Manual* (1st edition). CRC Press.

Gregory, 2010
Gregory P, 2010. *Manual of Clinical Paramedic Procedures.* Chichester: Wiley-Blackwell.

Guest, 2020
Guest J, Keating T, Gould D, et al., 2020. Modelling the Annual NHS costs and outcomes attributable to healthcare-associated infections in England. *BMJ Open*. Available at: https://bmjopen.bmj.com/content/10/1/e033367 [Accessed 21 January 2024].

Halliwell, 2011
Halliwell D, Jones P, Ryan L, et al., 2011. The revision of the primary survey: A 2011 review. *Journal of Paramedic Practice*, 3(7), 366–374. https://doi.org/10.12968/jpar.2011.3.7.366

Hart, 2006
Hart CA and Thomson APJ, 2006. Meningococcal disease and its management in children. *British Medical Journal*, 333(7570), 685–690.

Hasler, 2011
Hasler RM, Exadaktylos AK, Bouamra O, et al., (2011). Epidemiology and predictors of spinal injury in adult major trauma patients: European cohort study. *European Spine Journal*. https://doi.org/10.1007/s00586-011-1866-7

HCPC, 2020
Health and Care Professions Council, 2020. What equality, diversity and inclusion means to us. Available at: https://www.hcpc-uk.org/about-us/equality-diversity-and-inclusion/what-equality-diversity-and-inclusion-means-to-us/ [Accessed 22 January 2024].

Health and Safety at Work etc. Act 1974
UK Government, 1974. Health and Safety at Work etc. Act 1974. Available at: http://www.legislation.gov.uk/ukpga/1974/37 [Accessed 27 December 2014].

Health and Social Care Act 2008
UK Government, 2008. Health and Social Care Act 2008. Available at: http://www.legislation.gov.uk/ukpga/2008/14/contents [Accessed 27 December 2014].

Hettiaratchy, 2004
Hettiaratchy S and Papini R, 2004. Initial management of a major burn: II – assessment and resuscitation. *British Medical Journal*, 329(7457), 101–103.

Hickin, 2015
Hickin S, Renshaw J, Williams R, et al., 2015. *Respiratory System.* Mosby.

Hignett, 2015
Hignett S, 2015. Musculoskeletal injury risks for ambulance workers. *Journal of Paramedic Practice*, 7(6). https://doi.org/10.12968/jpar.2015.7.6.276

HMG, 2017
HM Government, 2017. FGM: mandatory reporting in healthcare. Available at: https://www.gov.uk/government/publications/fgm-mandatory-reporting-in-healthcare [Accessed: 08 May 2024].

HMG, 2023
HM Government, 2023. Definition of disability under the Equality Act 2010. Available at: https://www.gov.uk/definition-of-disability-under-equality-act-2010 [Accessed 18 December 2023].

HMG, 2023b
HM Government, 2023. Disability rights. Available at: https://www.gov.uk/rights-disabled-person/overview [Accessed 18 December 2023].

HO, 2023
Home Office, 2023. Fire statistics data tables. Available at: https://www.gov.uk/government/statistical-data-sets/fire-statistics-data-tables [Accessed 5 May 2024].

Holland, 2011
Holland K, 2011. Factsheet: learning disabilities. Available at: http://www.bild.org.uk/EasySiteWeb/GatewayLink.aspx?alId=2522 [Accessed 14 June 2015].

Holt, 2010
Holt TA, 2010. *ABC of Diabetes* (6th edition). ABC series. Chichester: Wiley-Blackwell/BMJ.

Howlett, 2011
Howlett JG, 2011. Acute heart failure: lessons learned so far. *Canadian Journal of Cardiology*, 27(3), 284–295. https://doi.org/10.1016/j.cjca.2011.02.007

HSCIC, 2014
Health and Social Care Information Centre, 2014. Accident and Emergency Attendances in England – 2012–13. Available

References

at: http://hscic.gov.uk/catalogue/pub13464/acci-emer-atte-eng-2012-13-data.xls [Accessed 23 December 2014].

HSE, 2009
Health and Safety Executive, 2009. Health and Safety Law. Available at: http://www.hse.gov.uk/pubns/law.pdf [Accessed 29 December 2014].

HSE, 2013a
Health and Safety Executive, 2013. Managing for Health and Safety. Available at: http://www.hse.gov.uk/pubns/priced/hsg65.pdf [Accessed 29 December 2014].

HSE, 2013b
Health and Safety Executive, 2013. Oxygen Use in the Workplace. Available at: https://www.hse.gov.uk/pubns/indg459.pdf [Accessed 27 April 2024].

HSE, 2015
Health and Safety Executive, 2015. Skin care at work. Available at: http://www.hse.gov.uk/healthservices/skin.htm [Accessed 23 November 2015].

HSE, 2016
Health and Safety Executive, 2016. Manual Handling Operations Regulations 1992: Guidance on Regulations (4th edition). Available at: https://www.hse.gov.uk/pubns/priced/l23.pdf [Accessed 21 January 2024].

HSE, 2017
Health and Safety Executive, 2017. Carriage of dangerous goods manual. Available at: https://www.hse.gov.uk/cdg/manual/index.htm [Accessed 20 April 2024].

HSE, 2020
Health and Safety Executive, 2020. Manual Handling at Work: A Brief Guide. Available at: https://www.hse.gov.uk/pubns/indg143.pdf [Accessed 29 January 2024].

HSE, 2022a
Health and Safety Executive, 2022. Hazard statements, precautionary statements and signal words. Available at: https://www.hse.gov.uk/chemical-classification/labelling-packaging/hazard-precautionary-statements-signal-words.htm [Accessed 20 April 2024].

HSE, 2022b
Health and Safety Executive, 2022. Hazard symbols and hazard pictograms – chemical classification. Available at: https://www.hse.gov.uk/chemical-classification/labelling-packaging/hazard-symbols-hazard-pictograms.htm [Accessed 20 April 2024].

HSE, 2023
Health and Safety Executive, 2023. UK mandatory classification and labelling and self-classification – chemical classification. Available at: https://www.hse.gov.uk/chemical-classification/classification/harmonised-classification-self-classification.htm [Accessed 20 April 2024].

HSE, 2024a
Health and Safety Executive, 2024. Managing risks and risk assessment at work. Available at: https://www.hse.gov.uk/simple-health-safety/risk/index.htm [Accessed 21 January 2024].

HSE, 2024b
Health and Safety Executive, 2024. Methods of decontamination. Available at: https://www.hse.gov.uk/biosafety/blood-borne-viruses/methods-of-decontamination.htm [Accessed 21 January 2024].

HSE, 2024c
Health and Safety Executive, 2024. Introduction to fire safety. Available at: https://www.hse.gov.uk/fireandexplosion/fire-safety.htm [Accessed 21 January 2024].

HSE, 2024d
Health and Safety Executive, 2024. Work-related stress and how to manage it. Available at: https://www.hse.gov.uk/stress/overview.htm [Accessed 21 January 2024].

HSE, 2024e
Health and Safety Executive, 2024. Managing risks and risk assessment at work. Available at: https://www.hse.gov.uk/simple-health-safety/risk/steps-needed-to-manage-risk.htm [Accessed 29 January 2024].

HSE, 2024f
Health and safety Executive, 2024. Risk factors associated with pushing and pulling loads. Available at: https://www.hse.gov.uk/msd/pushpull/risks.htm [Accessed 29 January 2024].

Human Rights Act 1988
UK Government. Human Rights Act 1998. Available at: http://www.legislation.gov.uk/ukpga/1998/42/contents [Accessed 31 October 2015].

Idris, 2003
Idris AH, Berg RA, Bierens J, et al., 2003. Recommended guidelines for uniform reporting of data from drowning. *Circulation*, 108(20), 2565–2574.

References

Innes, 2018
Innes JA, Dover AR, Fairhurst K., et al., 2018. *Macleod's Clinical Examination* (14th edition). Elsevier.

JESIP, 2023a
Joint Emergency Services Interoperability Programme, 2023. M/ETHANE. Available at: https://www.jesip.org.uk/downloads/m-ethane-full-version/ [Accessed 20 April 2024].

JESIP, 2023b
Joint Emergency Services Interoperability Programme, 2023. Initial Operational Response (IOR) to Incidents Suspected to Involve Hazardous Substances or CBRN Materials. Available at: https://naru.org.uk/wp-content/uploads/2023/05/IOR-2023-Accessible-Hi-res-No-Ticks-1.pdf [Accessed 5 May 2024].

JESIP, 2024
Joint Emergency Services Interoperability Programme, 2024. About JESIP. Available at: https://www.jesip.org.uk/about-jesip/ [Accessed 19 January 2024].

Johnson, 2012
Johnson G and Hill-Smith 2012. *The Minor Illness Manual*. London: Radcliffe Publishing.

Jolles, 2002
Jolles S, 2002. Paul Langerhans. *Journal of Clinical Pathology*, 55(4), 243–243.

JRCALC, 2023
Joint Royal Colleges Ambulance Liaison Committee and Association of Ambulance Chief Executives, 2023. JRCALC Clinical Guidelines. Cited from JRCALC Plus (Version 2.2) [Mobile application software] (2.2.1) [Computer software]. Bridgwater: Class Publishing Ltd.

Kehoe, 2015
Kehoe A, Smith JE, Edwards A, et al., 2015. The changing face of major trauma in the UK. *Emergency Medicine Journal*, 32(12), 911–915. https://doi.org/10.1136/emermed-2015-205265

Kerber, 2012
Kerber RE, 2012. Hands-on defibrillation – the end of 'I'm clear, you're clear, we're all clear'? *Journal of the American Heart Association*, 1(5), e005496.

King, 2014
King D, Morton R and Bevan C, 2014. How to use capillary refill time. *Archives of Disease in Childhood – Education & Practice Edition*, 99(3), 111–116.

King's Fund, 2024
The Kings Fund, 2024. What are health inequalities? Available at: https://www.kingsfund.org.uk/publications/what-are-health-inequalities#life [Accessed 22 January 2024].

Knight, 2008a
Knight J and Nigam Y, 2008. Exploring the anatomy and physiology of ageing. Part 2 – the respiratory system. *Nursing Times*, 104(32), 24–25.

Knight, 2008b
Knight J and Nigam Y, 2008. Exploring the anatomy and physiology of ageing. Part 1 – the cardiovascular system. *Nursing Times*, 104(31), 26–27.

Knight, 2008c
Knight J and Nigam Y, 2008. Exploring the anatomy and physiology of ageing. Part 5 – the nervous system. *Nursing Times*, 104(35), 18–19.

Knight, 2008d
Knight J and Nigam Y, 2008. Exploring the anatomy and physiology of ageing. Part 10 – muscles and bone. *Nursing Times*, 104(48), 22–23.

Knops, 2011
Knops SP, 2011. Comparison of three different pelvic circumferential compression devices: a biomechanical cadaver study. *The Journal of Bone & Joint Surgery (American)*, 93(3), 230. https://doi.org/10.2106/JBJS.J.00084

Knuuti, 2020
Knuuti J, Wijns W, Saraste A, et al., 2020. 2019 ESC Guidelines for the diagnosis and management of chronic coronary syndromes: the Task Force for the diagnosis and management of chronic coronary syndromes of the European Society of Cardiology (ESC). *European Heart Journal*, 41(3), 407–477. https://doi.org/10.1093/eurheartj/ehz425

Konstantinides, 2020
Konstantinides SV, Meyer G, Becattini C, et al., 2020. 2019 ESC Guidelines for the diagnosis and management of acute pulmonary embolism developed in collaboration with the European Respiratory Society (ERS): the Task Force for the diagnosis and management of acute pulmonary embolism of the European Society of Cardiology (ESC). *European Heart Journal*, 41(4), 543–603. https://doi.org/10.1093/eurheartj/ehz405

Kovacs, 2011
Kovacs G and Law JA, 2011. *Airway Management in Emergencies* (2nd edition). Shelton: McGraw-Hill Medical.

References

Krell, 2006
Krell J, McCoy M, Sparto P, et al., 2006. Comparison of the Ferno Scoop Stretcher with the long backboard for spinal immobilization. *Prehospital Emergency Care*, 10(1), 46–51.

Kumar, 2012
Kumar P and Clark M, 2012. *Kumar and Clark's Clinical Medicine* (8th edition). Edinburgh: Saunders.

Layon, 2009
Layon AJ and Modell JH, 2009. Drowning: update 2009. *Anesthesiology*, 110(6), 1390–1401.

Lee, 2007a
Lee C, Revell M, Porter K, et al., 2007. The prehospital management of chest injuries: a consensus statement. Faculty of pre-hospital care, Royal College of Surgeons of Edinburgh. *Emergency Medicine Journal*, 24(3), 220–224. https://doi.org/10.1136/emj.2006.043687

Lee, 2007b
Lee C, Porter KM and Hodgetts TJ, 2007. Tourniquet use in the civilian prehospital setting. *Emergency Medicine Journal*, 24(8), 584–587. https://doi.org/10.1136/emj.2007.046359

Lee, 2011
Lee JK and Vadas P, 2011. Anaphylaxis: mechanisms and management. *Clinical & Experimental Allergy*, 41(7), 923–938.

Leech, 2017
Leech C, Porter K, Steyn R, et al., 2017. The pre-hospital management of life-threatening chest injuries: a consensus statement from the Faculty of Pre-Hospital Care, Royal College of Surgeons of Edinburgh. *Trauma*, 19(1), 54–62. https://doi.org/10.1177/1460408616664553

Leenen, 2010
Leenen L, 2010. Pelvic fractures: soft tissue trauma. *European Journal of Trauma and Emergency Surgery*, 36(2), 117–123. https://doi.org/10.1007/s00068-010-1038-0

Leigh-Smith, 2005
Leigh-Smith S and Harris T, 2005. Tension pneumothorax – time for a re-think? *Emergency Medicine Journal*, 22(1), 8–16. https://doi.org/10.1136/emj.2003.010421

Leonard Cheshire, 2022
Leonard Cheshire, 2022. Disability hate crimes rise to record level. Available at: https://www.leonardcheshire.org/about-us/our-news/press-releases/disability-hate-crimes-rise-record-levels. [Accessed 23 December 2023].

Lewin, 2008
Lewin J and Maconochie I, 2008. Capillary refill time in adults. *Emergency Medicine Journal*, 25(6), 325–326.

Lipman, 2019
Lipman GS, Gaudio FG, Eifling KP, et al., 2019. Wilderness Medical Society Clinical Practice Guidelines for the Prevention and Treatment of Heat Illness: 2019 update. *Wilderness & Environmental Medicine*, 30(4S), S33–S46. https://doi.org/10.1016/j.wem.2018.10.004

Lissauer, 2007
Lissauer T and Clayden G, 2007. *Illustrated Textbook of Paediatrics* (3rd edition). Edinburgh: Mosby.

Lonnecker, 2001
Lonnecker S and Schoder V, 2001. Hypothermia after burn injury – influence of pre-hospital management. *Der Chirurg*, 72(2), 164–167. https://doi.org/10.1007/s001040051286

Lord, 2005
Lord SR and Davis PR, 2005. Drowning, near drowning and immersion syndrome. *Journal of the Royal Army Medical Corps*, 151(4), 250.

Lott, 2021
Lott C, Truhlář A, Alfonzo A, et al., 2021. European Resuscitation Council Guidelines 2021: cardiac arrest in special circumstances. *Resuscitation*, 161, 152–219. https://doi.org/10.1016/j.resuscitation.2021.02.011

Lunt, 2010
Lunt H, Florkowski C, Bignall M, et al., 2010. Capillary glucose meter accuracy and sources of error in the ambulatory setting. *New Zealand Medical Journal*, 123(1310), 74–85.

Lupsa, 2014
Lupsa BC and Inzucchi SE, 2014. Diabetic ketoacidosis and hyperosmolar hyperglycemic syndrome. In: Loriaux L (ed.), *Endocrine Emergencies*, Totowa, NJ: Humana Press.

Mackway-Jones, 2012
Mackway-Jones K, Carley S and Advanced Life Support Group, 2012. *Major Incident Medical Management and Support: The Practical Approach at the Scene*. Chichester: Wiley-Blackwell.

Management of Health and Safety at Work Regulations 1999
UK Government, 1999. The Management of Health and Safety at Work Regulations 1999. Available at: http://www.legislation.gov.uk/uksi/1999/3242/contents/made [Accessed 29 December 2014].

References

Mansfield, 2018
Mansfield A, Association of Ambulance Chief Executives and Joint Royal Colleges Ambulance Liaison Committee, 2018. *Emergency Birth in the Community* (1st ed.). Bridgwater: Class Professional Publishing.

Marieb, 2013
Marieb E and Hoehn K, 2013. *Human Anatomy and Physiology*. New York: Pearson.

Marieb, 2019
Marieb E and Hoehn K, 2019. *Human Anatomy and Physiology* (11th edition). Pearson.

McCormack, 2010
McCormack R, Strauss EJ, Alwattar BJ, et al., 2010. Diagnosis and management of pelvic fractures. *Bulletin of the NYU Hospital for Joint Diseases*, 68(4), 281.

McDonagh, 2021
McDonagh TA, Metra M, Adamo M, et al., 2021. 2021 ESC Guidelines for the diagnosis and treatment of acute and chronic heart failure: developed by the Task Force for the diagnosis and treatment of acute and chronic heart failure of the European Society of Cardiology (ESC) with the special contribution of the Heart Failure Association (HFA) of the ESC. *European Heart Journal*, 42(36), 3599–3726. https://doi.org/10.1093/eurheartj/ehab368

McGrath, 2012
McGrath BA, Bates L, Atkinson D, et al., 2012. Multidisciplinary guidelines for the management of tracheostomy and laryngectomy airway emergencies: tracheostomy management guidelines. *Anaesthesia*, 67(9), 1025–1041.

Mencap, 2023a
Mencap, 2023. https://www.mencap.org.uk/learning-disability-explained/what-learning-disability [Accessed 18 December 2023].

Mencap, 2023b
Mencap, 2023. Health Inequalities. Available at: https://www.mencap.org.uk/learning-disability-explained/research-and-statistics/health/health-inequalities [Accessed 23 December 2023].

Mencap, 2023c
Mencap, 2023. Communicating with people with a learning disability. Available at: https://www.mencap.org.uk/learning-disability-explained/communicating-people-learning-disability. [Accessed 23 December 2023].

Mental Capacity Act 2005
UK Government, 2005. Mental Capacity Act 2005. Available at: http://www.legislation.gov.uk/ukpga/2005/9/contents [Accessed 5 January 2015].

Merten, 2017
Merten H, van Galen LS and Wagner C, 2017. Safe handover. *British Medical Journal*. https://doi.org/10.1136/bmj.j4328

MHF, 2015
Mental Health Foundation, 2015. Mental health in later life. Available at: http://www.mentalhealth.org.uk/help-information/mental-health-a-z/o/older-people/ [Accessed 6 December 2015].

MHOR 1992
UK Government, 1992. The Manual Handling Operations Regulations 1992. Available at: http://www.hse.gov.uk/pubns/priced/l23.pdf [Accessed 29 December 2014].

Michael, 2008
Michael J, 2008. Healthcare for All. Available at: https://www.mencap.org.uk/sites/default/files/documents/Healthcare_for_all_0.pdf [Accessed 6 December 2015].

Mind, 2016
Mind, 2016. One in four emergency services workers has thought about ending their lives. Available at: https://www.mind.org.uk/news-campaigns/news/one-in-four-emergency-services-workers-has-thought-about-ending-their-lives/ [Accessed 19 January 2024].

Mind, 2024a
Mind, 2024. How to improve your mental wellbeing. Available at: https://www.mind.org.uk/information-support/tips-for-everyday-living/wellbeing/wellbeing/ [Accessed 19 January 2024].

Mind, 2024b
Mind, 2024. Managing stress and building resilience. Available at: https://www.mind.org.uk/information-support/types-of-mental-health-problems/stress/managing-stress-and-building-resilience/ [Accessed 19 January 2024].

Mind, 2024c
Mind, 2024. Supporting someone in the ambulance service. Available at: https://www.mind.org.uk/news-campaigns/campaigns/blue-light-programme/blue-light-information/supporting-someone-in-the-ambulance-service/ [Accessed 19 January 2024].

References

Monsieurs, 2015
Monsieurs KG, Nolan JP, Bossaert LL, et al., 2015. European Resuscitation Council guidelines for resuscitation 2015. Section 1. Executive summary. *Resuscitation*, 95, 1–80.

Moorhouse, 2007
Moorhouse I, Thurgood A, Walker N, et al., 2007. A realistic model for catastrophic external haemorrhage training. *Journal of the Royal Army Medical Corps*, 153(2), 99–101.

Moppett, 2007
Moppett IK, 2007. Traumatic brain injury: assessment, resuscitation and early management. *British Journal of Anaesthesia*, 99(1), 18–31. https://doi.org/10.1093/bja/aem128

Moritz, 1947
Moritz AR and Henriques FC, 1947. Studies of thermal injury. *The American Journal of Pathology*, 23(5), 695–720.

Muehlberger, 2010
Muehlberger T, Ottomann C, Toman N, et al., 2010. Emergency pre-hospital care of burn patients. *The Surgeon*, 8(2), 101–104. https://doi.org/10.1016/j.surge.2009.10.001

Müller, 2006
Müller D, Agrawal R and Arntz H-R, 2006. How sudden is sudden cardiac death? *Circulation*, 114(11), 1146–1150.

NAEMT, 2019
National Association of Emergency Medical Technicians and College of Paramedics, 2019. *Advanced Medical Life Support: UK Edition* (2nd edition). Burlington, MA: Jones & Bartlett Learning.

NAEMT, 2020
National Association of Emergency Medical Technicians (US) (ed.), 2020. *PHTLS: Prehospital Trauma Life Support* (9th edition). Burlington, MA: Jones & Bartlett Learning.

NARU, 2019
National Ambulance Resilience Unit, 2019. National Ambulance Service Command and Control Guidance. Available at: https://naru.s3.eu-west-2.amazonaws.com/wp-content/uploads/2021/03/03212229/NARU-COMMAND-AND-CONTROL-GUIDE-V3.1-07.2019.pdf [Accessed 19 January 2024].

NARU, 2022
National Ambulance Resilience Unit, 2022. Hazardous Area Response Teams (HART). Available at: https://naru.org.uk/the-interoperable-capabilities/hart/

NARU, 2024
National Ambulance Resilience Unit, 2024. Hazardous Area Response Teams. Available at: https://naru.org.uk/the-interoperable-capabilities/hart/ [Accessed 18 January 2024].

NCPC, 2013
The National Council for Palliative Care, 2013. Advance decisions to refuse treatment. A guide for health and social care professionals. Available at: https://www.england.nhs.uk/improvement-hub/wp-content/uploads/sites/44/2017/11/Advance-Decisions-to-Refuse-Treatment-Guide.pdf [Accessed 25 January 2024].

Neligan, 2010
Neligan A and Shorvon SD, 2010. Frequency and prognosis of convulsive status epilepticus of different causes: a systematic review. *Archives of Neurology*, 67(8), 931–940.

Nellist, 2013
Nellist E and Lethbridge K, 2013. The importance for paramedics to identify cauda equina syndrome. *Journal of Paramedic Practice*, 5(7), 310–313.

NHS, 2022a
NHS, 2022. Allergies. Available at: https://www.nhs.uk/conditions/allergies/ [Accessed 4 May 2024].

NHS, 2022b
NHS, 2022. Sunscreen and sun safety. Available at: https://www.nhs.uk/live-well/seasonal-health/sunscreen-and-sun-safety/ [Accessed 5 May 2024].

NHS, 2022c
NHS, 2022. Burns and scalds. Available at: https://www.nhs.uk/conditions/burns-and-scalds/ [Accessed 5 May 2024].

NHS, 2022d
NHS, 2022. Arthritis. Available at: https://www.nhs.uk/conditions/arthritis/ [Accessed 28 July 2024].

NHS, 2023a
NHS, 2023. MRSA. Available at: https://www.nhs.uk/conditions/mrsa/ [Accessed 21 January 2024].

NHS, 2023b
NHS, 2023. Broken hip. Available at: https://www.nhs.uk/conditions/broken-hip/ [Accessed 5 May 2024].

NHS, 2023c
NHS, 2023. Learning disabilities. Available at: https://www.nhs.uk/conditions/learning-disabilities/ [Accessed 18 December 2023].

References

NHS, 2023d
NHS, 2023. What is dementia? Available at: https://www.nhs.uk/conditions/dementia/about-dementia/what-is-dementia/ [Accessed 2 March 2024].

NHS Choices, 2015
NHS Choices, 2015. Causes of dementia. Available at: http://www.nhs.uk/conditions/dementia-guide/pages/causes-of-dementia.aspx [Accessed 29 November 2015].

NHS Choices, 2021a
NHS, 2021. What should I do if I injure myself with a used needle? Available at: https://www.nhs.uk/common-health-questions/accidents-first-aid-and-treatments/what-should-i-do-if-i-injure-myself-with-a-used-needle/ [Accessed 21 January 2024].

NHS Choices, 2021b
NHS, 2021. 10 stress busters. Available at: https://www.nhs.uk/mental-health/self-help/guides-tools-and-activities/tips-to-reduce-stress/ [Accessed 21 January 2024].

NHS Digital, 2022
NHS Digital, 2022. Data on written complaints in the NHS, 2021–22. Available at: https://digital.nhs.uk/data-and-information/publications/statistical/data-on-written-complaints-in-the-nhs/2021-22 [Accessed 28 January 2024].

NHS England, 2018
NHS England, 2018. The Ambulance Response Programme Review. Available at: https://www.england.nhs.uk/publication/the-ambulance-response-programme-review/ [Accessed 28 July 2024].

NHS England, 2019
NHS England, 2019. Confidentiality Policy. Available at: https://www.england.nhs.uk/wp-content/uploads/2019/10/confidentiality-policy-v5.1.pdf [Accessed 22 January 2024].

NHS England, 2020
NHS England, 2020. We are the NHS: People Plan 2020/21– action for us all. Available at: https://www.england.nhs.uk/wp-content/uploads/2020/07/We-Are-The-NHS-Action-For-All-Of-Us-FINAL-March-21.pdf [Accessed 22 January 2024].

NHS England, 2022
NHS England, 2022. NHS Emergency Preparedness, Resilience and Response Framework. Available at: https://www.england.nhs.uk/publication/nhs-emergency-preparedness-resilience-and-response-framework/ [Accessed 20 April 2024].

NHS England, 2023a
NHS England, 2023. Statistical Note: Ambulance Quality Indicators (AQI). Available at: https://www.england.nhs.uk/statistics/wp-content/uploads/sites/2/2023/04/20230413-Statistical-Note-AQI.pdf [Accessed 28 July 2024].

NHS England, 2023b
NHS England, 2023. National infection prevention and control manual for England. Available at: https://www.england.nhs.uk/wp-content/uploads/2022/04/PRN00908-national-infection-prevention-and-control-manual-for-england-v2.7.pdf [Accessed 21 January 2024].

NHS England, 2024a
NHS England, 2024. Freedom to speak up. Available at: https://www.england.nhs.uk/ourwork/freedom-to-speak-up/ [Accessed 22 January 2024].

NHS England, 2024b
NHS England, 2024. About information governance. Available at: https://www.england.nhs.uk/ig/about/ [Accessed 22 January 2024].

NHS England, 2024c
NHS England, 2024. What are healthcare inequalities? Available at: https://www.england.nhs.uk/about/equality/equality-hub/national-healthcare-inequalities-improvement-programme/what-are-healthcare-inequalities/ [Accessed 22 January 2024].

NHS England 2024d
NHS England, 2024. Safeguarding. Available at: https://www.england.nhs.uk/long-read/safeguarding/ [Accessed: 08 May 2024].

NHS Professionals, 2024
NHS Professionals, 2024. The 6Cs of care. Available at: https://www.nhsprofessionals.nhs.uk/nhs-staffing-pool-hub/working-in-healthcare/the-6-cs-of-care [Accessed 22 January 2024].

NHS Resolution, 2023
NHS Resolution, 2023. Advice for claimants. Available at: https://resolution.nhs.uk/services/claims-management/advice-for-claimants/#toc-item-0 [Accessed 22 January 2024].

NHS Scotland, 2024
NHS Scotland, 2024. Care Home Infection Prevention and Control Manual. Available at: https://www.nipcm.scot.nhs.uk/care-home-infection-prevention-and-control-manual-ch-ipcm/#a2821 [Accessed 21 January 2024].

References

NICE, 2013
National Institute for Health and Care Excellence, 2013. Falls: assessment and prevention of falls in older people. Available at: http://www.nice.org.uk/guidance/cg161/evidence/falls-full-guidance-190033741 [Accessed 29 November 2015].

NICE, 2015
National Institute for Health and Care Excellence, 2015. Meningitis (bacterial) and meningococcal septicaemia in under 16s: recognition, diagnosis and management. Available at: https://www.nice.org.uk/guidance/cg102 [Accessed 30 April 2024].

NICE, 2016
National Institute for Health and Care Excellence, 2016. Major trauma: assessment and initial management. Available at: https://www.nice.org.uk/guidance/ng39/chapter/recommendations#management-of-haemorrhage-in-prehospital-and-hospital-settings [Accessed 5 May 2024].

NICE, 2017
National Institute for Health and Care Excellence, 2017. Child maltreatment: when to suspect maltreatment in under 18s. Available at: https://www.nice.org.uk/guidance/CG89/ [Accessed 08 May 2024].

NICE, 2019
National Institute for Health and Care Excellence, 2019. Chronic obstructive pulmonary disease in over 16s: diagnosis and management. Available at: https://www.nice.org.uk/guidance/ng115 [Accessed 27 April 2024].

NICE, 2020
National Institute for Health and Care Excellence, 2020. Sprains and strains: scenario: Management. Available at: https://cks.nice.org.uk/topics/sprains-strains/management/management/ [Accessed 5 May 2024].

NICE, 2022a
National Institute for Health and Care Excellence, 2022. Type 1 diabetes in adults: diagnosis and management. Available at: https://www.nice.org.uk/guidance/ng17/chapter/Recommendations#diagnosis-and-early-care-plan [Accessed 28 July 2024].

NICE, 2022b
National Institute for Health and Care Excellence, 2022. Fractures (complex): assessment and management. Available at: https://www.nice.org.uk/guidance/ng37/chapter/Recommendations#pre-hospital-settings [Accessed 5 May 2024].

NICE, 2023
National Institute for Health and Care Excellence, 2023. Diabetes (type 1 and type 2) in children and young people: diagnosis and management. Available at: https://www.nice.org.uk/guidance/ng18 [Accessed 4 May 2024].

Nigam, 2008
Nigam Y and Knight J, 2008. Exploring the anatomy and physiology of ageing. Part 3 – the digestive system. *Nursing Times*, 104(33), 22–23.

Ninis, 2010
Ninis N, Nadel S and Glennie L, 2010. *Sections from Research for Doctors in Training* (3rd edition). Bristol: Meningitis Research Foundation.

Nolan, 2021
Nolan JP, Sandroni C, Böttiger BW, et al., 2021. European Resuscitation Council and European Society of Intensive Care Medicine Guidelines 2021: post-resuscitation care. *Resuscitation*, 161, 220–269. https://doi.org/10.1016/j.resuscitation.2021.02.012

Noppen, 2010
Noppen M, 2010. Spontaneous pneumothorax: epidemiology, pathophysiology and cause. *European Respiratory Review*, 19(117), 217–219. https://doi.org/10.1183/09059180.00005310

NPIS, 2022
National Poisons Information Service, 2022. Report 2021 to 2022. Available at: https://www.npis.org/Download/NPIS%20report%202021-22.pdf [Accessed 5 May 2024].

NSPCC, 2015
National Society for the Prevention of Cruelty to Children, 2015. Female genital mutilation (FGM): what is FGM? Available at: https://www.nspcc.org.uk/preventing-abuse/child-abuse-and-neglect/female-genital-mutilation-fgm/what-is-fgm/ [Accessed 6 November 2015].

NSPCC, 2020
National Society for the Prevention of Cruelty to Children, 2020. How safe are our children? 2020 report. Available at: https://learning.nspcc.org.uk/research-resources/how-safe-are-our-children [Accessed 08 May 2024].

NTSP, 2014
National Tracheostomy Safety Project (Great Britain), 2014. *Comprehensive Tracheostomy Care: The National Tracheostomy Safety Project Manual*. McGrath BA (ed.). Chichester: John Wiley & Sons.

References

Nutbeam, 2013
Nutbeam T and Boylan M, 2013. *ABC of Prehospital Emergency Medicine*. Chichester: John Wiley & Sons.

O'Brien, 2003
O'Brien E, Asmar R, Beilin L, et al., 2003. European society of hypertension recommendations for conventional, ambulatory and home blood pressure measurement. *Journal of Hypertension*, 21(5), 821–848.

O'Donnell, 2010
O'Donnell MJ, Xavier D, Liu L, et al., 2010. Risk factors for ischaemic and intracerebral haemorrhagic stroke in 22 countries (the INTERSTROKE study): a case-control study. *The Lancet*, 376(9735), 112–123.

O'Driscoll, 2017
O'Driscoll BR, Howard LS, Earis J, et al., 2017. BTS guideline for oxygen use in adults in healthcare and emergency settings. *Thorax*, 72(Supplement 1), ii1–ii90. https://doi.org/10.1136/thoraxjnl-2016-209729

Olasveengen, 2021
Olasveengen TM, Semeraro F, Ristagno G, et al., 2021. European Resuscitation Council Guidelines 2021: basic life support. *Resuscitation*, 161, 98–114. https://doi.org/10.1016/j.resuscitation.2021.02.009

ONS, 2021
Office for National Statistics, 2021. Deaths registered in England and Wales. https://www.ons.gov.uk/peoplepopulationandcommunity/birthsdeathsandmarriages/deaths/datasets/deathsregisteredinenglandandwalesseriesdrreferencetables [Accessed 25 April 2024].

ONS, 2022
Office for National Statistics, 2022. Voices of our ageing population: living longer lives. Available at: https://www.ons.gov.uk/peoplepopulationandcommunity/birthsdeathsandmarriages/ageing/articles/voicesofourageingpopulation/livinglongerlives. [Accessed 15 January 2024].

Osler, 2012
Osler W, 2012. Pneumonia part 1: pathology, presentation and prevention. *British Journal of Nursing*, 21(2), 103.

Papadopoulos, 2006
Papadopoulos IN, Kanakaris N, Bonovas S, et al., 2006. Auditing 655 fatalities with pelvic fractures by autopsy as a basis to evaluate trauma care. *Journal of the American College of Surgeons*, 203(1), 30–43. https://doi.org/10.1016/j.jamcollsurg.2006.03.017

Parkinson's UK, 2015
Parkinson's UK, 2015. What is Parkinson's? Available at: http://www.parkinsons.org.uk/content/what-parkinsons [Accessed 6 December 2015].

Parliament, 2021
Parliament, 2021. Down syndrome Bill Explanatory Notes. Available at: https://publications.parliament.uk/pa/bills/cbill/58-02/0017/en/210017en.pdf [Accessed 18 December 2023].

Paxton, 2003
Paxton S, Peckham M and Knibbs A, 2003. *The Leeds Histology Guide*. Available at: https://www.histology.leeds.ac.uk/skin/epidermis_layers.php

PHE, 2018
Public Health England, 2018. First stroke estimates in England: 2007 to 2016. GOV.UK. https://www.gov.uk/government/publications/first-stroke-estimates-in-england-2007-to-2016 [Accessed 30 April 2024].

PHE, 2019
Public Health England, 2019. Meningococcal disease: guidance on public health management. Available at: https://www.gov.uk/government/publications/meningococcal-disease-guidance-on-public-health-management [Accessed 30 April 2024].

PHE, 2020
Public Health England, 2020. Reasonable adjustments for people with a learning disability. Available at: https://www.gov.uk/government/collections/reasonable-adjustments-for-people-with-a-learning-disability [Accessed 23 December 2023].

PHE, 2022
Public Health England, 2022. Meningococcal: the green book, chapter 22. Available at: https://www.gov.uk/government/publications/meningococcal-the-green-book-chapter-22 [Accessed 30 April 2024]

PHE, 2023
Public Health England, 2023. Learning disability – applying all our health. Available at: https://www.gov.uk/government/publications/learning-disability-applying-all-our-health/learning-disabilities-applying-all-our-health [Accessed 18 December 2023]

Pickard, 2011
Pickard A, Karlen W and Ansermino JM, 2011. Capillary refill time: is it still a useful clinical sign? *Anesthesia & Analgesia*, 113(1), 120–123. https://doi.org/10.1213/ANE.0b013e31821569f9

References

PIE, 2014
Picker Institute Europe, 2014. NHS staff surveys – 2013 results. Available at: http://www.nhsstaffsurveys.com/page/1006/latest-results/2013-results/ [Accessed 8 December 2014].

Pilbery & Lethbridge, 2022
Pilbery R and Lethbridge K, 2022. *Ambulance Care Clinical Skills* (1st edition). Bridgwater: Class Publishing Ltd.

Porth, 2014
Porth C, 2014. *Essentials of Pathophysiology: Concepts of Altered States* (4th international edition). Philadelphia: Lippincott Williams & Wilkins.

Prien, 1988
Prien T and Traber DL, 1988. Toxic smoke compounds and inhalation injury – a review. *Burns, Including Thermal Injury*, 14(6), 451–460.

Purcell, 2016
Purcell D, 2016. *Minor Injuries: A Clinical Guide* (3rd edition). London: Churchill Livingstone.

Randle, 2009
Randle J, Coffey F and Bradbury M, 2009. *Oxford Handbook of Clinical Skills in Adult Nursing*. Oxford; New York: Oxford University Press.

RCEM, 2019
Royal College of Emergency Medicine, 2019. Paediatric Trauma – Stabilisation of the Cervical Spine. Available at: https://rcem.ac.uk/wp-content/uploads/2021/10/Paediatric_Trauma_Stabilisation_of_the_Cervical_Spine_Jan20.pdf [Accessed 5 May 2019].

RCN, 2023
Royal College of Nursing, 2023. Duty of care. Available at: https://www.rcn.org.uk/Get-Help/RCN-advice/duty-of-care [Accessed 22 January 2024].

RCUK, 2015
Working Group of the Resuscitation Council UK 2015. Guidance for safe handling during cardiopulmonary resuscitation in healthcare settings. Available at: https://www.resus.org.uk/EasysiteWeb/getresource.axd?AssetID=5194&type=Full&servicetype=Attachment [Accessed 2 May 2016].

RCUK, 2021a
Resuscitation Council UK, 2021. *Advanced Life Support* (8th edition). Resuscitation Council UK.

RCUK, 2021b
Resuscitation Council UK, 2021. *European Paediatric Advanced Life Support* (5th edition). London: Resuscitation Council.

RCUK, 2021c
Resuscitation Council UK, 2021. Emergency treatment of anaphylaxis. Available at: https://www.resus.org.uk/sites/default/files/2021-05/Emergency%20Treatment%20of%20Anaphylaxis%20May%202021_0.pdf [Accessed 5 May 2024].

Roberts, 2014
Roberts JR, 2014. *Roberts and Hedges' Clinical Procedures in Emergency Medicine* (6th edition). New York: Elsevier.

Rodgers, 2004
Rodgers H, Greenaway J, Davies T, et al., 2004. Risk factors for first-ever stroke in older people in the North East of England: a population-based study. *Stroke*, 35(1), 7–11.

Rothermel, 2016
Rothermel LD and Lipman JM, 2016. Estimation of blood loss is inaccurate and unreliable. *Surgery*, 160(4), 946–953. https://doi.org/10.1016/j.surg.2016.06.006

ROS, 2021
Royal Osteoporosis Society, 2021. About osteoporosis and weaker bones. Available at: https://strwebprdmedia.blob.core.windows.net/media/wazb1oxv/about-osteoporosis-and-weaker-bones-easy-print-version.pdf [Accessed 28 July 2024].

SAS, 2014
Scottish Ambulance Service, 2014. Dementia Learning Resource. Available at: https://www.nes.scot.nhs.uk/media/nlqdz3fn/scottish_ambulance_service.pdf [Accessed 28 July 2024].

Savage, 2011
Savage MW, Dhatariya KK, Kilvert A, et al., 2011. Joint British diabetes societies guideline for the management of diabetic ketoacidosis: diabetic ketoacidosis guidelines. *Diabetic Medicine*, 28(5), 508–515.

Scott, 2013
Scott I, Porter K, Laird C, et al., 2013. The prehospital management of pelvic fractures: initial consensus statement. *Emergency Medicine Journal*, 30(12), 1070–1072. https://doi.org/10.1136/emermed-2013-203211

References

Scott, 2015
Scott AR, the Joint British Diabetes Societies (JBDS) for Inpatient Care and the JBDS Hyperosmolar Hyperglycaemic Guidelines Group, 2015. Management of hyperosmolar hyperglycaemic state in adults with diabetes. *Diabetic Medicine*, 32(6), 714–724.

Semeraro, 2021
Semeraro F, Greif R, Böttiger BW, et al., 2021. European Resuscitation Council Guidelines 2021: systems saving lives. *Resuscitation*, 161, 80–97. https://doi.org/10.1016/j.resuscitation.2021.02.008

Seventer, 2017
Seventer J and Hochbery N, 2017. Principles of infectious diseases: transmission, diagnosis, prevention, and control. International Encyclopedia of Public Health. Available at: https://www.ncbi.nlm.nih.gov/pmc/articles/PMC7150340/ [Accessed 21 January 2024].

SG, 2009
Scottish Government, 2009. Review of Allergy Services in Scotland: A Report by a Working Group of the Scottish Medical and Scientific Advisory Committee. Available at: http://www.gov.scot/publications/2009/06/17135245/0 [Accessed 5 November 2014].

Shannon, 1949
Shannon CE and Weaver W, 1949. *The Mathematical Theory of Communication*. Champaign, IL: University of Illinois Press.

Sharma, 2008
Sharma A and Jindal P, 2008. Principles of diagnosis and management of traumatic pneumothorax. *Journal of Emergencies, Trauma and Shock*, 1(1), 34–41. https://doi.org/10.4103/0974-2700.41789

Sheridan, 2012
Sheridan R, 2012. *Burns: A Practical Approach to Immediate Treatment and Long-term Care*. London: Manson Publishing.

Shivaji, 2014
Shivaji T, Lee A, Dougall N, et al., 2014. The epidemiology of hospital treated traumatic brain injury in Scotland. *BMC Neurology*, 14, 2. https://doi.org/10.1186/1471-2377-14-2

Shorten, 1994
Shorten GD, Opie NJ, Graziotti P, et al., 1994. Assessment of upper airway anatomy in awake, sedated and anaesthetised patients using magnetic resonance imaging. *Anaesthesia and Intensive Care*, 22(2), 165–169. https://doi.org/10.1177/0310057X9402200208

SIA, 2020
Spinal Injuries Association, 2020. Spinal cord injury paralyses someone every four hours, new estimates reveal. Available at: https://spinal.co.uk/news/spinal-cord-injury-paralyses-someone-every-four-hours-new-estimates-reveal/ [Accessed 5 May 2024].

SIGN/BTS, 2019
Scottish Intercollegiate Guidelines Network and British Thoracic Society, 2019. British guideline on the management of asthma. https://www.brit-thoracic.org.uk/quality-improvement/guidelines/asthma/ [Accessed 27 April 2024]

Simon, 2010
Simon C, 2010. *Oxford Handbook of General Practice* (3rd edition). Oxford Handbooks. Oxford: Oxford University Press.

Simons, 2001
Simons FER, Gu X and Simons KJ, 2001. Epinephrine absorption in adults: intramuscular versus subcutaneous injection. *Journal of Allergy and Clinical Immunology*, 108(5), 871–873.

Singer, 2010
Singer AJ, Taira BR, Thode Jr HC, et al., 2010. The association between hypothermia, prehospital cooling, and mortality in burn victims. *Academic Emergency Medicine*, 17(4), 456–459. https://doi.org/10.1111/j.1553-2712.2010.00702.x

Singer, 2016
Singer M, Deutschman CS, Seymour CW, et al., 2016. The third international consensus definitions for sepsis and septic shock (sepsis-3). *JAMA*, 315(8), 801–810. https://doi.org/10.1001/jama.2016.0287

SJA, 2021
St John Ambulance, St Andrew's First Aid and British Red Cross, 2021. *First Aid Manual* (11th edition). Harlow: Dorling Kindersley.

Skills for Health, 2020
Skills for Health, 2020. Manual Handling Regulations: The Complete Employer's Guide. Available at: https://www.skillsforhealth.org.uk/article/manual-handling-regulations-the-complete-employers-guide/ [Accessed 29 January 2024].

Smith, 2011
Smith J (ed.), 2011. *The Guide to the Handling of People: A Systems Approach*. Teddington: BackCare.

References

Smithson, 2012
Smithson H and Walker MC, 2012. *ABC of Epilepsy* (1st edition). ABC series. Chichester: John Wiley & Sons.

Soar, 2021
Soar J, Böttiger BW, Carli P, et al., 2021. European Resuscitation Council Guidelines 2021: adult advanced life support. *Resuscitation*, 161, 115–151. https://doi.org/10.1016/j.resuscitation.2021.02.010

Stewart, 2013
Stewart M, 2013. BET 3: pelvic circumferential compression devices for haemorrhage control: panacea or myth? *Emergency Medicine Journal*, 30(5), 425–426. https://doi.org/10.1136/emermed-2013-202602.3

Sundstrøm, 2014
Sundstrøm T, Asbjørnsen H, Habiba S, et al., 2014. Prehospital use of cervical collars in trauma patients: a critical review. *Journal of Neurotrauma*, 31(6), 531–540. https://doi.org/10.1089/neu.2013.3094

Szpilman, 2012
Szpilman D, Bierens JJLM, Handley AJ, et al., 2012. Drowning. *New England Journal of Medicine,* 366(22), 2102–2110.

Talley, 2006
Talley NJ and O'Connor S, 2006. *Clinical Examination: A Systematic Guide to Physical Diagnosis* (5th edition). London: Elsevier.

Tapson, 2008
Tapson VF, 2008. Acute pulmonary embolism. *The New England Journal of Medicine*, 358(10), 1037–1052. https://doi.org/10.1056/NEJMra072753

TARN, 2017
Trauma Audit and Research Network, 2017. *Major Trauma in Older People – 2017 Report*. Manchester: University of Manchester.

TASC, 2024
The Ambulance Staff Charity, 2024. What does The Ambulance Staff Charity do? Available at: https://www.theasc.org.uk/what-we-do/ [Accessed 19 January 2024].

Teixeira, 2018
Teixeira PGR, Brown CVR, Emigh B, et al., 2018. Civilian prehospital tourniquet use is associated with improved survival in patients with peripheral vascular injury. *Journal of the American College of Surgeons*, 226(5), 769. https://doi.org/10.1016/j.jamcollsurg.2018.01.047

Thompson, 2006
Thompson MJ, Ninis N, Perera R, et al., 2006. Clinical recognition of meningococcal disease in children and adolescents. *The Lancet*, 367(9508), 397–403.

Thompson, 2006b
Thompson N, 2006. *Anti-Discriminatory Practice* (4th edition). Basingstoke: Palgrave Macmillan.

Thompson, 2008
Thompson G and Sciarra J (eds), 2008. *Wound Care Made Incredibly Visual*. Ambler, PA: Lippincott Williams & Wilkins.

Toon, 2010
Toon MH, Maybauer MO, Greenwood JE, et al., 2010. Management of acute smoke inhalation injury. *Critical Care and Resuscitation: Journal of the Australasian Academy of Critical Care Medicine*, 12(1), 53–61.

Tortora, 2017
Tortora GJ and Derrickson B, 2017. *Principles of Anatomy and Physiology* (15th edition). John Wiley & Sons.

UKHSA, 2021
UK Health Security Agency, 2021. Bloodborne viruses in healthcare workers: report exposures and reduce risks. Available at: https://www.gov.uk/guidance/bloodborne-viruses-in-healthcare-workers-report-exposures-and-reduce-risks [Accessed: 8 May 2024].

UKG, 2018
UK Government, 2018. First stroke estimates in England: 2007 to 2016. Available at: https://www.gov.uk/government/publications/first-stroke-estimates-in-england-2007-to-2016 [Accessed 28 July 2024].

UKST, 2024
UK Sepsis Trust, 2024. *The Sepsis Manual*. Available at: https://sepsistrust.org/wp-content/uploads/2024/02/Sepsis-Manual-7th-Edition-2024-V1.0.pdf [Accessed 2024-05-04].

UNICEF, 2023
UNICEF, 2023. What is female genital mutilation? Available at: https://www.unicef.org/protection/female-genital-mutilation [Accessed: 08 May 2024].

Vaidya, 2016
Vaidya R, Scott AN, Tonnos F, et al., 2016. Patients with pelvic fractures from blunt trauma. What is the cause of mortality and when? *American Journal of Surgery*, 211(3), 495–500. https://doi.org/10.1016/j.amjsurg.2015.08.038

References

Valensi, 2011
Valensi P, Lorgis L and Cottin Y, 2011. Prevalence, incidence, predictive factors and prognosis of silent myocardial infarction: a review of the literature. *Archives of Cardiovascular Diseases*, 104(3), 178–188.

Van Ness-Otunnu, 2013
Van Ness-Otunnu R and Hack JB, 2013. Hyperglycemic crisis. *Journal of Emergency Medicine*, 45(5), 797–805.

Vassallo, 2024
Vassallo J, Cowburn P, Park C, et al., 2024. Ten second triage: a novel and pragmatic approach to major incident triage. *Trauma*, 26(1), 3–6. https://doi.org/10.1177/14604086231156219

Voorde, 2021
Voorde PV de, Turner NM, Djakow J, et al., 2021. European Resuscitation Council Guidelines 2021: paediatric life support. *Resuscitation*, 161, 327–387. https://doi.org/10.1016/j.resuscitation.2021.02.015

Wallace, 2018
Wallace J and Raven D, 2018. Silver trauma. *RCEMLearning*. Available at: https://www.rcemlearning.co.uk/foamed/silver-trauma/ [Accessed 5 May 2024].

Walls, 2012
Walls RM and Murphy MF (eds), 2012. *Manual of Emergency Airway Management* (4th edition). Philadelphia: Wolters Kluwer/Lippincott Williams & Wilkins Health.

Wardrope, 2008
Wardrope J, Driscoll P, Laird JC, et al., 2008. *Community Emergency Medicine* (1st edition). London: Churchill Livingstone.

Watson, 2001
Watson RS, Cummings P, Quan L, et al., 2001. Cervical spine injuries among submersion victims. *Journal of Trauma*, 51(4), 658–662.

Wells, 2001
Wells LC, Smith JC, Weston VC, et al., 2001. The child with a non-blanching rash: how likely is meningococcal disease? *Archives of Disease in Childhood*, 85(3), 218.

Weston, 2014
Weston D, 2014. *Fundamentals of Infection Prevention and Control: Theory and Practice* (2nd edition). Chichester: John Wiley & Sons.

White, 2023
White A, Sheehan R, Ding J, et al., 2023. *LeDeR Annual Report Learning from Lives and Deaths: People with a Learning Disability and Autistic People 2022*. Available at: https://www.kcl.ac.uk/ioppn/assets/fans-dept/leder-2022-v2.0.pdf [Accessed 28 July 2024].

WHO, 2009
World Health Organization, 2009. WHO Guidelines for Safe Surgery 2009: Safe Surgery Saves Lives. Available at: http://apps.who.int/iris/bitstream/10665/44185/1/9789241598552_eng.pdf [Accessed 19 January 2015].

WHO, 2024a
World Health Organization, 2024. Infection prevention and control. Available at: https://www.who.int/health-topics/infection-prevention-and-control#tab=tab_1 [Accessed 21 January 2024].

WHO, 2024b
World Health Organization, 2024. WHO COVID-19 dashboard. Available at: https://data.who.int/dashboards/covid19/cases?n=c [Accessed 21 January 2024].

WHO, 2024c
World Health Organization, 2024. Infection prevention control: hand hygiene. Available at: https://www.who.int/teams/integrated-health-services/infection-prevention-control/hand-hygiene [Accessed 21 January 2024].

Wijdicks, 2010
Wijdicks EFM, 2010. The bare essentials: coma. *Practical Neurology*, 10(1), 51–60.

Williams, 2013
Williams TA, Finn J, Celenza A, et al., 2013. Paramedic identification of acute pulmonary edema in a metropolitan ambulance service. *Prehospital Emergency Care*, 130313131857002.

Williams, 2018
Williams B, Mancia G, Spiering W, et al., 2018. 2018 ESC/ESH guidelines for the management of arterial hypertension: the Task Force for the management of arterial hypertension of the European Society of Cardiology (ESC) and the European Society of Hypertension (ESH). *European Heart Journal*, 39(33), 3021–3104. https://doi.org/10.1093/eurheartj/ehy339

References

Yarmus, 2023
Yarmus L and Akulian J, 2023. Pneumothorax – symptoms, diagnosis and treatment. *BMJ Best Practice*. Available at: https://bestpractice.bmj.com/topics/en-gb/3000083 [Accessed 5 May 2024].

Yoon, 2023
Yoon JS, Choi SY, Suh JH, et al., 2013. Tension pneumothorax, is it a really life-threatening condition? *Journal of Cardiothoracic Surgery*, 8, 197. https://doi.org/10.1186/1749-8090-8-197

Young, 2024
Young GB, 2024. Assessment of coma. Available at: https://bestpractice.bmj.com/topics/en-gb/417 [Accessed 30 April 2024]

Zideman, 2021
Zideman DA, Singletary EM, Borra V, et al., 2021. European Resuscitation Council Guidelines 2021: first aid. *Resuscitation*, 161, 270–290. https://doi.org/10.1016/j.resuscitation.2021.02.013

Glossary

Medical terminology can be rather overwhelming at first. This glossary will provide an explanation of various terms.

Anterior
The front surface of the body, or situated nearer to the front of the body (particularly if comparing the position of one structure to another).

Arrhythmia
A problem with the rate or rhythm of the heartbeat.

Aspiration
Fluid or solid entering the lower respiratory tract (larynx and below).

Aspirin
Aspirin has an anti-platelet action which reduces clot formation and has analgesic (pain-relieving), antipyretic (temperature reducing) and anti-inflammatory actions.

Auscultation
The technique of listening to sounds within the body using a stethoscope.

Autoimmune disease
Autoimmune diseases arise from an abnormal immune response of the body against itself, i.e. against substances and tissues that are normally present in the body.

Battle's sign
Bruising behind the ears, which can indicate a skull fracture.

Body mass index
Body mass index (BMI) is defined as a persons weight divided by the square of their height in metres (kg/m^2). This can be adjusted for age and gender, and supplemented with waist circumference measurements, if appropriate. A patient with a BMI of 25–29.9 kg/m^2 is considered to be overweight, and if over 30 kg/m^2, obese.

Bradycardia
Slow heart rate.

Brittle asthma
Brittle asthma is a rare form of severe asthma which can result in very serious and often life-threatening attacks.

BVM
Bag-valve-mask.

Care Quality Commission
An independent health and adult social care regulator for England. Their job is to make sure health and social care services provide people with safe, effective, compassionate, high-quality care. They do this by monitoring, inspecting and regulating services to make sure they meet fundamental standards of quality and safety.

Cartilage
Cartilage is a flexible connective tissue found in areas of the body, including the joints between bones, the ribcage, the ear, the nose, the bronchial tubes and the intervertebral discs. It is not as hard and rigid as bone but is stiffer and less flexible than muscle. It does not contain blood vessels, so grows and repairs slowly.

Catastrophic haemorrhage
Bleeding severe enough to cause exsanguination, i.e. blood loss causing death, typically within minutes, or less.

Choking
A mechanical obstruction of the airway occurring anywhere between the mouth and carina.

Circadian rhythms
Circadian rhythms are physical, mental and behavioural changes that follow an approximate 24-hour cycle, responding primarily to light and darkness in a persons environment.

Cognitive function
A persons ability to process thoughts. It encompasses memories, perception, thinking and reasoning.

Connective tissue
Basic tissue type that binds, supports and separates other tissue and organs.

Crepitus
The grating, crackling or popping sounds and sensations experienced under the skin and joints, or a crackling sensation due to the presence of air under the skin. A type of crepitus, bone crepitus, can be heard and felt when two fragments of a fracture are moved against each other.

Distal
Further from the point of attachment of a limb.

Glossary

Fetal maceration
Tissue degeneration that occurs once an undelivered fetus dies.

Focal
Affecting a specific region of the body. For example, a focal neurological deficit may result in a weakness or paralysis of a limb following an impairment of nerve, spinal cord, or brain function.

Furosemide
A commonly used diuretic drug (water tablet) from the group known as *loop diuretics*.

Glasgow Coma Scale score
The Glasgow Coma Scale (GCS) was developed in 1974 as a way of objectively testing the level of consciousness in brain-injured patients and to improve communication between healthcare professionals. It was originally a 14-point score, but the division of limb flexion into withdrawal and abnormal flexion led to the 15-point score familiar today. Although designed for in-hospital use, it is now routinely used by the ambulance service and is an important marker for the early management of traumatic brain injury (TBI).

Haematoma
A blood clot that has formed outside a blood vessel (artery or vein).

Haemoptysis
Coughing up or spitting of blood from the lungs.

Humerus
The long bone of the upper arm.

Ileus
A partial or complete blockage of the bowel.

Intercostal
Between the ribs.

Ketonaemia
The presence of ketone bodies in the blood.

Korotkoff sounds
Turbulent blood flow that can be heard when using the manual auscultatory technique to record blood pressure. Named after a Russian surgeon, Nikolai Korotkoff, who first described them in 1905.

Kussmaul breathing
Breathing that is abnormally deep and rapid, sighing. Named after the nineteenth century Strasbourg physician Adolph Kussmaul.

Lateral
Of, at, towards, or from the side or sides.

Medial
Towards or at the midline of the body.

METHANE
The mnemonic METHANE is designed to provide the initial communication surrounding details of a major incident. It consists of:
- **M**ajor incident declared or standby. The person making the report should be explicit whether this is a major incident declaration or a standby in anticipation of the occurrence of a major incident.
- **E**xact location of the incident. Where possible the grid reference or GPS co-ordinates should be included, along with any landmarks or iconic sites.
- **T**ype of incident. What is the exact nature of the incident? For example rail, chemical, road or terrorist.
- **H**azards. What hazards are known to be present or could potentially manifest themselves?
- **A**ccess and egress. What are the agreed or best routes to and from the scene?
- **N**umber of casualties. How many casualties are there and, if possible to determine, what are the level and severity of injuries?
- **E**mergency services. Which emergency services are present and which are required? Include specialist resource request if known.

Micro-organism
A very small organism that lives outside and inside larger organisms such as the human body.

Oedema
An abnormal build-up of fluid, mainly water, in the body. People with kidney failure are prone to fluid overload, leading to oedema.

Oliguria
Abnormally reduced production of urine.

OPA
Oropharyngeal airway. A curved plastic tube, with a reinforced flange at one end and designed so that it fits between the tongue and hard palate to help keep the airway open.

Panda eyes
Bruising around both eyes that can be a sign of skull fracture.

Partial pressure
In a mixture of gases, each gas has a partial pressure which is the hypothetical pressure of that gas if it alone occupied

the volume of the mixture at the same temperature. The total pressure of the gas mixture is the sum of the partial pressures of each individual gas in the mixture.

Percussion
A method of tapping on a surface to determine the underlying structure. It is used in clinical examinations to assess the condition of the thorax or abdomen.

Pleuritic chest pain
Chest pain that is usually sharp and stabbing, localised to a specific area of the chest (the patient can often point to the pain with a finger) and made worse by coughing and deep inspiration.

Posterior
Further back in position; of or nearer the rear or hind end.

Primary assessment
A swift patient assessment and management process, which can be completed within 60–90 seconds. It is designed to be a stepwise approach, meaning that any abnormalities identified in one step should be addressed before moving on to the next.

Precordium
The area over the heart and lower thorax.

Proximal
Located nearer to the centre of the body or the point of attachment.

Psychomotor
Physical behaviour that is the result of conscious mental processes.

Pulse oximetry
The technique of measuring the oxygen saturation of the haemoglobin in the blood.

Recession
In an anatomical context, the drawing away of a tissue (or part of a tissue) from its normal position.

Rigors
Shaking or exaggerated shivering which usually occurs in response to a high temperature.

SADs
Supraglottic airway devices. Airway devices that sit just above the glottis. The most common SAD is the laryngeal mask airway.

SAMPLE
An acronym for:
- **S** Signs and symptoms of the presenting complaint.
- **A** Allergies (particularly to medication but food allergies might be relevant).
- **M** Medications.
- **P** Past medical history.
- **L** Last oral intake.
- **E** Events that led to the current illness or injury.

Scope of practice
The area or areas of a persons profession where they have the knowledge, skill and experience to practise safely and effectively.

SOCRATES
- **S** Site.
- **O** Onset.
- **C** Character. Same as Quality above.
- **R** Radiation.
- **A** Association. Are there any other signs and symptoms associated with the presenting complaint?
- **T** Timing.
- **E** Exacerbating/relieving factors.
- **S** Severity.

Stridor
High-pitched (usually) inspiratory breath sound, indicating upper airway narrowing.

Superior
Located above or directed upward. In human anatomy, situated nearer to the top of the head (vertex). Opposite of inferior.

Supine
Lying face up, usually referring to a patient who is lying on their back.

Surfactant
A substance made up of lipids and proteins and produced in the lungs. It lines the surface of the alveoli and decreases the surface tension, making it much easier to inflate the lungs.

Tachycardia
Rapid heart rate.

Tachypnoea
Rapid breathing rate.

Glossary

TILEE
- **T**ask. Consider if the lift:
  - involves holding the load away from the body
  - involves long distances
  - requires strenuous effort or twisting.
- **I**ndividual. Consider whether the lift:
  - requires specialist training
  - presents a hazard
  - if you and your colleagues are capable of performing the lift.
- **L**oad. Is the load:
  - heavy
  - difficult to get hold of
  - unstable
  - unpredictable
  - harmful
  - likely to grab out when alarmed at being carried down the stairs.
- **E**nvironment. Determine the presence of:
  - constraints on posture, e.g. low ceiling, confined spaces
  - poor, uneven flooring
  - hot/cold/wet weather
  - poor lighting
  - noise.
- **E**quipment: Consider what equipment:
  - is available
  - will reduce the risk to you and the patient
  - is safe to use
  - you are trained and competent in the use of.

Turgor
Condition of normal tension in a cell or group of cells, such as the skin.

Urticaria
(Also called nettle rash or hives.) Swelling of the superficial layers of the skin, usually as a result of an allergic reaction. The characteristic itchy lumps (called weals or hives) last for only a few hours.

Index

Abbey Pain Scale 276, 277
abdomen
    assessment 92
    trauma 205–206, 219, 220
abdominal thrusts
    choking adult 112
    choking child 114
abrasion 213
absence convulsions 175
abuse 59–64
    learning disabilities 266
    management 63
    psychological 61
accessory muscles, respiration 117, 260
accusations of abuse 63
acrocyanosis 259
acute coronary syndrome 165–166
acute heart failure 166–167
acute poisoning 201
acute smoke inhalation injury 249
adolescents. see teenagers
adrenaline
    blood sugar regulation 193
    intramuscular 188
ADRT (advance decision to refuse treatment) 29, 297
adult basic life support 292–295
    with AED 292–293
Adults with Incapacity (Scotland) Act 2000 28
advance decision to refuse treatment 29, 297
advanced practitioners 8–9
AEDs (automated external defibrillators) 3–4, 284
age
    communication 18
    discrimination 34, 273
ageing 269–271
ageism 278
agonal breathing 293
agonal rhythm 283
air pressure 116–117
aircraft, in-flight defibrillation 284
airwaves pager 21
airway 93–114
    assessment 88–89, 96–107, 215
    child 113, 259, 288–292
    convulsions 176
    infant 113, 259, 285–288
    lower 95–96
    management 96–107
    smoke inhalation 249
airway adjuncts 104–107
    oropharyngeal airway 104

alcohol
    hypothermia and 182
    toxidromes 200
alcohol-based hand rub 45–46
    medical gases and 121
alkalis, burns 250
allergies, history taking 90
alternative care pathways/providers 7
alveoli, lungs 116
Alzheimer's disease 275
ambient light, capillary refill time 156
Ambulance Response Programme 5, 6
ambulance service 5–13
    at scene 82
ambulance trusts, role in NHS response to emergencies 82
amylin 192
anaphylaxis 187–190
anatomy
    airway 93–96
    cardiovascular system 147–153
    nervous system 169–173
    pancreas 192–193
aneroid sphygmomanometer 158
angina 164
angioedema 187
anterior (term) 319
anticholinergic toxidromes 199
aorta, physiology 150–151
aprons 47, 48–49
    removing 49–50
arachnoid mater 171
arrhythmia 292, 319
arterial bleeding 207
arterial blood gas 138
arteries 151
    ageing 270
    brain 176
arterioles 150
arthritis 272
aspiration 319
aspirin 165–166, 319
    on blood glucose 196
assessment, at major incidents 82
assisted ventilation 124–129
associate ambulance practitioners 8
asthma 140–142
    assessing severity 141
    brittle 319
asystole 282, 283
atherosclerosis 164, 275
ATMIST model, handovers 20

Index

atria, heart 148
atrial systole 151–152
atrioventricular node 149
atrioventricular valve 151–152
auscultation 319
    blood pressure 158
autoimmune disease 319
auto-injectors, adrenaline 188–190
automated blood pressure measurement 158, 161
automated external defibrillators 3–4, 284
autonomic nervous system 172–173
autonomy, personal 28
AVPU (level of consciousness) 89, 262
axilla, thermometers 183
axillary temperature measurement 183–184

Baby P (Connelly), abuse case 60
Bachmann bundles 148–149
back blows 112
    infant 113
back injury 65
    see also spine
backup 29
bacteria 41
bag-valve-mask ventilation 125–129, 319
balance, ageing 271
'bare below elbows' policy 47
barotrauma 218
basic life support 3–4
    see also cardiopulmonary resuscitation
batch label, gas cylinders 120, 121
Battle's sign (panda eyes) 217, 319
beclometasone 140
behavioural dementia 275
best-interest decisions 28
'big bang' incidents 81
biomechanics 68
bleeding 207–214
    see also haemorrhage
blood 150
blood gas, arterial 138
blood loss, estimation 208
blood pressure 158–163
    anaphylaxis 187
    children 254
    pulse oximetry 139
blood sugar measurement 89, 196
blood vessels 150
    ageing 270
blood volume, children 254
blood-borne viruses 53, 55
blunt trauma 203
body fluids
    management 53
    splash contamination 55
body mass index (BMI) 319

bones
    ageing 269
    trauma 216
box splints 227–229
Boyle's law 116
brachial pulse 154
    blood pressure measurement 160
bradycardia 155, 319
    children 261
brain 170–171
    ageing 270–271
    arteries 176
    children 255, 262
    damage 264
    dementia 274–278
    haemorrhage 176
    trauma 204, 217
brain damage 264
brain stem 170
breach of duty 25
breath, smell of 92
breathing 115–143
    ageing 270
    assessment 89, 96, 137–139, 215
    children 253–254, 258, 259–261, 290
    control 118
    forceful 117
    infants 254, 287
    Kussmaul 320
    mechanics 116–117
    physiology 115–118
    tracheostomy 109
    see also assisted ventilation; oxygen
British Standard, gas cylinder 119
brittle asthma 319
broad arm sling 224–225
bronchi 95
    rupture 218
bronchodilators, COPD 143
bronchopneumonia 144
budesonide 140
bullets. see gunshot wounds
bundle of His 149
burns 214, 247–251
    chemical 250
    classification 248, 249
    radiation 250–251
    thermal 248
business continuity incident 81
'but for' principle, negligence 25
buttons, laryngectomy 110
BVM (bag-valve-mask ventilation) 125–129, 319

call handler 5
capacity (mental) 28–29
    learning disabilities 264

Index

capillaries 150
    bleeding from 208
capillary refill time 156–158, 261
carbon monoxide
    poisoning 201
    pulse oximetry and 139
cardiac arrest 3, 281–298
    anaphylaxis 188
    basic life support 284–295
    decisions 296–298
    defibrillation 282–284
    drowning 186
    post-resuscitation care 296
    pregnancy 295
cardiac cycle 151
cardiac failure
    children 258
cardiac output 89
    children 254
cardiogenic shock 168
cardiopulmonary resuscitation (CPR) 281
    infants 285–288
    paediatric 284–292
    procedures 285–295
    starting and stopping 296–297
    see also defibrillation
cardiovascular system
    ageing 270
    anatomy 147–153
    disorders 164–168
    physiology 147–153
Care Act 264
care environment, management 51
care equipment, management 51–52
Care Quality Commission 319
carotid pulse 155
cartilage 319
catastrophic haemorrhage 88, 208–209, 215, 319
cauda equina 171
causation of harm, negligence 25
CBRNe. *see* chemical, biological, radiological, nuclear and explosives
central nervous system 169
    control of breathing 118
    see also brain; spinal cord
cerebellum 171
cerebral spinal fluid (CSF) 171
cerebrum 171
cervical collars 241–244
cervical spine, trauma 204, 241
chain of infection 41–42
chain of survival 281–282
chairs, use for moving 71–76
challenging behaviour 279
channel, communication 16
charities 12

chemical, biological, radiological, nuclear and explosives (CBRNe) 82
chemical burns 250
chemoreceptors, respiration 118
chest compressions 294
    choking adult 112
    choking infant 112
    CPR *vs* 281
    techniques 285–295
chest pain 3, 164, 165
    pleuritic 321
child abuse 60
children 253–262
    asthma 141
    basic life support 288–292
    capillary refill time 156
    cardiac arrest 282, 288–292
    choking 112–114
    Entonox 135
    meningococcal disease 177
    oxygen 129, 253, 260
chin lift 285, 289
choking 319
    in adults 111–112
    child 112–114
cholinergic toxidromes 200
chordae tendineae 148
chronic bronchitis 142
chronic obstructive pulmonary disease (COPD), oxygen and 130, 132, 142
circadian rhythms 319
circle of Willis 176
circulation 147–168
    assessment 89, 153–163, 216
    children 254, 261–262
    post-resuscitation care 296
    trauma 208
circum-rescue collapse, drowning 186
Civil Contingencies Act 2004 81
Classification, Labelling and Packaging Regulation 85
cleaning 51–52
Climbié, Victoria, abuse case 60
Clinell wipes 52
clinical leadership roles 9
clinical risk, defined 39
closed fractures 221, 222
clothing
    contamination 47
    hygiene 51
'cloud on the horizon' 81
CLP pictograms, danger labels 85–86
cognitive dementia 274
cognitive development, children 255
cognitive function 319
cognitive impairment. *see* dementia
colleagues, caring for 11–13

Index

colonisation, by pathogens 40
coma 179
    see also Glasgow Coma Scale; unconsciousness
combustion, triangle of 55–56
command and control 9–10, 82
comminuted fractures 221, 222
commitment 24
communication 2, 15–21, 24
    barriers 18–19
    confidentiality 30
    consent 28
    dementia 278–279
    learning disabilities 266
    at major incidents 82
community acquired pneumonia 144
community first responders 1, 7–8
    illnesses of 40
co-morbidities 273–274, 276
compassion 24
compensated circulatory failure, children 261
compensated respiratory failure, children 258
competence 24
complaints 26
complex partial convulsions 175
compound fractures 221, 222
compression injuries, spine 205
conducting portion of respiratory system 115
    see also specific structures
conduction 181
conduction pathway, heart 148–149
conduction system, heart 270
confidentiality 30–33
connective tissue 319
Connelly (Baby P), abuse case 60
consciousness, level of 89, 261, 262
consent 27–30
    learning disabilities and 264
    maintenance 28
    reporting abuse 63
    to sharing information 31
    valid 28
constipation, ageing 271
consultant paramedic 9
contact dermatitis 46
contents gauge, gas cylinders 120, 121, 134
contusion 213
conus medullaris 171
convection 181
convulsions 175–176
cooling
    heat-related illness 183
    thermal burns 250
COPD. see chronic obstructive pulmonary disease
coping strategies, stress 58
coronary arteries 149–150
coronary artery disease (CAD) 164

coroner 32
coughing
    choking child 113
    hygiene 46
courage 24
CPR. see cardiopulmonary resuscitation
crepitus 319
crew arrival 4
critical care, specialist practitioner for 8
critical incident 81
cuffed tracheostomy tubes 108
cultural influences, abuse and 60
Cushing's triad 217
cyanide 249
cyanosis 259
cyber security incident 82
cylinders (medical gases) 118
    after use 133–134
    anatomy 119–120
    components 119–120
    oxygen 122–124
    preparing for use 121–122
    safety 121
    storage 119

damages, negligence 25
danger, CLP pictograms 85
death
    from burns 251
    signs 297
decannulation caps, tracheostomies 109
decapitation 297
decoder, communication 16
decompensated cardiac failure, children 258
decompensated respiratory failure, children 260
decompensated shock 168
decomposition/putrefaction 296
decompression sickness, Entonox and 135
decontamination 51–52
    chemical burns 250
deep dermal burns 249
deep vein thrombosis 144
defibrillation 3–4, 282–284
    early 281
    oxygen and 130, 284
defibrillators 3, 284
degenerative arthritis 272
delirium 278
demand valve, Entonox 135, 136
dementia 273, 274–278
    delirium vs 278
    progression 275–276
depression 273
dermatitis 46
dermis 206–207
    ageing 271
detergents, wipes 52

Index

diabetes mellitus 194
    type 1 194
    type 2 194
diabetic ketoacidosis 195
diaphragm 117
    infants 254
diastole 152
diastolic blood pressure 158, 161
diencephalon 171
diffusion, gases 117
digestive system, ageing 271
direct contact burns 248
disability 169–179
    assessment 89, 173–174, 216
    healthcare 265–267
    see also learning disabilities
disability (Equality Act 2010) 263
    dementia as 276
    hate crimes 266
disclosures
    of abuse 63
    information 32
discrimination 34–35, 273
discs, intervertebral 66
disinfection. see decontamination
dislocations 221–223
dissociative shock 168
distal (term) 319
distributive shock 168
diversity (of people) 33–35
diving, Entonox and 135
do not attempt CPR (DNACPR) 297–298
documentation. see record-keeping
doffing PPE 49–50
domestic waste 53
donning PPE 48–49
double-cannula tracheostomy tubes 108
Down Syndrome Bill 264
Down's syndrome 264
DRA model 79, 80
dressings 209, 212
    burns 250
drinking, last oral intake 90–91
drowning 185–186
    cardiac arrest 295
dura mater 171
duty of candour 27
duty of care 24–25
dynamic risk assessments 39, 79, 80

ears, assessment 91
eating, last oral intake 90–91
education
    learning disabilities and 263
elastic recoil 117
elderly people 269–279
electrical conduction pathway, heart 148–149, 270

electrical injuries 251
electrocardiograms 152–153
    ST segment 153, 165
    ventricular fibrillation 282
    ventricular tachycardia 282
electronic communication devices 21
elevated arm sling 225–226
embolism, pulmonary 144–145
emergencies, medical 187–201
emergency call 1–4
emergency operations centre 1–2, 5
    communication with 21
emergency preparedness, resilience and response (EPRR) 81
emergency services 38
emotional abuse 61
emotions, communication and 18
emphysema 142
employers
    health and safety regulations 37
    structured risk assessments 39
    support 12
employment rights, learning disabilities and 263
encircling technique, chest compressions 287
encoding, communication 16
end of life decisions, advance decision to refuse treatment 297–298
endocardium 147–148
endocrine system disorders 192–198
end-organ perfusion 261
enhanced triage 5
enteric nervous system 172
Entonox 118, 134–137
    temperature 121
entry route, of infection 42
environment
    risks from 80
    temperature 181–185
enzymes, COPD 142
epicardium 147
epidermis 206
    ageing 271
    burns 249
epiglottis, infant 113
epilepsy 175
epinephrine. see adrenaline
EPRR. see emergency preparedness, resilience and response
equality, in healthcare 33–34
Equality Act 2010 263, 276
escalating safeguarding concerns 64
evaporation 181
events leading to illness, history taking 91
exit route, of infection 42
expiration (breathing) 117
explosives, CLP pictogram 86
exposure, assessment 89, 216
extended skills 4
extension (movement), spinal trauma 205

Index

external bleeding 207
extra resources, scene assessment 80
eye contact 17
eye protection 47, 48–49
    removing 49–50

face, arm, speech test 173–174
face masks (oxygen delivery) 123
    children 260
    infants 253
face masks (PPE) 47, 52
facial shields, mouth-to-mouth ventilation 124
failure to achieve standards 26
falls, spinal trauma 217
fascia, superficial. *see* hypodermis
febrile convulsions 175
feedback, communication 16
female circumcision 62
female genital mutilation (FGM) 61, 62–63
fenestrated tracheostomy tubes 108
Ferno stretcher 67
fetal maceration 297, 320
fever, meningococcal disease 178
FFP3 masks 48–49, 52
fibrillation, ventricular 282
filtering face piece masks 48–49, 52
financial abuse 62
fire 55–56, 118–119
    thermal burns 249
fire marshals 56
fire safety 55–57
Firesafe 124
first-aid techniques 224–226
firtree, gas cylinders 120, 122
fissures, lungs 115
flail chest 219
flame burns 248
flammable substances, CLP pictogram 86
flaring, nose 258, 260
flexion (movement), spinal trauma 204
floor
    getting up from 71–76
    moving patient on to 76–78
flow selector, gas cylinders 120, 122, 134
fluticasone 140
focal (term) 320
food, last oral intake 90–91
forceful breathing 117
foreign objects, wounds 214
fractures 221–223
fragile X syndrome 264
freedom to speak up (FTSU)
    policy 27
friction burns 249
full thickness burns 249
fungi 41
furosemide 320

gas exchange 115, 117
gases, CLP pictogram 86
gases (medical) 118–137
gastric distension 124
gauge, gas cylinders 120, 121, 134
gauze
    wound cleansing 214
    wound packing 209
general impression 215
generalised convulsions 175
genetics, learning disabilities and 264
getting up from floor 71–76
ghrelin 192
Glasgow Coma Scale (GCS) 320
gloves 46–47, 48–49
    removing 49–50
glucagon 192
glucose
    blood level 89
    blood regulation 193–194
glycaemic emergencies 194
glyceryl trinitrate (GTN) 166
greenstick fractures 221, 222
grooming, for sexual abuse 61–62
grunting, infants 260
GTN 166
gunshot wounds 214
    head 203
gurgling, airway 97

haematoma 320
haemoptysis 145, 320
haemorrhage
    assessment 218
    brain 176
    catastrophic 88, 208–209, 215
    non-catastrophic 209
    trauma 208–209
    see also bleeding
haemostatic agents 209
haemothorax 218
HALO (mnemonics) 10
hand hygiene 42–46
handling 65–78
    aids 70–71
    healthcare waste 54
    see also manual handling
handovers 4, 19–20
handwashing 43–44
handwheel, gas cylinders 120, 121, 133, 136
harassment, learning disabilities 263
harm
    defined 59
    negligence 25
HART teams 9, 85
hate crimes, learning disabilities 267
hazard, defined 39

Index

hazardous manual handling operations, legislation 38
hazardous materials (HAZMAT) 82, 84–86
hazardous mixture 85
head, trauma 204, 217
head bobbing 260
head tilt–chin lift 100–101, 286, 290
'headline news' 81
'head-to-toe' assessment 91–92
health and safety 37–58
    legislation on infections 40
Health and Safety at Work etc. Act 1974 37
    personal protective equipment 40
Health and Social Care Act 2008 40
healthcare, equality 33–34
healthcare linen, management 52
healthcare waste, handling 54
healthcare-associated infections 40
'hear and treat' responses 5
heart
    ageing 270
    anatomy 147–150
    electrical conduction pathway 148–149
    electrical conduction system 270
    see also entries beginning cardiac
heart failure 166–167
    children 258
heart rate. *see* pulse rate
heat exhaustion 182, 183
heat stress 182, 183
heat stroke 182–183
heat-loss mechanisms 181
heat-promoting mechanisms 181
heat-related illness 182–183
helicopters, in-flight defibrillation 284
helmet removal 239–241
help, seeking 12
Help Fall checklist 74, 75
hemicorporectomy 296
hemiplegia 179
herniation, intervertebral discs 66
history taking 89–91
    asthma 141
    musculoskeletal injuries 220–221
    patient 3
hormones 193
hospital ambulance liaison officer 10
hosts, infections 42
Human Rights Act 1998 34
humerus 320
hydrogen cyanide 249
hygiene waste 53
hyperactive delirium 278
hyperflexion injuries, spine 204
hyperglycaemia, severe 195
hyperglycaemic crisis 195
hyperosmolar hyperglycaemic state 195
hypertension, defined 158

hypoactive delirium 278
hypodermis 207
    ageing 271
hypoglycaemia 89, 193, 194–195
hypostasis 297
hypotension
    children 262
    defined 158
hypothalamus 171, 181
hypothermia 181–182, 216
    burns patients 250
    cardiac arrest 295
hypovolaemia 292
hypovolaemic shock 168
hypoxaemia, oxygen and 131
hypoxia
    cardiac arrest 282
    COPD 143

ice 223
ice packs 183
ileus 320
immobilisation
    MILS 238–239
    spine 238
    trauma patients 217, 223–246
immune system, ageing 271
impaired mental capacity, dementia 277
incineration 297
incision (trauma) 213
inclusion (of people) 33
inequality in healthcare 265–266
infants 253
    airways 113, 253, 259, 285–288
    assessment 256
    basic life support 285–288
    bradycardia 261
    breathing 254, 287
    choking 112–114
    circulation 254
    cognitive development 255
infections
    mechanisms 41–42
    older people 271
    pneumonia 143–144
    prevention and control 40–55
infectious waste 53
inflammatory arthritis 272
in-flight defibrillation 284
information governance 30–33
inhalation injury. *see* smoke inhalation
inhalers, asthma 140
injections, waste disposal after 54
injuries
    mechanism of (MOI) 79, 203–206
    to staff 65
    see also physical abuse; trauma

Index

in-line stabilisation (manual) 215
inner cannulas, tracheostomy tubes 108
inspiration 117
insulin 192, 193
integrated valve cylinders 119, 120
integumentary system. see skin
intercostal (term) 320
intercostal muscles, children 254
intercostal recession 254, 258, 260
internal bleeding 207
    see also haemorrhage
inter-scapular blows, choking child 114
intervertebral discs 66
ipratropium bromide 140
irrigation of wounds 214
ischaemia, myocardial 164, 281
ischaemic strokes 177
islets of Langerhans 192
isovolumetric contraction, heart 152

J point, electrocardiograms 153
jaw thrust 101–102, 286
    with head tilt 101–102
Jext auto-injector 189
Joint Emergency Services Interoperability Programme 9
joints
    ageing 270
    arthritis 272
    see also specific joints
JRCALC clinical guidelines 201
judgements (pre-judgements) 23

keratinocytes 206, 260
ketoacidosis 195
ketonaemia 195, 320
kidneys, children 261
Korotkoff sounds 158–159, 320
Kussmaul breathing 196, 320
kyphosis 270

labels
    gas cylinders 120, 121
    hazardous substances 85–86
laceration 213
language 16–17, 18
laryngectomy 107, 110–111
laryngopharynx 94
laryngospasm, drowning 185
larynx 95
last oral intake 90–91
lateral (term) 320
learning culture 26
learning disabilities 263–267
left anterior descending artery 150
left atrium 148
left bundle branch 149
left coronary artery 150

left ventricle 148
legal issues 23–35
    health and safety 37
    manual handling 67
level of consciousness 89, 262
levers 68
lifting
    chairs 74–76
    see also manual handling
lightning strikes 251
line manager 11
listening 17
living wills (advance decision to refuse treatment) 297
loads 66, 67–68, 69–70
    see also manual handling
lobar pneumonia 144
lobes, lungs 115, 116
lobules, lungs 116
LOC (level of consciousness) 261
local authorities, disclosure 32
lumbar spine 66
Lund and Browder charts 248
lungs
    anatomy 95–96
    physiology 115–116
lying position, rising from 71–76

major incidents 81–82
    terrorism 81
maltreatment, defined 59
Management of Health and Safety at Work Regulations 1999 38
mandible 94
    see also jaw thrust
manual airway manoeuvres 97–103
manual handling 65–71
    abusive 61
    legislation on 39, 67
    risk assessment 39, 66–68
Manual Handling Operations Regulations 1992 38, 67
manual in-line stabilisation 215
marauding terrorist attack (MTA) 82
masks. see face masks
mass casualty 82
mechanically powered stretchers 67
mechanism of injury (MOI) 79, 203–206
medial (term) 320
mediastinum 95
medical director 9
medical emergencies 187–201
medical handover 20
medical support 12
medication
    current 4
    history taking 90
medium concentration face mask 123
medulla oblongata 170
melanocytes 206

Index

Mencap 265
meninges 171
meningococcal disease 177–178
mental capacity 28–29
    learning disabilities 264
mental illness, older people 273
mental well-being 12
metal surfaces, defibrillation and 284
METHANE (mnemonic) 320
M/ETHANE model 82, 83
microbial filters, Entonox 135
micro-organism 320
micro-organisms 40
midbrain 170
mid-dermal burns 249
MILS, immobilisation 238–239
misunderstandings
    avoidance 21
    clarifying 19
mitral valve 148
mixed, delirium 278
mobile phone 21
MOI. *see* mechanism of injury
monoplegia 179
motor function 169
mottling, children 259
mouth
    anatomy 94
    assessment 91
    infants 253
mouth-to-mask ventilation 125
mouth-to-mouth ventilation 124, 290
movement
    musculoskeletal system 220, 269
    spine 204–205
moving
    getting up from floor 71–76
    see also handling; manual handling
Munchausen's syndrome by proxy 61
municipal waste 53
muscles
    ageing 270
    respiratory 117
musculoskeletal system 220–223
myocardium 147
    infarction 152, 292
    ischaemia 164, 281

nail varnish, pulse oximetry and 139
nasal cannulae, oxygen delivery 123, 130
nasopharynx 94
National Health Service
    ambulance service 7
    values and attitudes 24
National inter-agency liaison officer 10
nature of illness (NOI) 79
nebuliser 123

neck
    assessment 92
    trauma 217
neck of femur fractures 223
neglect 62
negligence 25
nervous system 169–173
    ageing 270–271
    control of breathing 118
    disorders 174–179
neurological dementia 275
neurons 169
    ageing 270
NILO (mnemonics) 10
999 calls
    fire 56
    response to 5–7
NOI. *see* nature of illness
non-accidental injury 61
non-catastrophic haemorrhage 209
non-invasive blood pressure measurement 158
non-rebreathe mask 123
    respiratory rate and 138
non-shockable rhythms 282–283
non-ST-segment elevation myocardial infarction 165
non-verbal communication 17
norovirus 40
nose
    anatomy 93
    flaring 258, 260
    infants 253
    oxygen cannulae 123, 130
number of patients 80, 215

obesity
    body mass index 194
    burn assessment 248
    diabetes mellitus 194
oblique fractures 221, 222
observations 19
obstructive shock 168
obturators, tracheostomies 109
oedema 320
offensive waste 53
older adults, trauma 203
older people 269–279
    care for 271–274
oliguria 320
one-chair method, rising from floor 71–73
onward care 6–7
OPA. *see* oropharyngeal airways
open fractures 221, 222
operational commanders 9–10
opioid, toxidromes 200
oropharyngeal airways 104, 320
    children 259
oropharynx 94

Index

osteoarthritis 272
osteoporosis 272–273
over-the-counter medicines 90
oxidiser, CLP pictogram 86
oxygen
    administration 129–134
    bag-valve-mask ventilation 125
    children 129, 253, 260
    concentrations for combustion 55–56
    convulsions 176
    COPD and 130, 132, 142
    defibrillation and 130, 284
    delivery devices 122–124
    dosage 130–131, 132–133
    fire 118–119
    hyperglycaemic crisis 196
    partial pressures 117, 118, 320–321
    post-resuscitation care 296
    saturations 138–139
    tracheostomy 109

P wave, electrocardiograms 152
pacemaker
    defibrillation and 284
    heart 148–149
packaging, waste disposal 54
packing, wounds 209
pad placement, defibrillation 284
paediatric assessment triangle (PAT) 258
paediatrics. see children
pager 21
pain
    Abbey Pain Scale 276, 277
    acute coronary syndrome 165
    angina 164
    assessment 90
    dementia 276
    learning disabilities 266
    patient history 2–3
pallor 259
pancreas 192, 193
pancreatic islets, cells of 192
pancreatic polypeptide 192
Panda eyes 320
panda eyes (Battle's sign) 217
papillary dermis 206
paracetamol, on blood glucose 196
paralinguistics 17
paralysis 179
paramedics 8
paraplegia 179
paraquat poisoning, oxygen and 132–133
parasites 41
parasympathetic divisions 173
paresis 179
Parkinson's disease 272
partial convulsions 175

partial pressures 117, 118, 320–321
past medical history 90
PAT. see paediatric assessment triangle
pathogen 41
patient assessment 3, 87–92
    burns 248
    general impression 88
    paediatrics 256–262
patient-identifiable information 30–31
Pelka, Daniel, abuse case 60
pelvic splints 231–235
pelvis
    assessment 92
    trauma 206, 220
penetrating injuries 203
    abdomen 219
    thorax 205
percussion 321
pericardium 147–148
peripheral nervous system 170
peritoneal organs 219
personal protective equipment 46
    for decontamination 52
    Health and Safety at Work etc. Act 1974 40
    scene assessment for 2, 82
    for waste disposal 54
petechial non-blanching rash 178
pharmaceutical adviser 9
pharynx 94
    infants 253
phones, mobile 21
physical abuse 61
physical response, 999 calls 6
pia mater 171
pictograms, danger labels 85–86
pilot balloon, tracheostomy tube 108
plasma 150
platelets 150
pleura 95, 217–218
pleuritic chest pain 321
pneumonia 143–144
pneumothorax 217–218
pocket masks, mouth-to-mask ventilation 125
poisoning 199–201
police
    disclosure 32
    learning disabilities and 263
    reporting abuse 63
pons 170
positioning, respiratory failure 258, 260
positive-pressure ventilation
    children 253
    infants 253
post-cardiac arrest syndrome 296
posterior (term) 321
posterior descending artery (coronary) 149–150
post-ictal phase 175

Index

post-resuscitation care 296
posture
    ageing 270
    cardiac arrest in pregnancy 295
    for manual handling 69
PPE. *see* personal protective equipment
PR segment, electrocardiograms 152
practical communication 19–21
precordium 321
pregnancy, cardiac arrest 295
pre-hospital screening tool 191
pre-judgements 23
pre-school children 253
    assessment 257
    cognitive development 255
presenting complaint 89–90
pressure (physical), air 116–117
pressure (psychological), stress *vs* 57
preventer inhalers 140
PRICE (mnemonic) 223
primary assessment 321
primary survey 87–89, 215–216
    children 258–262
protection, defined 59
proximal (term) 321
psychological abuse 61
psychomotor (term) 321
public interest 32
pulmonary embolism 144–145
pulse 89, 153–156
    assessment 155
    children 261
    measurement 155–156
pulse oximetry 138–139, 321
    children 260
pulse rate 155
    pulmonary embolism 145
pulse volume 261
pulseless electrical activity 283
puncture (stab) 214
    see also stab wounds
pupils 89, 91
    children 262
Purkinje fibres 149

QRS complexes, electrocardiography 153, 282
QRS wave, electrocardiography 152, 282
quadriplegia 179

radial pulse 154
radiation 181
radiation burns 250–251
rashes 89
    meningococcal disease 178
'reasonably practicable' (term) 39
reassessment 92
receiver, communication 16

recession 258, 260, 321
    intercostal 254, 258, 260
record-keeping 17, 19
    abuse and 64
    confidentiality 30–33
    information governance 30–33
recovery position 97–100
    children 261
red blood cells 150
    dissociative shock 168
red flag sepsis 190
reflexes 172
    infants 255
rehydration 183
relationships (working relationships) 11
relaxation period, cardiac cycle 152
reliever inhalers, asthma 140
removing PPE 49–50
rescue, from drowning 186
reservoirs of infection 42
resilience 12
respiratory centres 118
respiratory failure
    children 258
    tripod position 96, 260
respiratory rate 137–138
    asthma 141
    children 254, 260
    pulmonary embolism 145
respiratory system
    ageing 270
    anatomy 93–96
    hygiene 46
    physiology 115–118
responsiveness 88
resuscitation. *see* cardiopulmonary resuscitation
reticular dermis 206
retroperitoneal space 219
return of spontaneous circulation
    (ROSC) 281, 296
rheumatoid arthritis 272
rhythm
    for defibrillation 282–283
    pulse 155
ribs
    assessment 92
    children 254
    flail chest 219
right atrium 148
right bundle branch 149
right coronary artery 149–150
right ventricle 148
rights, learning disabilities and 264
rigor mortis 297
rigors 321
rising from lying position 71–76
'rising tide' incidents 81

Index

risk assessment 38–39
    manual handling 39, 66–68
    scene assessment 79
    trauma 215
risk to well-being 32
risks, defined 39
rotation, spinal trauma 204
rule of nines 248

SADs (supraglottic airway devices) 321
safeguarding 59–64
safeguarding referrals 64
safety
    defibrillators 284
    gas cylinders 121
    at major incidents 82
    at scene 79, 215, 249, 250
    see also health and safety
salbutamol 140
SAM pelvic sling 231–233
Samaritans charity 12
SAMPLE acronym 321
SAMPLE history 90
scalds 248
scene assessment 2, 39, 79–86, 215
SCENE mnemonic 79
school-age children 253
    assessment 257
    cognitive development 255
Schrader outlet 120, 134
    after use 134
scoop stretcher 244–247
scope of practice 25, 321
Scotland, Adults with Incapacity (Scotland) Act 2000 28
secondary survey 91–92
security, patient-identifiable information 31
sedative-hypnotic toxidromes 200
seizures 175
sender, communication 15
sensory function (perception) receptors 169
sensory problems 18
sepsis 190–191
    meningococcal disease 178
    screening tool 190
serial halving 248
serotonin syndrome 200
sexual abuse 61–62
sharps 53, 54–55
shields (facial), mouth-to-mouth ventilation 125
shivering 181
shock 167–168
    children 261
    meningococcal disease 178
    septic 190
shockable rhythms 282
shortness of breath on exertion, ageing 270
SICPs. see standard infection control precautions

signs (clinical) 90
    death 297
sildenafil, GTN and 166
simple partial convulsions 175
single-handed BVM ventilation 126–127
sinoatrial node 148–149
skeleton
    injuries to 66
    see also bones
skin 206–207
    ageing 271
    care 46
    circulation in children 259, 261
    physiology 207
    trauma 206–207
skin irritation, CLP pictogram 86
skull, assessment 91
sleeve protectors 47
smoke inhalation 249
smoking
    COPD 142
    fire prevention 39
snoring 97
social context, communication 18
social services, safeguarding and 64
SOCRATES 321
SOCRATES (acronym) 90
soft palate 94
somatic nervous system 171–172
somatostatin 192
spacer device 140
speaking valves, tracheostomies 109
specialist practitioner 8
sphygmomanometer 158
spigots, Venturi masks 123
spinal cord 171
    trauma 217
spinal nerves 172
spine 66
    immobilisation 238
    trauma 204–205, 217, 223
spiral fractures 221, 222
splash contamination 55
splints 227–238
sprains 223
sputum, pneumonia 144
ST segment, electrocardiograms 153, 165
stab wounds
    abdomen 206, 219
    see also puncture
stabilisation (manual in-line) 215
stable angina 164
standard infection control precautions (SICPs) 42
standards for responders 25
Staphylococcus 41
status epilepticus, convulsive 175
stereotyping 23, 34

Index

sterilisation 51
stigma, dementia 277
stoma patency, laryngectomy 110
stomach, distension 124
storage
    gas cylinders 119
    patient record 31
straddle injuries 220
strains 223
stranger anxiety 255, 256
strategic commanders 10
Streptococcus 41
stress 57–58
    communication and 16
stretchers 67
stridor 97, 260, 321
stroke 176–177
    face, arm, speech test 173
    types 177
stroke volume, children 254
structured risk assessments 39
ST-segment elevation myocardial infarction 165
sublingual spray, GTN 166
suction, airway 103–104
sugar. *see* glucose
sunburn 251
superficial dermal burn 249
superficial fascia. *see* hypodermis
superior (term) 321
supine (term) 321
support, learning disabilities and 267
support structures 11
    capacity assessment 29
    discrimination and 34
    errors and 26
support workers 8
supraglottic airway devices 321
supraglottic airway devices (SADs) 321
surfactant 321
surgical face masks 47
susceptible hosts, infections 42
swallowing 94
sympathetic divisions 173
sympathomimetic toxidromes 199
symptoms 90
systole, atrial 151–152
systolic blood pressure 158, 161

T wave, electrocardiograms 153
tachycardia 155, 321
    children 261
    ventricular 282
tachypnoea 321
tactical commanders 10
TASC (mnemonics) 12

teenagers 253
    assessment 257
    cognitive development 255
temperature
    assessment of 183–185
    body 181
    capillary refill time 156
    drowning 186
    Entonox 121
    environment 181–185
ten second triage 83–84
tension pneumothorax 217
terrorism 81
tetraplegia 179
thalamus 171
The Ambulance Staff Charity 12
thermal burns 248
thermometers 181, 183
thermoregulation 181
think the unthinkable, on abuse 60
thorax, trauma 205, 217–218
thrombosis, deep vein 144
TICLS (mnemonic) 258
TILEE 67
TILEE acronym 322
time-critical factors, burns 247
tiotropium bromide 140
toddlers 253
    assessment 256–257
    cognitive development 255
tongue 94
tonic-clonic convulsions 175
total body surface area 248
tourniquets 209–212
toxic substances, danger labels 86
toxidromes 199–200
    signs 201
T-POD stabilisation device 233–235
trachea 95
tracheo-oesophageal puncture valve 110
tracheostomy 107–111
    patency 109–110
tracheostomy tubes 108–109
traction splints 235–238
transient ischaemic attacks 176
transmission of infections 42
transport, at major incidents 82
transverse fractures 221, 222
trauma 203–251
    brain 204, 217
    handover 20
    head 204, 217
    primary survey 87–88
    spine 204–205, 217
    see also physical abuse
traumatic brain injury 217
treatment, at major incidents 82

Index

triage 5
    at major incidents 82
triangle of combustion 39
triangle of paediatric assessment (PAT) 258
tricuspid valve 148
tripod position 96, 260
tunica externa 151
tunica media 150
turbinates, nose 93
turgor 322
twisting, for manual handling 70
two-chair method, rising from floor 73–74
two-handed BVM ventilation 128–129, 290
tympanic temperature measurement 184–185
tympanic thermometers 181

unconsciousness
    airway 259
    see also coma
unstable angina 164
upper limbs, weakness 175
urgent care, specialist practitioner for 8
urgent concern, in safeguarding 63
urticaria 322

vacuum splints 229–231
valid consent 28
values-based healthcare 23–24
valve
    atrioventricular 151–152
    Entonox 135, 136
    heart 148
vascular dementia 275
vehicles, fire 56–57
veins 150, 151
    bleeding from 207
venous bleeding 207
venous thromboembolism 144–145
ventilation (respiratory function) 115, 116, 281
    ageing 270
    assisted. *see* assisted ventilation
    children 290
    pregnancy 295
    trauma 216
Ventolin (salbutamol) 140
ventricles, heart 148
ventricular fibrillation 282
ventricular systole 152
ventricular tachycardia 282
Venturi masks 123
venules 150
verbal communication 16–17
vertebral column. *see* spine
vicarious liability 25
viruses 41
    blood-borne 53, 55
vital signs 91
vitamin C, on blood glucose 196
vocabulary 16–17
volume
    air pressure *vs* 116
    pulse 155
volunteers, health and safety responsibilities 37
vomiting
    airway management 103
    diabetic ketoacidosis 196
    from gastric distension 124
vulnerability to abuse 60

warning, CLP pictograms 85
waste disposal 53–54
weight, maximum safe handling 68, 69
wet surfaces, defibrillation and 284
wheeze 97, 260
whistleblowing 26
white blood cells 150
Winterbourne View hospital, abuse in 59
wipes 52
work of breathing, children 258, 259–261
working relationships 11
wounds 206, 207–214
written communication 17

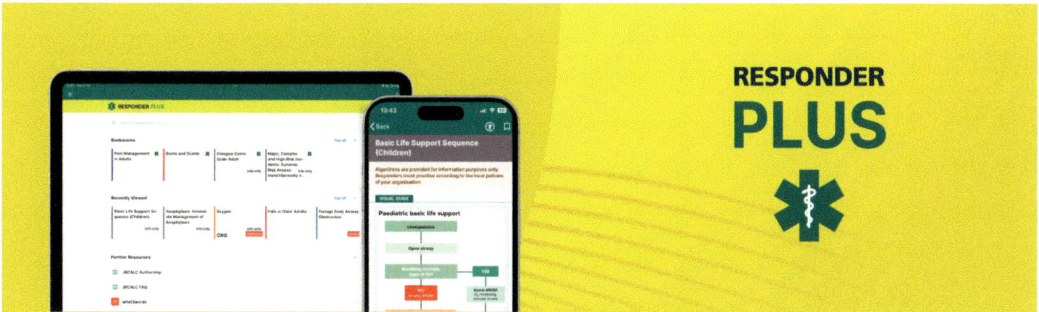

Introducing the Responder Plus App

Reference and Reassurance for Community First Responders

Key Features

- Reference to the latest legislation, guidance and policy.
- Updates published in real time as new guidance is issued.
- Access to First Responder Care Essentials.
- 'Quick Look' view to highlight important algorithms, diagrams and tables.
- Clinical skills photographs and anatomical diagrams to aid understanding.

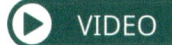

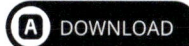

Developed in collaboration with CFR teams across the UK, Responder Plus contains guidance to support you in attending medical emergencies, resuscitation situations and trauma injuries.

T. +44 (0) 1278 427800 | E. apps@class.co.uk | W. classprofessional.co.uk